Differential Diagnosis in Pediatrics

Differential Diagnosis in Pediatrics

R Arvind
MBBS DCH DNB
Consultant Pediatrician and Neonatologist
Proprietor and Medical Director
Vathsalya Speciality Clinic
Bengaluru, Karnataka, India

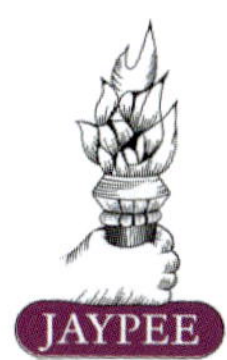

JAYPEE BROTHERS MEDICAL PUBLISHERS
The Health Sciences Publisher
New Delhi | London

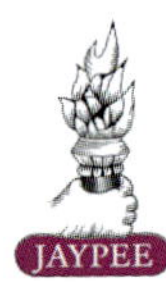

Jaypee Brothers Medical Publishers (P) Ltd

Headquarters
EMCA House, 23/23-B
Ansari Road, Daryaganj
New Delhi 110 002, India
Landline: +91-11-23272143, +91-11-23272703
+91-11-23282021, +91-11-23245672
e-mail: jaypee@jaypeebrothers.com

Corporate Office
4838/24, Ansari Road, Daryaganj
New Delhi 110 002, India
Phone: +91-11-43574357
Fax: +91-11-43574314
e-mail: jaypee@jaypeebrothers.com

Overseas Office
JP Medical Ltd
83 Victoria Street, London
SW1H 0HW (UK)
Phone: +44-20 3170 8910
e-mail: info@jpmedpub.com

EU GPSR Authorised Representative
Logos Europe, 9 rue Nicolas Poussin
17000, La Rochelle, France
Phone: +33 (0) 6 67 93 73 78
e-mail: contact@logoseurope.eu

Website: www.jaypeebrothers.com
Website: www.jaypeedigital.com

Inquiries for bulk sales may be solicited at: jaypee@jaypeebrothers.com

Differential Diagnosis in Pediatrics

First Edition: **2026**

ISBN: 978-93-6616-259-1

Printed at Nutech Print Services Pvt. Ltd.

Dedicated to

My beloved grand daughter
Isha Chaitanya

Preface

In this book, all the signs and symptoms related to pediatrics have been indexed in an alphabetical order. All of them have been discussed in detail up to the clinical diagnosis level. This includes definition, pathophysiology, causes, the technique to elicit, and impression of respective symptoms and signs. Wherever possible, these have been illustrated with photographs.

This book acts as ready reckoner to the reader to search for any symptoms or signs and to go through it completely in a single place. This is useful to undergraduates, postgraduates, residents, and practicing pediatricians as a reference book and as well as preparing for competitive examinations.

R Arvind

Acknowledgments

I thank my wife Dr Chetana for her suggestions and professional help. I am thankful to my children Rachana and Shikhar for their cooperation and encouragement.

I express my deep gratitude to Abhishek for typing the manuscript. I am grateful to Ramesha c/o Anubandha Studio for the photo work of the book.

My special thanks are due to Shri Jitendar P Vij (Group Chairman), Mr Ankit Vij (Managing Director), Mr Sabyasachi Hazra (Director—PG and PNR Content), Ms Nikita Chauhan (Publishing Manager), and staff of M/s Jaypee Brothers Medical Publishers (P) Ltd, New Delhi, India.

Contents

SECTION 1

SECTION 3

SECTION 4

SECTION 5

SECTION 6

SECTION 7

SECTION 8

SECTION 9

SECTION 10

SECTION 11

SECTION 12

SECTION 13

SECTION 14

SECTION 15

SECTION 16

SECTION 17

SECTION 18

SECTION 19

SECTION 20

SECTION 21

SECTION 22

SECTION 1

Abdominal Distention

Contour is the abdominal profile from the rib margin to the pubis, viewed on the horizontal plane. In newborn, the abdomen is normally prominent; in toddler, it is protuberant, while in adolescent, it is flat. Thin individuals have scaphoid abdomen while obese persons have prominent belly.

Abnormalities of the shape of the abdomen lie more with the generalized distension on one hand and scaphoid abdomen on the other hand. Distension of the abdomen is generalized with ascites, obesity, and flatus. Localized distension is seen in individual with visceromegaly and due to neoplasm. Scaphoid or sunken abdomen is seen in severe dehydration, starvation, and malignancy.

Abdominal distention is an important sign of intestinal obstruction. The lower the obstruction in the gut, the more marked the distention. Also, associated symptoms will be present, including vomiting and abdominal pain/irritability. Peristalsis may be visible through the abdominal wall in patients with intestinal obstruction. This peristalsis is most commonly observed in the upper abdomen in infants with hypertrophic pyloric stenosis. A depressed scaphoid abdomen in a newborn suggests a diaphragmatic hernia with some abdominal organs sitting in the chest cavity.

The potbelly contour of the abdomen is normal in infants. It should not be considered as an evidence of liver disease. Progressive abdominal distension is due to enlargement of the abdominal viscera, tumor, or gaseous distension.

Distension of the abdomen is usually caused by air (due to malabsorption, lactose intolerance, anticholinergic drugs, etc.) and fluid in the bowel or peritoneal cavity, but it may also be caused by atonic abdominal musculature, paralysis of the abdominal musculature, feces in the bowel, abnormal enlargement of organs, intestinal duplication, or tumors.

Abdominal distension due to laxity of the abdominal wall is seen in rickets, celiac disease, and hypothyroidism. Flat abdomen is seen in normal thin children, malnutrition, failure to thrive, and anorexia nervosa. Scaphoid abdomen in the newborn is due to diaphragmatic hernia. Complete absence of the muscles of the abdominal wall gives the skin a wrinkled appearance and is called as prune belly syndrome.

Look for any distension or bulges. Real distention of the abdomen is usually caused by air (due to malabsorption, lactose intolerance, anticholinergic drugs, etc.) or fluid in the bowel or peritoneal cavity, but it may also be caused by atonic abdominal musculature, paralysis of the abdominal musculature, feces in the bowel, abnormal enlargement of organs, intestinal duplication, or tumors. Distention is frequently noted in children with pancreatic fibrosis, rickets, hypothyroidism, bowel obstruction, constipation, ileus (following septicemia, drug intake, uremia, etc.), ascites, or protein energy malnutrition. Localized bulge is seen in phantom hernia as seen in acute polio.

Neonate's abdomen is naturally rounded due to poor muscle tone. An excessive protuberance can indicate pathology. Eliciting a thorough bowel history can help to differentiate the etiology of abdominal distention. Loose and/or grossly bloody stools in the setting of a well appearing infant with a normal examination may indicate cow's milk protein intolerance. This may be seen even in breastfed infants whose mothers are ingesting large volumes of dairy products. In addition to cow's milk protein, other dietary proteins may cause gastrointestinal upset in the infant.

The differential diagnosis includes functional and anatomic obstructions, infection, organomegaly, formula intolerance, and masses. The abdomen should be examined while the infant is quiet, i.e., after feeding.

Radiographic studies such as ultrasound (prenatal and postnatal) and abdominal plain films are helpful diagnostic aids. In addition, water-soluble contrast enemas and abdominal computed tomography (CT) scans may be necessary to differentiate an etiology. Surgical consultation may be warranted.

SWELLINGS IN THE ABDOMINAL WALL

Abdominal wall swellings are superficial, adherent to skin, subcutaneous tissue, and muscles.

Ask the patient to take a deep breath and hold it. The contour should remain smooth and symmetric. This maneuver lowers the diaphragm and compresses the organ so that the abdominal cavity, may cause previously unseen bulges or masses will appear. Next, ask the patient to raise his or her head from the table. This contracts the rectus abdominis muscles, which produces muscle prominent in thin or athletic adults. Superficial abdominal wall masses may become visible. If a hernia is present, the increased abdominal pressure may cause it to protrude.

Diastasis of the rectus muscle may be noted as a protrusion in the midline, usually from the xiphoid to the umbilicus but occasionally down to the symphysis pubis. Ordinarily, the protrusion is ½–2 inches size; it is usually common normal variant but may be caused by a congenital weakness of the musculature in a chronically distended abdomen. Diastasis of rectus abdominis ordinarily resolves by 6 years of age.

COMMON CAUSES OF ABDOMINAL DISTENSION

Newborn

- Septicemia
- Pneumonia
- Aerophagy
- Phototherapy
- Necrotizing enterocolitis
- Cardiac failure and congenital heart diseases
- Distended bladder
- Hypertrophic pyloric stenosis
- Imperforate anus
- Intussusception
- Meconium ileus
- Hydronephrosis

Infants

- Septicemia
- Aerophagy
- Cardiac failure
- Hypertrophic pyloric stenosis
- Distended bladder
- Necrotizing enterocolitis
- Intussusception

- Hydronephrosis
- Hypokalemia

Older Children (Preschool Group)

- Normal pot belly
- Malnourished children
- Chronic diarrhea and hypokalemia
- Aerophagy
- Enlargement of liver or spleen—Beta thalassemia
- *Abdominal ascites:*
  - Cirrhosis
  - Tuberculosis
  - Nephrosis
  - Kwashiorkor and congestive cardiac failure (CCF)
- Excessive feeding
- Chronic constipation
- Intestinal obstruction—intussusception
- Hydronephrosis
- Bladder distension
- Mesenteric cyst and dermoid cyst
- Ovarian tumors
- Rickets

Older Children (School Groups) and Adolescents

- Excessive feeding
- Malnutrition
- Muscle weakness
- Chronic constipation
- *Ascitic fluid*:
  - CCF and nephrotic syndrome
  - Tuberculous peritonitis
  - Kwashiorkor
  - Hepatic cirrhosis
  - Portal obstruction
- *Prominent liver:*
  - Downward displacement in chest deformities
  - Subacute hepatitis
  - CCF
  - Thalassemia
  - Sickle cell disease
  - Liver abscess
  - Leukemia
- *Prominent spleen:*
  - Malaria
  - Typhoid
  - Subacute bacterial endocarditis
  - Portal obstruction
  - Thalassemia
  - Sickle cell disease
  - Hemolytic anemias
- Malabsorption syndrome
- *Abdominal masses:*
  - Tuberculous mesenteric adenitis (plastic peritonitis)
  - Hydronephrosis
  - Mesenteric cyst
  - Hydatid cyst
- Acquired intestinal obstruction as:
  - Worm obstruction
  - Fecal impaction
  - Intussusception
  - Incarcerated hernia
- Bladder distension
- Rickets and hypokalemia
- Pregnancy

Causes of Nonobstructive Acquired Abdominal Distension

- Ileus
- Hypokalemia
- Hypercalcemia
- Hyperthyroidism
- Sepsis
- Necrotizing enterocolitis
- Hirschsprung's enterocolitis

Causes of Transient Abdominal Masses

- Hernia
- Intussusception

- Urinary bladder
- Rectal masses
- Round worm
- Spleen

HISTORY

Child with the history of fever, rigors, sweating, and toxemia will give clue to pyonephrosis, perinephric abscess, amebiasis, leukemia, and splenic infection.

History suggestive of gastroenteritis with the redcurrant jelly stool indicates the intussusception.

History of vomiting, abdominal distention, and not passed meconium suggests meconium ileus, intestinal obstruction, and congenital megacolon.

History of projectile vomiting, not gaining weight and presence of mass after feed, indicates congenital pyloric stenosis.

History of fever and chills with jaundice indicates cholangitis. History of bleeding diathesis indicates hemolytic type of anemia and leukemia.

EXAMINATION

When dealing with the child with mass per abdomen, many peripheral signs should be looked for the probable which has been arrived at the history level.

Hemolytic facies indicates diagnosis of the hemolytic type of anemia. Conjunctival pallor will give clues for the diagnosis of the leukemia, lymphomas, renal tuberculosis, and Meckel's diverticulum. Presence of jaundice indicates hemolytic anemia, early phase of the cirrhosis and cholangitis. Periorbital edema gives clue to the CCF. Gum hypertrophy indicates the leukemia. Raised jugular venous pressure (JVP) indicates CCF due to some causes.

ASCITES

It is the accumulation of fluid in peritoneal cavity.

Causes of Ascites

- Congestive cardiac failure
- Acute glomerulonephritis
- Nephritic syndrome
- Tuberculosis
- Protein energy malnutrition
- Malabsorption syndrome
- Portal hypertension

General Examination Findings in a Case of Ascites

- *Jaundice, palmar erythema, and spider nevi:* Hepatic cause
- *Elevated JVP:* Cardiac cause
- *Clubbing:* Cirrhosis
- *Edema:*
  - Pitting in cirrhosis
  - Nonpitting in hypothyroidism

Pathogenesis

Ascitic fluid may be transudate with low protein or exudates with high protein. The pathogenesis includes:

- *Increased hydrostatic pressure in the portal vessels:* This is associated with portal hypertension. There is filtration of fluid from the blood vessels to the interstitial space.
- *Decreased oncotic pressure:* This occurs due to the increased protein loss from the renal or gastrointestinal tract (GIT). There is decreased production by the liver. Ascites due to hypoalbuminemia
- *Increased capillary endothelial permeability:* Here, there is flow of fluid out of capillaries. It happens in inflammatory neoplastic causes.

- *Stimulation of rennin angiotensin-aldosterone system:* This results from increase in aldosterone and antidiuretic hormone levels leading to sodium and water retention. This results in increased osmatic tension of interstitial fluid.

Clinical Features

There is uniform distension of abdomen with the fullness in the flanks. Skin over the abdomen is tense. Abdominal strokes are present secondary to chronic stretching of the skin. Shifting dullness, fluid thrill may be elicited. Umbilical hernia and scrotal or perineal edema are present.

Investigations

Ascitic Fluid Tap and Ascites Fluid Analysis

The appearance of ascitic fluid gives some clues. Clear, transparent yellow-tinged fluid is seen among chronic liver diseases, hypoproteinemia, and renal causes. Straw-colored fluid is present in tuberculosis. In other, in infections, the fluid is cloudy and turbid. Xanthochromic fluid is seen among the jaundice, opaque and chylous fluid in lymphatic obstruction.

Specific Gravity of the Ascitic Fluid

It is <1.016 in transudate and >1.016 in exudates.

Serum–Ascites Albumin Gradient

It is calculated by subtracting ascitic fluid albumin value from the serum albumin value. It is used to assess the causes of ascites as it correlates with portal pressure. High serum-ascites albumin gradient (SAAG), i.e. (>1.1 g/dL) with high protein >2.5 g/dL are seen in hepatic congestion. Low SAAG (<1.1 g/dL) ascites with high protein are seen with malignancy.

Biochemical Analysis

It includes the estimation of total protein and albumin. Raised amylase level in the fluid is seen in pancreatitis and intestinal perforation. Lactate dehydrogenase is increased in infection. The decreased glucose is seen in infection. Triglycerides are increased in chylous ascites.

Liver Function Tests

Total serum protein is decreased due to decreased albumin production. Liver enzymes are increased. Serum glutamic-oxaloacetic transaminase (SGOT) is increased in hepatocellular injury. SGDP is increased in liver cell injury. Prothrombin time is increased especially in liver cell failure due to decreased vitamin K absorption. Alkaline phosphatase is increased in cholestasis due to biliary obstruction. Serum bilirubin is increased. Serum blood urea and creatinine are increased in hepatorenal failure.

Ultrasound Abdomen

It is useful to detect fluid in peritoneal cavity.

CT Scan

This will detect 100 mL of fluid in peritoneum. It helps to detect the other types of fluid such as hemoperitoneum.

Liver Biopsy

This is done to ascertain etiology and for prognostic value.

CHAPTER 2

Abdominal Movements

Normally, all the quadrants of the abdomen move equally during respiration. It moves upward during inspiration and moves inward during expiration.

But in diaphragmatic paralysis, abdomen moves upward during expiration and inward in inspiration, i.e., paradoxical respiration. The causes are phrenic nerve injury in newborn, poliomyelitis, and Guillain-Barre syndrome in older children.

With outlet obstruction of the stomach, a succussion splash is at times detectable because of the presence of fluid and gas in the distended organ. This is easily appreciated by placing the stethoscope diaphragm over the epigastrium and shaking the patient vigorously from side to side. A characteristic splashing and gurgling sound is readily identified. It is important to determine the interval since the previous meal, as it is possible to elicit this sign in a normal person immediately after ingestion of a large quantity of fluid.

Bulging of abdominal wall during crying: Phantom hernia is seen in abdominal wall paralysis during acute poliomyelitis.

In generalized peritonitis, this movement is absent or markedly diminished, which helps to limit further spread of infection within the peritoneal cavity and pain of peritoneal irritation. The degree of movement of the abdominal wall is compromised by the localized masses.

Peristalsis contributes to the abdominal movement in babies. Visible gastric peristalsis may be seen in premature infant's obstruction and in congenital hypertrophic pyloric stenosis.

Visible pulsation of the abdominal aorta may be noticed in the epigastrium and is a frequent finding in nervous and thin patients. It must be distinguished from an aneurysm of the abdominal aorta, where pulsation is more obvious and a widened aorta is itself on palpation.

Visible peristalsis of the stomach or small intestine may be observed in three situations described below.

OBSTRUCTION AT THE PYLORUS

Visible peristalsis may occur where there is obstruction at the pylorus produced either by fibrosis following chronic duodenal ulceration. Peristalsis will be seen as a slow wave either passing across the upper abdomen from left to right hypochondria, or if gross gastric dilatation is present, passing own to the suprapubic region ascending to terminate in the right epigastrium. In pyloric obstruction, a diffuse swelling may be seen in the left upper abdomen but, where obstruction is longstanding with severe gastric destruction, this swelling may occupy the left mid and lower quadrants.

CONGENITAL PYLORIC STENOSIS OF INFANCY

Visible gastric peristalsis is apparent, but also the grossly hypertrophied circular muscle of

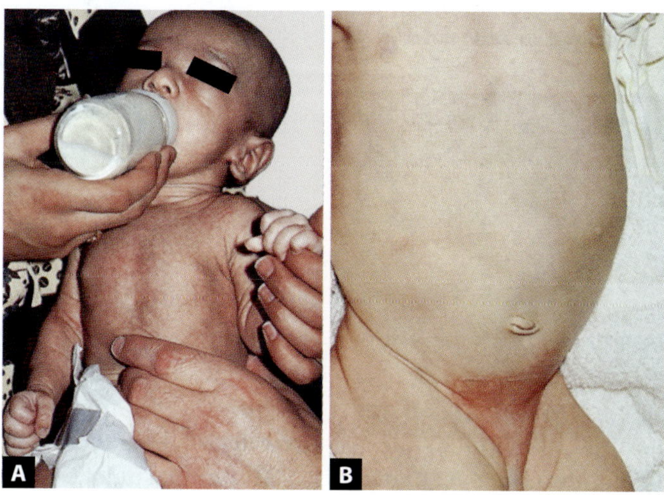

Figs. 1A and B: Congenital hypertrophic pyloric stenosis.

the antrum and pylorus may be felt as a tumor to the right of the midline in the epigastrium. Both these signs may be elicited more easily after the infant has been given a fed. Standing behind the child's mother with the child held on her lap may allow the child's abdominal musculature to relax sufficiently to feel the walnut-sized swelling as shown in **Figures 1A and B**.

OBSTRUCTION IN THE DISTAL BOWEL

Peristalsis may be seen where there is intestinal obstruction in the distal small bowel hold-up produced in the distal small bowel hold-up produced by distal colonic obstruction, with an incompetent ileocecal valve allowing reflux of gas and liquid feces into the ileum.

Step ladder type of obstruction, i.e., small intestine type: Here, the bowel loops are seen in the central position of the abdomen. The abdomen is distended and tympanic. The distended coils of intestine may be visible in a thin patient and tend to appear in step ladder pattern.

Large bowel type of obstruction is seen in the periphery of the abdomen, e.g., Hirschsprung's disease.

CHAPTER 3

Abdominal Pain

Abdominal pain in children may be either acute or chronic. Abdominal pain may originate in a gut or in other abdominal and thoracic organs. Intestinal pain is often due to distension or due to inflammation. A surgical abdominal cause should be ruled out in any child presenting with acute abdominal pain.

PATHOPHYSIOLOGY

Abdominal pain is of two types. They are visceral and parietal abdominal pain. Parietal pain is somatic pain.

Visceral Pain

Serosal surface, the mesentery, intestinal muscle, and mucosa of hollow organs contain pain receptors. Excessive contraction, stretching, tension or ischemia of the walls of hollow viscera, the capsule of a solid organ (liver, spleen, and kidney), or of the mesentery will initiate pain. Unmyelinated afferent C-fibers enter spinal cord bilaterally. This produces dull poorly localized pain.

Parietal Pain

Inflammatory noxious stimulation of the parietal peritoneum or the diaphragm produces parietal pain. This is seen in appendicitis and splenic rupture, subdiaphragmatic abscess respectively.

Delta fibers transmit pain to specific dorsal root ganglia. This pain is sharp and more intense. There will be tenderness over the site of the organ. Pain is exacerbated by cough or movement. Parietal pain will identify the anatomical location of organ involved.

Abdominal pain is usually associated with other symptoms such as vomiting, diarrhea, constipation, and fever. Vomiting is with gastroenteritis, intestinal obstruction, severe gastritis, in peptic ulcer disease and urinary tract infection. Diarrhea is present in viral or bacterial infection, acute appendicitis or pelvic infections, tubo-ovarian abscess. Diarrhea is caused by the irritation of colon adjacent to inflammatory mass. Constipation indicates other gastrointestinal dysfunction. Fever is seen in appendicitis and common in other diseases.

HISTORY

History should focus on the onset of pain, i.e., gradual or sudden nature, i.e., colicky or constant **(Box 1)**. Location of exact site of pain and progression, i.e., worsening or improving, should be ascertained. Usually, visceral pain tends to be poorly localized, somatic structural pain is generally better defined, coming from well-circumscribed area. Other aspects in the history should include presence of fever, vomiting, diarrhea, cough, dysuria, constipation, and anorexia. Presence of rashes over the body, history of trauma, and menstruation should be noted. Any history of contact with infectious disease should be noted. Loss of appetite is

BOX 1: Red flag symptoms and signs in chronic abdominal pain.

Symptoms:
- Localized pain away from umbilicus
- Pain disturbing sleep in night
- Altered bowel habits
- Frequent vomiting
- Dysphagia
- Recurrent oral ulcer
- Weight loss
- Delayed puberty
- Extraintestinal symptoms (fever, rash, and arthralgia)
- Positive family history (peptic ulcer, celiac disease, and inflammatory bowel disease)

Signs:
- Poor growth
- Anemia
- Digital clubbing
- Nonfecal abdominal mass
- Perianal disease
- Extraintestinal sign (fever, rash, and arthralgia)

an important indicator of acute inflammatory abdominal disorder in children.

EXAMINATION

Presence of sunken eyes, depressed anterior fontanelle, and dry tongue indicate the signs of dehydration due to gastroenteritis and intussusception.

Tenderness at certain anatomical region gives clue to cause of acute abdomen. Generalized tenderness indicates peritonitis, intestinal obstruction, and porphyries. Tenderness in right hypochondrium indicates hepatitis, pneumonia, cholangitis, infectious mononucleosis, and intussusception. Tenderness in left hypochondrium suggests splenic infarction and splenic rupture. Tenderness in epigastrium indicates peptic ulcer. Umbilical tenderness indicates peritonitis, parasitoses, and amebiasis. Right iliac fossa tenderness indicates appendicitis, Meckle's diverticulitis. Left iliac fossa tenderness indicates fecalith and colitis.

Abdominal Examination

The abdomen is inspected. Underlying peritoneal irritation will cause failure of abdominal movement with respiration.

High-pitched tinkling bowel sounds or rushes are present with an obstructive process. Bowel sounds are very active and loud in gastroenteritis but may be normal. Acute appendicitis is accompanied by normal sounds in the early stages, but bowel sounds disappear with diffuse peritonitis.

The examiner should focus on finding the location of pain and the presence or absence of guarding or rebound tenderness.

Voluntary contraction of abdominal wall on palpation is called guarding. Fear of pain is the most common cause for voluntary guarding while involuntary guarding results from reflexive spasms of the abdominal musculature in the setting of peritoneal irritation.

Rebound pain indicates peritoneal irritation. It is elicited during examination of the anterior abdominal wall. It occurs when an inflamed focus within the abdomen is compressed and the pressure is then quickly released, resulting in sudden and sometimes severe pain. The standard method to elicit rebound is to palpate deeply, then suddenly remove the palpating hand.

ABDOMINAL PAIN IN INFANTS AND TODDLERS

Excessive crying is the primary manifestation of abdominal pain in infants and toddler. Paroxysm of irritability, fussing, or crying that starts and stops without obvious cause in a thriving baby from birth to 4 months of age suggests infant colic. This crying peaks at 6 weeks of age and tends to resolve spontaneously by 12 weeks of age. Crying may also be a result of pain due to acid reflux and gut inflammation in infants with cow's milk allergy.

Other causes of acute abdominal pain will lead to loss of interest in feeding or vomiting, along with irritability and inconsolable crying. Localizing signs are often absent. Systemic disorders such as sepsis and meningitis should be considered. Urinary tract infection is the common cause and occurs without any symptoms.

CHRONIC ABDOMINAL PAIN

Ninety percent of chronic abdominal pain is functional or nonorganic in nature **(Boxes 2 and 3)**. The term functional means that no specific anatomic, metabolic, infections, inflammatory or neoplastic cause can be found. The pain can vary in frequent duration and severity. It is typically periumbilical or lower epigastric, nonradiating, and rarely occurs in night. The child is well in-between the episodes and physical examination is typically normal.

Organic causes of chronic abdomen are uncommon. The features of organic causes include localized pain in non-periumbilical region, referred pain, and wakens the child from sleep by sudden onset with severe pain. It will be associated with jaundice burning micturition and high-grade fever. There will be specific physical finding. There will be anorexia and weight loss.

The organic causes include gastrointestinal hepatobiliary, pancreatic, and urinary disorders. Gastrointestinal causes include esophagitis, peptic ulcer, celiac disease, Crohn's disease, lactose intolerance, and constipation **(Box 4)**.

Upper abdominal pain with regurgitation and chest discomfort suggests

BOX 2: Causes of abdominal pain in childhood.

- Intussusception
- Volvulus
- Strangulated hernia
- Appendicitis
- Meckle's diverticulum
- Urinary tract infection
- Gastroenteritis
- Migraine

BOX 3: Causes of acute abdomen.

Medical causes:
- Gastroenteritis
- Colic
- Pneumonias
- Hepatitis
- Pancreatitis
- Urinary tract infection
- Mesenteric lymphadenitis
- Inflammatory bowel disease
- Functional

Surgical:
- Appendicitis
- Intussusception
- Malrotation
- Necrotizing enterocolitis
- Volvulus
- Peritonitis
- Trauma
- Strangulated hernia

BOX 4: Common organic causes of chronic recurrent abdominal pain.

- Recurrent subacute intestinal obstruction
- Cholecystitis
- *Urinary tract:*
  - Infection
  - Pelvic ureteric obstruction
  - Stone
- Aerophagy
- Splenic infarction
- Tuberculosis
- Crohn's disease
- Pancreatitis
- Porphyries
- Peptic ulcer

gastroesophageal reflux disease. Bloating and flatulence with the abdominal pain suggest lactose intolerance. Biliary pain is right sided, usually colicky, and may be associated with vomiting and jaundice. Pancreatic disorders usually present with acute abdomen. Crohn's disease and celiac disease are two common disorders in which patient may have no symptoms other than abdominal pain.

FEATURES OF ORGANIC ABDOMINAL PAIN

- Growth failure
- Gross abdominal distension
- Pain distant from umbilicus
- Failure to respond to regular medial management

FEATURES OF INORGANIC ABDOMINAL PAIN

- Usually periumbilical
- Often severe
- Rarely interfere with sleep
- Common among school days
- Associated symptoms include:
  - Nausea
  - Pallor
  - Low-grade fever
  - Headache
  - Constipation

CAUSES OF COLICKY INTERMITTENT PAIN

- *Without palpable abdominal mass:*
  - Gastroenteritis
  - Roundworm infestation
  - Renal colic
  - Biliary colic
  - Tuberculosis
  - Henoch–Schonlein (HS) purpura
- *With the palpable mass*:
  - Intussusception
  - Tuberculosis
  - Roundworm mass

CAUSES OF CONTINUOUS DULL ACHING PAIN

- Appendicitis
- Mesenteric adenitis
- Hepatitis
- Pyelonephritis
- Pancreatitis

DIFFERENTIAL DIAGNOSIS

Intussusception

Intussusception is an important disorder that occurs most commonly in mid to late infancy. It usually presents suddenly with pain. The child screams, draws both legs up, and inconsolable. This is intermittent with the period of calm in-between. Blood-tinged stool may be passed. Most common intussusception is ileocolic. The right lower quadrant may be empty. Sausage-like mass may be felt in the right upper quadrant. The diagnosis should be suspected with the typical history of sudden, severe pain in an infant and should be confirmed by imaging studies.

Appendicitis

Pain will be present in the periumbilical region. It may be localized to right iliac fossa. The localization of the pain is again dependent upon the position of the appendix.

Pancreatitis

Pancreatitis is an acute inflammatory condition of the pancreas. It occurs as a result of obstruction of the pancreatic duct. Clinical feature includes intense epigastric abdominal pain that may be described as steady, boring, constant, achelike, knifelike, and exacerbated by recumbency, that radiates to the back, upper abdominal quadrants, or the scapula. Vomiting is common, often protracted, and occasionally bilious. The diagnosis is proved by an elevated serum amylase and/ or lipase level (lipase levels may be elevated initially with normal amylase values). Ultrasonography and CT scan are helpful in identifying the acutely inflamed pancreas, the degree of necrosis, and the later development of a pancreatic pseudocyst.

Viral Hepatitis

It is associated with the pain in the right upper quadrant. It may be associated with anorexia, jaundice, and vomiting. Tender hepatomegaly may be present. Urine is tested for bile salts and bile pigments. This should follow the liver function tests.

Subphrenic Abscess

Pain and tenderness are present at the right or left hypochondrium. Pain is radiating to the shoulder. The child may be toxic. Ultrasonography will help in the diagnosis. Aspiration of the pus will confirm the diagnosis.

Anaphylactoid Purpura

It occurs most frequently between 5 and 6 years of age. It is associated with abdominal pain, urticaria, and petechiae over the lower limbs and buttocks. There may be bleeding from the gut and nephritis.

Pyelonephritis

Pain in the flanks or suprapubic region is associated with high temperature associated with chills. There will be dysuria, vomiting, and anorexia. Demonstrations of the pus cells microscopically will confirm the diagnosis.

Pleurodynia

It may produce severe colicky abdominal pain. This is mainly viral disease. There will be positive history of family member suffering from viral disease.

Mesenteric Lymphadenitis

It is more common among children above 3 years. It follows an upper respiratory tract infection. This has to be differentiated from appendicitis. In doubtful cases, laparotomy is preferred. Both conditions may also coexist.

Liver Abscess

Child is febrile. Pain is in the right hypochondrium. Sometimes, pain will be referred to right shoulder. The liver is enlarged and tender. Demonstration of *E. histolytica* in stool and aspiration of characteristic chocolate-colored pus, i.e., anchovy sauce from the liver swelling establishes the diagnosis of amoebic liver abscess.

Cholecystitis

It is caused by inflammation of the gallbladder wall. It occurs as a result of duct obstruction (i.e., calculus) or nonobstructing (i.e., acalculous) conditions. Clinical features include fever, mild jaundice, severe abdominal pain, nausea, and vomiting. The Murphy sign is demonstrated by palpating an acutely inflamed gallbladder, which causes the patient to halt respiration and feel the pain.

Abdominal Paracentesis

It is the puncture of abdominal wall with the needle for aspiration of peritoneal cavity fluid.

Puncture site is cleaned and sterilized in a wider area. Puncture is made on the umbilical–iliospinal line in right or left lumbar fossa. It is done on lateral side of the lateral border of the rectus muscle, when the patient is lying supine.

A wide base needle, i.e., 18–20 G, is inserted attached to a syringe at the desired site horizontally into the abdominal wall. Then the direction of the needle is changed to put needle into the abdominal cavity through the zig-zag tract.

The continuous negative pressure draws the fluid into the catheter or syringe, once the abdominal cavity is reached. The fluid is then drained and puncture site is sealed with tincture benzoin.

Abdominal paracentesis can provide symptomatic relief and may be a diagnostic of the cause of ascites. Determining serum–ascites albumin gradient can help to determine the cause of ascites. A gradient >1.1 g/dL (high-gradient ascites) is consistent with ascites caused by portal hypertension, whereas a gradient <1.1 g/dL (low-gradient ascites) indicates ascites of nonportal-hypertensive etiology.

Chapter 5 Abdominal Pulsations

In infants with good subcutaneous tissue, veins are rarely visible. Visible but not distended veins are usually seen until puberty in healthy children and are especially noticeable in malnourished children.

Distended veins are seen with heart failure, peritonitis, and venous obstruction. Above the umbilicus, venous return should be toward the head; below the umbilicus, it should be toward the feet.

To determine the direction of venous return, use following procedure. Place the index finger of each hand, side by side over a vein. Press laterally, separating the fingers and milking empty a section of the vein. Release one finger and time the refill. Release the other finger and time the refill. The flow of venous blood is in the direction of the faster filling. Flow patterns are altered in some disease states.

In portal hypertension, there are peri-umbilical engorged veins (caput medusae) with flow of blood away from the umbilicus. In inferior vena cava obstruction, the direction of blood flow is from below upward, and in superior vena caval obstruction, it is from above downward. Bidirectional blood flow is seen in longstanding dilated veins (incompetence of venous valves) and in case of congenital absence of valves in the veins. In normal individuals, venous flow is away from umbilicus.

PROMINENT AORTA

The pulsations of the normal aorta may be felt in thin subjects along a line extending from the xiphoid to the bifurcation of the aorta at the level of the fourth lumbar vertebra. This is on a line joining the iliac crests, about 2 cm below and a little to the left of umbilicus.

ABDOMINAL AORTIC ANEURYSM

The aneurysm may be symptomless or the patient may complain of epigastric or central abdominal discomfort which radiates into the lumbar region.

6 CHAPTER

Abdominal Rigidity

During this preliminary examination, one (well-warmed) hand may be laid gently on the abdomen and passed over its surface with a light touch that cannot possibly hurt; this maneuver will help to allay the patient's anxiety still further and give the examiner an idea of the extent, intensity, and constancy of the rigidity which he or she must later investigate in more detail.

The abdominal rigidity due to a lesion in the chest or chest wall usually involves a wide area limited to one side—a distribution most unusual with intraabdominal pathology, which, if it has spread widely but not everywhere, tends to be limited to the upper or lower half. The extent and degree of rigidity in chest affections also vary widely during examination. Other things such as a flushed face, rapid respiration, movement of the alae nasi, or a temperature of >39°C (102°F) may suggest that the lesion is not abdominal and a friction rub may be felt or heard in the chest.

Auscultation and rectal examination dispel any remaining doubts, for in chest conditions peristaltic sounds remain normal and there is no tenderness in Douglas's pouch.

Examination of the blood may show a high leukocytosis (up to 30,000 or 40,000 per mm^3), whereas in peritonitis, the count is seldom over 12,000 per mm^3. Chest X-rays (including a lateral film) will demonstrate the intrathoracic lesion.

Causes of abdominal rigidity:

- Perforation of peptic ulcer
- Acute cholecystitis
- Rupture of gallbladder
- Acute pancreatitis
- Meckel's diverticulum
- Peritonitis
- Ruptured aneurysm

7 CHAPTER Abdominal Tenderness

Abdominal tenderness may be generalized or localized. Rebound tenderness is one of the forms of generalized tenderness. It is the tenderness on the withdrawal of finger. It indicates peritoneal irritation. This is usually associated with guarding.

Localized abnormal tenderness is related to corresponding organs. Tenderness in the upper abdominal quadrant indicates splenic rupture and infarct. Tenderness in the left upper and lower quadrant indicates ulcerative colitis and amebiasis. Tenderness in the loin indicates perinephric abscess.

Use superficial palpation to detect areas of tenderness. Watch the child's face for any expression of discomfort. If the child presents with complaints in a specific area, begin palpation away from that area, then move gradually toward the site of pain. Check for guarding and rebound tenderness whenever you discover an area of tenderness on palpation. Deep palpation should be followed by quick release of pressure. If the patient has more pain when the hand is released of pressure. If the patient has more pain when the hand is released, rebound tenderness is present. Rebound tenderness is an important sign of peritoneal irritation but can be difficult to demonstrate in very young children.

Deeper palpation should follow to detect any masses or organ enlargement. In newborns, a large mass is usually of renal origin. Fecal masses can be felt in the hypogastrium and left lower quadrant. Sometimes, their massive size can be alarming. Fecal masses often are indentable and nontender. Ovaries normally are not palpable in healthy girls. The possibility of pregnancy should always be considered in any pubertal female with abdominal symptoms. You can get your hand above an ovarian or uterine mass, confirming its pelvic origin.

CHAPTER 8

Abdominal Swellings

Abdominal wall swellings are superficial, adherent to skin, subcutaneous tissue, and muscles.

Ask the patient to take a deep breath and hold it. The contour should remain smooth and symmetric. This maneuver lowers the diaphragm and compresses the organ so that the abdominal cavity, which may cause previously unseen bulges or masses to appear. Next, ask the patient to raise his or her head from the table. This contracts the rectus abdominis muscles, which produce muscle prominent in thin or athletic adults. Superficial abdominal wall masses may become visible. If a hernia is present, the increased abdominal pressure may cause it to protrude.

Diastasis of the rectus muscle may be noted as a protrusion in the midline, usually from the xiphoid to the umbilicus but occasionally down to the symphysis pubis. Ordinarily, the protrusion is ½–2 inches size; it is usually common normal variant but may be caused by a congenital weakness of the musculature in a chronically distended abdomen. Diastasis of rectus abdominis ordinarily resolves by 6 years of age.

HISTORY

Child with the history of fever, rigors, sweating, and toxemia will give clue to pyonephrosis, perinephric abscess, amebiasis, leukemia, and splenic infection.

History suggestive of gastroenteritis with the redcurrant jelly stool indicates the intussusception.

History of vomiting, abdominal distention, and not passed meconium suggests meconium ileus, intestinal obstruction, and congenital megacolon.

History of projectile vomiting, not gaining weight and presence of mass after feed, indicates congenital pyloric stenosis.

History of pain abdomen with the painless bleeding per rectum indicates Meckel's diverticulum.

History of fever and chills with jaundice indicates cholangitis. History of bleeding diathesis indicates hemolytic type of anemia and leukemia.

EXAMINATION

When dealing with the child with mass per abdomen, many peripheral signs should be looked for the probable which have been thought at the history level. The degree of the severity produced by the mass is to be judged as quick as possible. Differential diagnosis of parietal and intra-abdominal mass is mentioned in **Table 1**.

Hemolytic facies indicates diagnosis of the hemolytic type of anemia. Conjunctival pallor will give clues for the diagnosis of the leukemia, lymphomas, renal tuberculosis, and Meckel's diverticulum. Presence of jaundice indicates hemolytic anemia, early

TABLE 1: Differential diagnosis of parietal and intra-abdominal mass.

Parietal mass	*Intra-abdominal mass*
Right and left hypochondrium: • Boils • Carbuncle • Abscess • Lipoma • Cold abscess	*Right hypochondrium:* • Hepatomegaly • Gallbladder • Subphrenic abscess • Intussusception *Left hypochondrium:* • Splenomegaly
Epigastrium: • Above causes • Epigastric hernia	*Epigastrium*: • Congenital hypertrophic pyloric stenosis • Intestinal tuberculosis • Intussusception • Aortic aneurysm
Right and left lumbar region: • Lumbar hernia	*Right and left lumbar:* • Renal mass
Umbilical region: • Umbilical hernia • Umbilical polyp • Umbilical granuloma	
Right and left iliac fossa: • Inguinal hernia • Lymphomas • Undescended testes • Psoas abscess	*Right iliac fossa:* • Renal mass *Left iliac fossa:* • Fecalith

phase of the cirrhosis, and cholangitis. Periorbital edema gives clue to the congestive cardiac failure. Gum hypertrophy in the mouth indicates the leukemia.

Raised jugular venous pressure indicates congestive cardiac failure due to some causes. Abdomen is inspected for the anomalous site of the mass. Distention of the abdomen along with the position of the umbilicus is inspected.

The palpation of the child with the mass per abdomen should be started with vital parameters such as temperature and the blood pressure. A child with the fever and chills helps to diagnose amebiasis, cholangitis subphrenic abscess, perinephric abscess, and malaria. Presence of the hypertension indicates neuroblastoma, polycystic kidney, and hydronephrosis. Presence of the chloroma indicates the leukemia. Enlarged lymph nodes clinch the diagnosis of leukemia and lymphoma.

CAUSES OF ASCITES

- Congestive cardiac failure
- Acute glomerulonephritis
- Nephritic syndrome
- Tuberculosis
- Protein energy malnutrition
- Malabsorption syndrome
- Portal hypertension

CAUSES OF TRANSIENT ABDOMINAL MASSES

- Hernia
- Intussusception
- Urinary bladder
- Rectal masses
- Round worm
- Spleen—mobile

9

CHAPTER

Acanthosis Nigricans

Acanthosis nigricans is characterized by hyperpigmentation and hyperkeratosis in intertriginous areas and over bony prominences. Skin lines are accentuated, and the skin surface of involved areas may have a velvety, leathery, or warty appearance **(Fig. 1)**. Four main forms of the disorder exist. The benign/idiopathic form is the most common and is related to hyperinsulinemia and/or insulin resistance; insulin is a skin growth factor, so high levels lead to proliferation of keratinocytes. Onset is usually at puberty but can occur in childhood in concert with development of obesity. Interestingly, the prominence of lesions tends to lessen when the patients lose weight. An inherited form, transmitted as an autosomal dominant trait, usually presents in infancy or early childhood but becomes more prominent during adolescence. This form is unassociated with other underlying disorders. In endocrine-associated acanthosis nigricans, the condition may antedate or appear in association with insulin resistance with or without polycystic ovary disease. More rarely, it is seen in patients with pituitary tumors. Malignancy-related acanthosis nigricans is extremely rare in childhood.

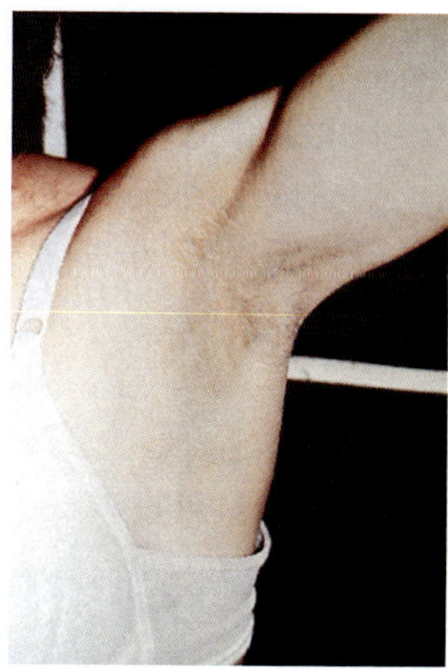

Fig. 1: Acanthosis nigricans.

CHAPTER 10

Accommodation Reflex

ACCOMMODATION REFLEX (ACCOMMODATION-CONVERGENCE SYNKINESIS)

It is elicited by having the patient shift his gaze to some near object after having relaxed his accommodation by gazing into the distance.

This is followed by:

- Thickening of the lens
- Convergence of the eyes
- Constriction of the pupils

Afferent limb:

- Optic nerve
- Proprioceptive fibers from intraocular muscles

Center: Nucleus of Perlia

Efferent: Oculomotor nerve illustrates the pathways involved in accommodation reflex.

Significance: This reflex is lost in—

- Post-diphtheritic paralysis of ciliary mechanism
- Encephalitis
- Parkinsonism

CHAPTER 11

Achalasia

Achalasia is uncommon cause of dysphagia in children. It is often diagnosed by esophagram and confirmed by esophageal manometry. It is a primary dysmotility disorder of the esophagus. It is marked by high pressure of lower esophageal sphincter (LES) at rest. There will be incomplete relaxation of LES during swallowing and uncoordinated peristalsis of esophageal smooth muscles.

Treatment is esophageal dilatation and/or injection of botulinum toxin into the LES. Both the procedures need to be repeated when symptoms return. The Heller myotomy is a surgical procedure which is a permanent treatment.

CHAPTER 12 Achondroplasia

It is the common skeletal cause of dwarfism. It is an autosomal dominant disorder affecting the bone growth. Clinical features include prominent forehead, flattened nasal bridge, midfacial hypoplasia, short limbs, broad hands with short metacarpals, phalanges, and frontal bossing. Microcephaly is present in most of them. Stenosis of foramen magnum causes otitis media, obstructive sleep apnea, and hydrocephalus.

13 CHAPTER

Acne Vulgaris

Acne is a very common condition in adolescents, but all age groups can be affected. Open and closed comedones, inflammatory papules, pustules, and nodules are characteristic primary lesions. Scarring and sinus tracts are present in moderate-to-severe forms. Androgens stimulate the hair follicle unit leading to hyperkeratosis of the follicular epithelium and increased sebum production resulting in follicular plugging. The microscopically plugged follicle is clinically apparent as a comedo. With further accumulation of keratin and sebum, the follicle wall may rupture and elicit an inflammatory reaction as contents are released into the surrounding dermis. Clinically, this corresponds to inflammatory lesions ranging from inflammatory papules and pustules to nodules or cysts. *Propionibacterium acnes*, an anerobic follicular diphtheroid, contributes to the inflammatory process.

The diagnosis of acne is a clinical one; skin biopsies and other diagnostic studies are not necessary. In some cases of mid-childhood acne (1–7 years of age), or associated signs or symptoms of androgen excess (e.g., hirsutism and irregular menses), endocrinologic evaluation may be needed to further elucidate the hormonal factors contributing to formation of acne lesions. Medication-induced acne can be seen in all age groups; the offending medications include glucocorticoids, androgens, hydantoin, and isoniazid.

CHAPTER 14

Acrocyanosis

Acrocyanosis is a common, transient, and self-limiting condition seen after the birth, disappearing over the next few hours. This typically occurs in association with crying or cold stress and can be seen in >30% of infants.

Here, central portion (chest) of the body appears pink but the extremities, particularly the palms and soles, are blue. The skin and mucus are spared. The normal newborn usually displays a bluish-purple discoloration of the hands, feet, and lips.

It results from increased peripheral arteriolar tone, which leads to vasospasm and subsequent venous pooling. Acrocyanosis should be differentiated from central cyanosis, which is noted on mucosal surfaces. Physiologic acrocyanosis gradually resolves spontaneously during the neonatal period.

It must be differentiated from central cyanosis, bluish color of skin, and mucous membrane. It requires urgent evaluation.

CHAPTER 15

Adie Tonic Pupil

Tonic pupil may develop after the acute stage of partial or complete iridoplegia. It can be seen after trauma to the eye or orbit and may occur in association with toxic or infectious conditions. Infectious processes (primarily viral syndromes) and trauma are the primary causes. The occurrence of tonic pupil in association with decreased deep tendon reflexes in young women is referred to as Adie syndrome.

Age-independent Growth Measurements

BANGLE TEST

A fiber glass bangle is used for this. The diameter is 4 cm. In malnutrition, bangle passes above the elbow. It is the quick assessment of midarm circumference.

SHAKER TAPE

This is the tape which has got three colors. Green indicates >13.5 cm of midarm circumference. Yellow indicates 12.5–13.5 cm. Red indicates <12.5 cm, i.e., malnutrition. This is useful for paramedical staff to assess the nutritional status.

QUACK STICK

It is a height measuring rod calibrated in midarm circumference, rather than height. Value of 80% of expected midarm circumference for height is marked on the stick to the corresponding height levels. If the child is taller than his arm circumference level, on the stick, it indicates malnourishment.

17 CHAPTER

Albinism

It occurs in an X-linked ocular form (in which the skin appears clinically normal) and several different autosomal recessive oculocutaneous forms.

In oculocutaneous albinism (OCA), both sexes and all races are affected equally. This form of the disorder is subdivided into a number of variants on the basis of clinical findings and biochemical markers. In the past, tyrosinase-negative and tyrosinase-positive subtypes were identified on the basis of the ability of plucked hairs to produce pigment when incubated in tyrosine. Now, deoxyribonucleic acid (DNA) markers allow for identification of specific mutations. In classic tyrosinase-negative OCA, children are born without any trace of pigment. Affected individuals have snow-white hair, pinkish-white skin, and translucent or blue irises. Nystagmus is common, as is moderate-to-severe strabismus and poor visual acuity. Although children with tyrosinase-positive OCA may be clinically indistinguishable from their tyrosinase-negative counterparts at birth, they usually develop variable amounts of pigment with increasing age. Eye color may vary from gray to light brown, and hair may change to blond or light brown. The subtypes can be distinguished by genetic testing.

CHAPTER 18

Alopecia

Alopecia (hair loss) is the most common hair abnormality seen in children. Hair loss can have a number of presentations ranging from focal patches to diffuse thinning. An accurate history alone can often lead to a presumptive diagnosis. Information regarding duration of loss, rate of shedding, medications, trauma, family history of hair disorders, symptoms such as pruritus or burning, breakage, and hair care is particularly important. The scalp should be examined for the pattern and distribution of hair loss, erythema, scaling, scarring, pustules, and crusts. Abnormal or broken hairs, as well as texture, length, and color should be noted. Associated abnormalities of the teeth, nails, and sweat glands may occur. Hair pulls (gentle pulling on small tufts of hair) and microscopic examination of removed hairs should be performed. Appropriate tests (KOH, fungal culture, and scalp biopsy) may be necessary to confirm the clinical suspicions. Classification of alopecia is somewhat arbitrary, but it is helpful to determine whether hair loss is acquired or congenital and localized or diffuse. Congenital alopecia usually results from aplasia cutis, intrauterine injury, or nevus sebaceous. Five common disorders responsible for most cases of childhood hair loss are (1) alopecia areata, (2) tinea capitis, (3) traction alopecia, (4) trichotillomania, and (5) telogen effluvium.

ALOPECIA AREATA

Alopecia areata is a common disorder that affects all ages, particularly children. Although several hypotheses have been proposed, it is generally thought to be an autoimmune condition linked to specific genetic mutations. There is a family history of alopecia areata for approximately 20% of affected individuals. Clinically, there is acute onset of hair loss that is occasionally preceded by burning or itching of the scalp. In most cases, well-demarcated, localized areas of alopecia result, and the scalp is usually normal without epidermal changes. The examination point hairs are pathognomonic and are caused by breakage of abnormally growing hairs. Exclamation point hairs, when pulled out, appear as a tapered or attenuated bulb secondary to atrophy of that portion. When the disease is active, dystrophic anagen hairs can be easily pulled from the periphery of lesions. Nail pitting, often seen in rows, is seen in some cases. Factors that portend a poor prognosis for regrowth include extensive loss, early onset, nail involvement, atopic background, and an ophiasis pattern (involvement of the temporal and occipital hairline).

Alopecia areata is a form of localized alopecia that usually presents with round or oval patches of smooth alopecia that may be located anywhere on the scalp, eyebrows, lashes, or body. On occasion, hair loss is more diffuse or generalized. Its origin is autoimmune, and scalp biopsies in cases of alopecia areata will demonstrate a swarm of lymphocytes around the hair follicles as well as increased numbers of telogen hairs. Clinical clues to diagnosis include absence of inflammation and scaling in the involved areas of scalp and the presence of short (3–6 mm), easily epilated hairs at the margins of the patch. Under magnification, these hair stubs resemble exclamation points, because the hair shaft narrows just before its point of entry into the follicle. Another finding in many patients with alopecia areata is Scotch-plaid pitting of the nails, consisting of rows of pits crossing in a transverse and longitudinal fashion. The clinical course of alopecia areata is difficult to predict. The disorder may resolve spontaneously; it may persist, with the appearance of new patches while the old patches regrow; or it may progress to total scalp *(alopecia totalis)* or even generalized whole-body alopecia *(alopecia universalis)*, either of which can be permanent. In severe cases, it is helpful to perform a thorough search to exclude coexistent autoimmune disease, such as autoimmune thyroiditis or pernicious anemia.

TINEA CAPITIS

Tinea capitis (*ringworm*) is another common cause of alopecia in children, although it may not always be associated with hair loss or breakage. The "seborrheic" type of tinea capitis is manifested by diffuse scaling without scalp inflammation. Alopecia is often not noted, but broken hairs are occasionally present. This type of alopecia is frequently misdiagnosed as dandruff. Tinea capitis can also manifest as localized scaly patches, kerions, and "black-dot" patches **(Fig. 1)**. This latter type features hairs that have broken at the surface of the scalp, resulting in a black-dot appearance.

Kerions are boggy, inflammatory plaques on the scalp that are caused by hypersensitivity to the offending dermatophyte. Pustules and drainage are common, but the purulent material is often sterile. Cervical lymphadenopathy, fever, and elevated

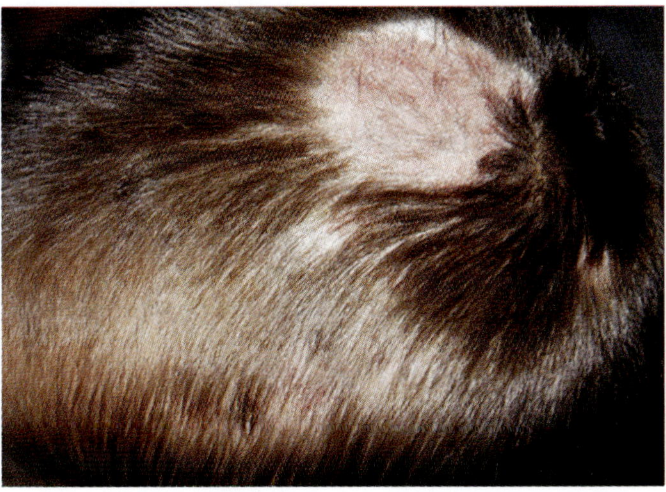

Fig. 1: Tinea capitis.

white blood cell counts may accompany kerions. The differential diagnosis of tinea capitis includes psoriasis, alopecia areata, trichotillomania, folliculitis, and seborrheic dermatitis.

The most common etiologic agent of tinea capitis is *Trichophyton tonsurans*, a dermatophyte that produces endothrix infections. Because spores are not present on the surfaces of the hair shafts, Wood lamp examination is not useful. If the infection is caused by *Microsporum canis* or another dermatophyte that produces an ectothrix infection, Wood lamp examination results in positive fluorescence. Fungal cultures should be performed in all suspected cases of tinea capitis. Fungal culture can be performed with a standard toothbrush and Petri dish. KOH preparations can be useful if positive, but false-negative results are common. Some children may be asymptomatic carriers.

CHAPTER 19

Ambiguous Genitalia

Ambiguous genitalia is a discrepancy between actual sex and the external genitalia. External genitalia are the characteristics of neither a male nor a female **(Fig. 1)**.

High adrenocorticotropic hormone (ACTH) levels cause increased nipple and labial or scrotal pigmentation. But in some, newborn darkening is expected because of exposure to maternal estrogen. Urethral opening and length of phallus are noted. Labial and scrotal areas are looked for testicles. If they are not palpable, groin should be looked for. When the external genitalia appear ambiguous and testicles are palpable, the differential diagnosis is narrowed and 21-hydroxylase or 11-hydroxylase deficiencies are excluded.

In newborn, enlarged clitoris may resemble a male phallus. The female child with hyperandrogenism due to congenital adrenal hyperplasia (CAH) has an enlarged clitoris with normal internal female sexual organs.

Perineum is carefully looked to see whether there is urethral orifice separation from and anterior to the hymenal ring. When the lower end of the vagina has not formed, there will be fistula from vagina to urethra with a common external opening.

The anatomic malformations include clitoral hypertrophy with the partial fusion of posterior labia. The joining skin is thickened and transparent. Boys with the CAH have an enlarged penis. These children will mature rapidly and develop increased muscle bulk because of the excessive testosterone secretion.

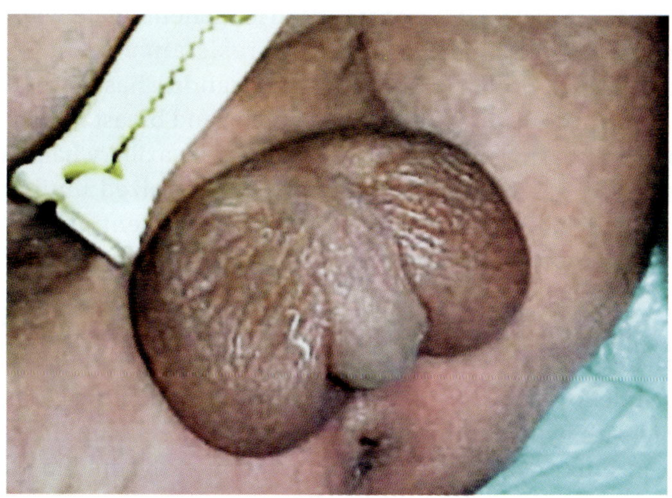

Fig. 1: Ambiguous genitalia.

The perineal hypospadias is used to describe a urethral openings the perineal surface. This occurs because of androgen receptor abnormality. This occurs in normal XY karyotype who has ambiguous genitalia.

Testicular feminization is condition where there is genetic male with complete androgen resistance. He has normal female external genitalia and breast development but little or no pubic or axillary hair. The condition may be recognized only at puberty because of primary amenorrhea. This is due to the absence of uterus and upper two-thirds of vagina. Testicular swelling may be palpated in the loin or groin. This will be missed in the childhood because of large size at the onset of puberty.

APPROACH TO THE PHYSICAL EXAMINATION OF A CHILD WITH AMBIGUOUS GENITALIA

High ACTH levels cause increased nipple and labial or scrotal pigmentation, yet in normal neonates, some darkening is expected because of exposure to maternal estrogen. Measure the phallus length, and check the terminal urethral position. Examine the labial or scrotal area for testicles. If they are not palpable, check the groin areas for an undescended testicle, which occurs in about 3% of full-term newborns. Undescended testicles may be unilateral, but most commonly the testicles are partially descended. 1 year ago, <1% of testes remain undescended.

When the external genitalia appear ambiguous and testicles are palpable, the differential diagnosis is narrowed, and 21-hydroxylase or 11-hydroxylase deficiencies are excluded.

The female child with hyperandrogenism due to CAH has an enlarged clitoris and normal internal female sexual organs. In a newborn, the enlarged clitoris may resemble a male phallus so closely as to be indistinguishable.

Look at the perineum carefully to see whether there is a urethral orifice separate from and anterior to the hymenal ring. When the lower end of the vagina has not formed, as occurs in some females with CAH, there is a fistula from vagina to urethra, with a common external opening. A milder anatomic abnormality may be clitoral hypertrophy with partial fusion of the posterior labia; in this abnormality, the joining skin is thickened, not grayish and transparent as in benign labial agglutination, a common phenomenon in female infants.

Boys with the common forms of CAH have an enlarged penis. If the condition is diagnosed after infancy, such children will mature rapidly and develop increased muscles bulk because of the excessive testosterone secretion.

At the other extreme is the child with a normal XY karyotype who has ambiguous genitalia because of an androgen receptor abnormality. The term used to describe a urethral opening on the perineal surface in boys is perineal hypospadias.

The genetic male with complete androgen resistance (also called testicular feminization) has normal female external genitalia and breast development but little or no public or axillary hair. The condition may not be recognized until the patient comes to medical attention because of primary amenorrhea, which is due to the absence of in the patient, which were missed in early childhood but are now larger because of the uterus and the upper two-thirds of the vagina. Palpation the groin and labia reveals testicular swelling in the patient, which was missed in early childhood but is now larger because of the onset of puberty.

CHAPTER 20

Amblyopia

This is also known as lazy eye. It is characterized by indistinct or poor vision in normal or structural abnormal eye. Visual image is not transmitted to the visual cortex, or it is poor. This is usually seen in one eye. Visual cortex should receive focused images simultaneously from both the eyes. If this does not occur, image from dysfunctional eye is suppressed and amblyopia occurs. Later in due time, irreversible loss of vision occurs in defective eye. Amblyopia occurs in congenital cataract, strabismus, and in anisometropia.

21 CHAPTER Amenorrhea

Absence of menstruation is amenorrhea. It may be primary or secondary.

Primary amenorrhea is defined as absence of menses by 13 years of age with no visible secondary sexual characteristic development, or absence of menses by 15 years of age in the presence of normal secondary sexual characteristics.

The etiology of primary amenorrhea as menstruation is an end result of coordinated activity of hypothalamic pituitary ovarian uterine axis with normal outflow tract with normal thyroid, adrenal and metabolic function.

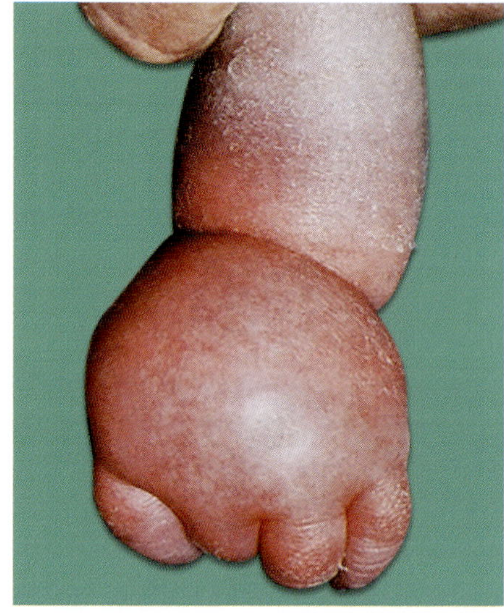

Fig. 1: Turner's syndrome.

Primary amenorrhea can be classified as:

- Delayed puberty
- Anatomical defect
- *Chromosomal abnormalities:* Turner's syndrome **(Fig. 1)**
- Endocrinal abnormalities

In Turner's syndrome (gonadal dysgenesis), there is also dwarfism, web-neck, cubitus valgus, and an XO sex-chromosome pattern **(Fig. 1)**. This is the most common form of gonadal dysgenesis. These women may develop spontaneous menstruation. Premature ovarian failure is common. The gonadotrophin levels may be raised, and these individuals may require hormone replacement therapy (HRT). Spontaneous conception has been reported, but many would require some form of assisted conception in order to have an intrauterine pregnancy.

- *Hypothalamus/CNS cause:* Kallmann syndrome; idiopathic
- *Pituitary cause:* Hyperprolactinemia, Sheehan syndrome, and empty sella syndrome
- *Ovarian cause:* Gonadal dysgenesis and Turner's syndrome
- Congenital adrenal hyperplasia
- Juvenile hypothyroidism

Secondary amenorrhea is absence of menstruation for 6 months in a patient who had previously regular menses or absence for at least three previous cycles in a women with previous irregular cycles.

Physiological causes include lactation, pregnancy, and menopause.

CAUSES OF SECONDARY AMENORRHEA

- *Hypothalamic:* Trauma, chronic illness, tuberculosis, and sarcoidosis
- *Pituitary:* Hyperprolactinemia, Sheehan's syndrome, and pituitary adenoma
- *Ovarian:* Polycystic ovary syndrome (PCOS) and arrhenoblastoma
- *Uterine*: Tuberculosis
- *Others*: Congenital adrenal hyperplasia (CAH), Cushing's syndrome, Addison's disease, adrenal tumor, and hypothyroidism.

CHAPTER 22

Amniocentesis

Amniocentesis involves the process of sampling of amniotic fluid under ultrasound guidance through the abdominal wall into the amniotic cavity. It is a transabdominal process. It is indicated in prenatal diagnosis of genetic disorders to assess the severity of Rh hemolytic disease and for biochemical assessment. Amniocentesis is advised at 16 weeks to all the mothers. Over the age of 35 years, most enzyme assay as well as DNA analysis can also be carried out that indicates the severity of the Rh hemolytic disease. α-fetoprotein (AFP) levels are measures. Raised levels indicate the neural tube defects. Cystic fibrosis, congenital nephrotic syndrome, and mucopolysaccharidosis can be diagnosed from the products excreted into the fluid by the fetus.

It is best performed between 15 and 20 weeks. Placenta should be localized by ultrasonography **(Fig. 1)**. Patient should pass the urine before the procedure. Spinal needle with the stylet is used, fetal parts are palpated and puncture site is determined. The ideal place is the concavity or hollowness between the head and the limbs. Sometimes, uterus contracts when the needle passes. If it contracts, the needle is withdrawn 1–2 cm, procedure should be started only when contraction stops. If, in case, fish blood is aspirated, the procedure is abandoned.

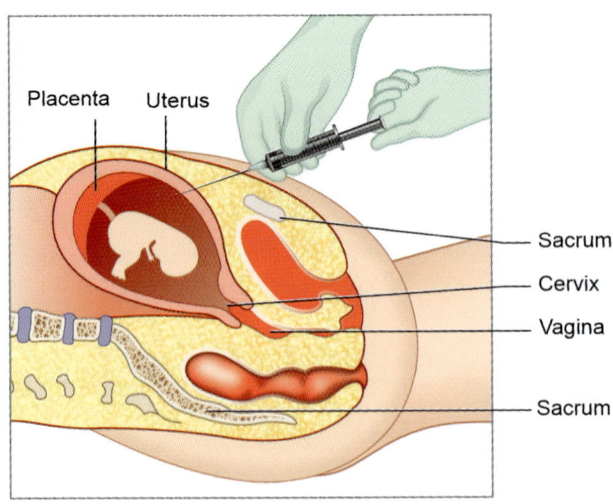

Fig. 1: Transabdominal amniocentesis.

23 CHAPTER

Amniotic Bands

A number of serious structural deformations can result from early in utero amniotic rupture and subsequent band-line compression or amputation **(Fig. 1)**. The band-induced abnormalities generally affect the limbs, digits, and craniofacial structures. This phenomenon is usually sporadic.

Amniotic bands may disrupt the skin, extremities (amputation, ring constriction, and syndactyly), face (clefts), or trunk (abdominal or thoracic wall defects). Their cause is uncertain but may be related to amniotic membrane rupture or vascular compromise with fibrous band formation

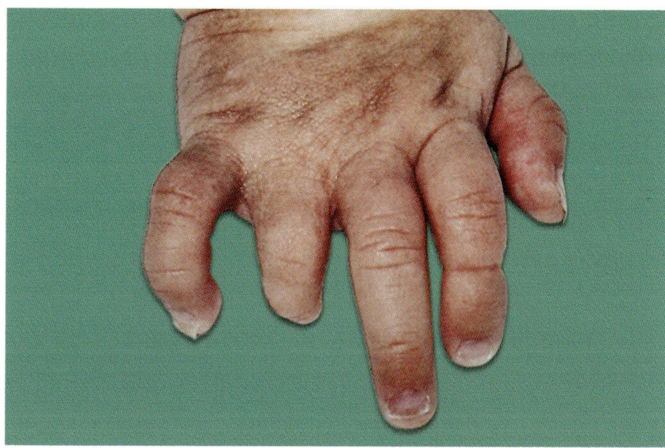

Fig. 1: Amniotic band.

CHAPTER 24

Anaphylaxis

Anaphylaxis results from widespread degradation of mast cells after cross-linking of IgE on mast cell surface. Onset is typically rapid and often explosive after bee stings, drug administration, or food indigestion. The pattern of organ system involvement is based on an antigen, dose, and route of administration, and can range from isolated urticarial to cardiovascular collapse. Airway obstruction and hypotension are the most severe manifestations of anaphylaxis. Upper airway obstruction is due to laryngeal edema, whereas lower airway obstruction is due to edema bronchospasm. Hypotension is caused by vasodilation, which may be complicated by loss of intravascular fluid volume. Vascular collapse may be aggravated by disease in myocardial function. The skin is most commonly involved organ, with urticaria. Angioedema is often present. Gastrointestinal (GI) involvement produces vomiting, diarrhea, and abdominal pain due to gut edema.

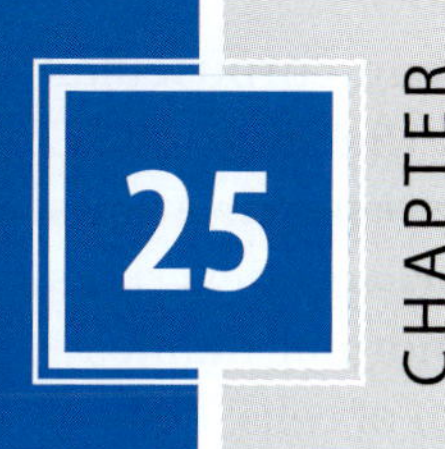

Anemia

It is a reduction in red blood cell (RBC) volume. Anemia causing pallor is appreciated when hemoglobin concentration is <8–9 g/dL.

Anemia occurs as the result of one or a combination of three pathophysiologic mechanisms:

1. Acute blood loss
2. Impaired bone marrow production of RBCs
3. Increased peripheral destruction of RBCs (hemolysis)

CLINICAL FEATURES

It is due to tissue hypoxia and its consequences. Tiredness, easy fatigability, lassitude, poor feeding, muscle weakness, lack of concentration, and dyspnea on exertion are the common symptoms. Pallor is seen in skin, oral mucosa, palmar creases, nails, and conjunctiva.

INVESTIGATIONS

Reticulocyte Count

The reticulocyte count, reported as a percentage of total RBCs, is essential in categorizing anemia. An elevated reticulocyte count implies a bone marrow response to either increased RBC destruction (hemolysis) or acute or chronic blood loss. In cases of acute blood loss, there is an average delay in bone marrow response of 3–4 days. Thus, in the setting of acute blood loss, the reticulocyte count is most helpful when the bleeding and subsequent anemia have been present for more than a few days.

Anemias are categorized on the basis of the adequacy of the reticulocyte response. The reticulocyte count is expressed as a percentage of the total number of RBCs. In the setting of a normal hemoglobin, the reticulocyte count is about 1–2%. In patients with moderate or severe anemia, the reticulocyte count may appear elevated, but in absolute terms, it may be insufficient for the degree of anemia. Therefore, the reticulocyte count must be corrected using the following formula:

$$\text{Corrected reticulocyte count} = \frac{\text{Reticulocyte count hemoglobin}}{\text{(Normal hemoglobin for age)}}$$

CLINICAL ASSESSMENT OF THE CHILD WITH POSSIBLE IRON DEFICIENCY

Parent of iron-deficient infants often report that the baby refuses all solid food. In each infants, severe reduction or temporary elimination of milk intake, coupled with discontinuation of bottle feeding, invariably results in rapid acceptance of solid foods. Severe restriction of milk intake not only increases the child's appetite for solid foods but also removes the dietary cause of gastrointestinal mucosal alteration that may result in erythrocyte and protein losses into the gut, which further aggravate the iron deficiency state and may cause hypoalbuminemia and edema.

It is also important to ask whether the child had a history of pica (i.e., ingestion of foreign materials such as dirt and starch). For reasons that are poorly understood, iron deficiency states are sometimes associated with pica. The pica usually disappears when the iron deficiency is corrected.

DIFFERENTIAL DIAGNOSIS

Anemia Secondary to Acute Blood Loss

When severe acute blood loss occurs, intravascular volume depletion is the primary concern, which cannot be assessed by hemoglobin level. Therefore, in the setting of severe blood loss, blood pressure, heart rate, adequacy of peripheral perfusion, and mental status are the best ways to assess patients. In most instances, an obvious history of blood loss is apparent (epistaxis, hematemesis, lower gastrointestinal bleeding, and trauma). Large amounts of blood may accumulate in the gastrointestinal tract before the development of hematemesis, hematochezia, or melena. Intra-abdominal bleeding may occur after trauma or may result from an ulcer and may be associated with progressive anemia in the absence of an obvious source of bleeding.

Anemia Secondary to Underproduction

Microcytic Anemias

Hemoglobin, the chief intracellular component of the RBC, is composed of heme (iron and protoporphyrin IX) and globin chains (α and β). Any factor that diminishes the availability or utilization of these components results in microcytic anemia. The automated mean corpuscular volume (MCV) represents the mean RBC volume and does not address variations in cell size. The RDW, however, describes variation in RBC size and, if normal, defines a relatively uniform population of cells. Review of the peripheral blood smear also provides additional evidence regarding variability in cell size and shape. It is important to note that MCV is age related.

Iron deficiency anemia: Iron deficiency results when nutritional intake is insufficient to meet demands associated with growth and/or blood loss. Iron is a key component of the hemoglobin molecule; its deficiency leads to anemia associated with reduced hemoglobin production (hypochromia) and small RBCs (microcytosis). Infants are at particular risk for the development of iron deficiency since their rapid growth and expanding blood volume impose considerable iron demands. Premature infants are at the highest risk because most in utero iron is transferred to the fetus during the last trimester of pregnancy and postnatal growth rate is rapid. When iron deficiency occurs outside of the setting of infancy, toddlers, or adolescent females, a pathologic source of blood loss must be strongly considered.

Thalassemia syndromes: The thalassemia syndromes represent a heterogeneous group of inherited disorders of decreased globin production that lead to microcytic anemia, which can be mistaken for iron deficiency. The child with microcytic anemia, without evidence of iron deficiency, should be evaluated for thalassemia.

Two genes, one inherited from each parent, code for the production of the β-globin chains of hemoglobin. When one gene is affected by the β-thalassemia mutation, a moderate diminution in the production of the β-globin chain occurs, resulting in mild microcytic anemia of underproduction.

Lead poisoning: The occurrence of elevated serum and total body burdens of lead is a major public health problem. This is of particular importance for infants and young children from lower socioeconomic families living in old housing with lead-based paint. Elevated lead levels may decrease erythropoiesis because lead inhibits several enzymes along the path of protoporphyrin synthesis. Lead may also produce hemolysis.

Anemia is usually seen in association with lead levels of 60–70 μg/dL or higher. Anemia is mild, variably microcytic, and associated with prominent basophilic stippling of RBCs. Coexistent iron deficiency is common because iron deficiency promotes increased lead absorption.

Anemia of inflammation: In a wide variety of chronic inflammatory or infectious disorders, mild-to-moderate anemia, termed anemia of inflammation (previously known as anemia of chronic disease), may be present. The MCV is usually normal to mildly decreased. Chronic inflammation or infection impairs the transfer of iron from reticuloendothelial cells within the marrow to developing erythroid elements. This results in some degree of iron-deficient erythropoiesis despite adequate marrow stores of iron. This impaired transfer of iron is thought to be due in part to the molecule hepcidin that is elevated during times of inflammation.

Sideroblastic anemias: These are a group of very rare congenital (often X-linked) inherited diseases associated with impairment of protoporphyrin synthesis and variable microcytic anemia. The bone marrow examination demonstrates evidence of developing erythroid cells with excess iron deposited in mitochondria that tend to form a circular appearance around the nucleus; hence, the term ringed sideroblast.

Normocytic Anemia

Normocytic anemia secondary to underproduction: When normocytic anemia secondary to underproduction is identified in a patient, the key issue is whether anemia is occurring in isolation or is associated with other cytopenias. Normocytic anemia with an inadequate reticulocyte response and pancytopenia raises the possibility of serious primary or secondary bone marrow disease including malignancy. The history and physical examination findings are often predictive of the presence of thrombocytopenia (easy bruising, petechiae, and ecchymosis) and/or neutropenia (fever and signs of infection). Adenopathy and hepatosplenomegaly are suggestive of bone marrow infiltration caused by malignancy.

Macrocytic Anemia

Diamond–Blackfan anemia is a constitutional pure RBC aplasia syndrome that manifests during the 1st year of life with isolated severe anemia and reticulocytopenia. The remainder of the CBC is unremarkable. Because synthesis of RBCs containing adult hemoglobin is markedly impaired, RBCs generally manifest fetal characteristics, including elevated MCV, increased levels of fetal hemoglobin, and the "i" surface antigen. Bone marrow aspirate demonstrates pure RBC aplasia.

Fanconi anemia usually manifests with macrocytic anemia secondary to underproduction and pancytopenia. It is a constitutional disorder frequently, but not invariably, associated with physical stigmata. Most patients do not present with overt hematologic manifestations until 4 or 5 years of age. Thumb and radial anomalies should alert the clinician to possible Fanconi anemia even in the absence of cytopenias. RBCs tend to have fetal characteristics including increased MCV and elevated fetal hemoglobin level.

Megaloblastic Anemia (Vitamin B_{12} Deficiency or Folate Deficiency)

Megaloblastic anemia, characterized by macrocytic RBCs with variable abnormalities of WBCs and platelets, is usually caused by vitamin B_{12} deficiency or folate deficiency. Albeit rare in children, it can occur secondary to nutritional or congenital etiologies. If severe, associated pancytopenia can occur. In addition to large ovoid RBCs, hypersegmented neutrophils (>5 lobes/cell) are often seen on the peripheral smear; large platelets can be present. It is appropriate to suspect vitamin B_{12} deficiency or folate deficiency in patients with otherwise unexplained macrocytic anemia. Documenting the presence of vitamin B_{12} deficiency or folate deficiency requires an exhaustive etiologic search, including assessment of nutrition and gastrointestinal absorption.

CHAPTER 26

Angioedema

Hereditary angioedema (HAE) is an autosomal dominant disorder characterized by the absence or abnormal function of a protein in the complement cascade known as C1 esterase inhibitor. Inhibitors of the complement system are part of the complement pathway and are capable of blocking activated complement components. C1 esterase inhibitor binds to activated C1 and thereby prevents further activation of the classical pathway. It also serves to regulate other blood protein cascades, including the bradykinin system. In the absence of C1 inhibitor, these cascades can proceed unchecked. This results in increased vascular permeability and the observed clinical features of angioedema. This disorder is characterized by recurrent bouts of swelling that involve any part of the body with the face, extremities, genitals, and respiratory and GI tracts most frequently involved **(Fig. 1)**. The swelling is generally self-limited, episodic, and commonly triggered by minor trauma. The swelling is distinguished from idiopathic angioedema (which is frequently accompanied by urticaria) by its longer duration (1–3 days) and the absence of urticaria. Laryngeal edema is a frightening, life-threatening complication that may result in asphyxiation. Involvement of the gastrointestinal (GI) tract is characterized by severe abdominal pain, bloating, vomiting, and rarely intestinal obstruction resulting from intussusception. Other components of the complement system affected in HAE are C2 and C4: C4 levels are consistently low in 95% of patients, and C2 levels are decreased during attacks. The diagnosis of HAE can be confirmed by measuring the C1 esterase level and function. Until more recently, anabolic steroids were prescribed widely as treatment for HAE, with problems with efficacy, side effects, and toxicity. Fortunately, there are now different forms of purified C1 esterase inhibitor, kallikrein inhibitors, and bradykinin receptor antagonists available for treatment, with options for both prophylactic and acute use, and other products are under investigation.

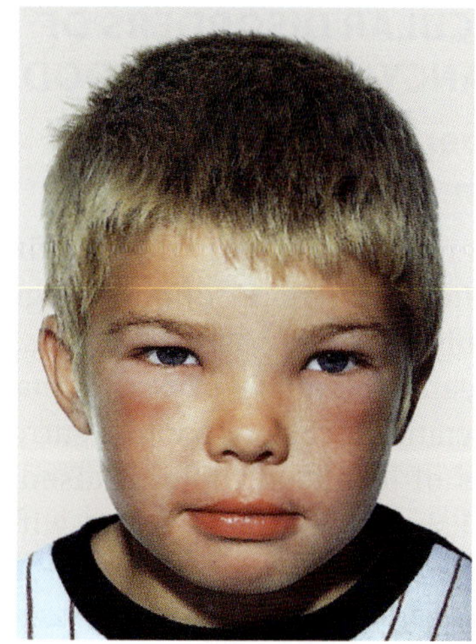

Fig. 1: Angioedema.

CHAPTER 27 Angiomata and Telangiectasia

VASCULAR DISORDERS OF INFANCY AND CHILDHOOD

Strawberry Hemangiomas (Capillary Hemangioma)

They generally develop during first few weeks after birth, more common in girls and commonly seen over head and trunks.

Appearance initially as well-demarcated, telangiectatic macules or papules surrounded by areas of localized pallor. Raised bright or purplish red lobulated lesion with well-defined borders and minute capillaries protruding from its surface, compressible but seldom blanches completely.

Cavernous Hemangiomas

These represent deep seated strawberry hemangiomas with little penetration of the overlying skin. They are present at birth, grow in proportion to the growth of the individual, bluish red masses with less distinct border. In 90% of cases, they disappear by 9 years.

Salmon Patch (Nevus Simplex, Telangiectatic Nevus)

It is most common vascular lesion of infancy.

Clinical features: Flat, dull pink, macular lesion often with telangiectasia on the nape of the neck, glabella, forehead, upper eyelids, and nasolabial folds. When seen over the nape of the neck, they are referred as stork bite. 95% resolve within 1st year.

Nevus Flammeus (Portwine Stains)

It is a congenital vascular malformation composed of dilated capillary-like vessels. It presents at birth, persists throughout the life, and does not grow out of proportion. It is part of Sturge-Weber syndrome. Lesions, reddish purple and flat, are barely elevated, and do not fade and associated with other syndromes. Color is pale pink to bright red or bluish purple. It commonly involves the face.

When hemangiomas are present, look for amblyopia, myopia, astigmatism, strabismus, ptosis, retrobulbar involvement, optic nerve atrophy, neurologic stridor caused by laryngeal hemangioma, lumbosacral hemangiomas may be associated with spina bifida, spinal dysraphism, meningomyelocele, imperforate anus, rectoscrotal-rectovaginal fistulas, gastrointestinal, genitourinary, and skeletal anomalies.

CHAPTER 28

Aniridia

It is an autosomal condition. There is an absence of iris. This occurs as a result of failure of mesoderm to grow onward from the root of the iris. This occurs in 4th month of gestation. The iris and cornea are rudimentary findings. Pupils appear of same size. Photophobia and nystagmus are present. It is associated with Wilms' tumor, corneal opacities, dislocation of lens, and cataract.

CHAPTER 29

Anisometropia

In patients with anisometropia, the refractive error of one eye differs significantly from that of the other eye. The difference in refraction can be spherical (hyperopia or myopia) or cylindric (unequal amounts of astigmatism). Mild degrees of anisometropia usually cause no visual symptoms and do not lead to amblyopia. Amblyopia develops with higher degrees of anisometropia because the child uses the less ametropic eye and suppresses vision in the other. Strabismus frequently coexists with anisometropia, and both conditions may be involved in the pathophysiologic mechanisms of amblyopia. Anisometropia may initially be detected by comparison of the red reflex between the two eyes (Brückner test). The affected eye has the duller red reflex. Early detection and treatment of anisometropia are essential for the development of optimal visual function.

30 CHAPTER Antimongoloid Slant

Antimongoloid slant refers to downward slanting of eyes. The outer canthi below the line join inner canthi. Here, the nasal corners of the palpebral fissure are higher than the temporal corners. This occurs when the lateral palpebral ligament is inserted lower than the medial palpebral ligament. The zygomatic bones are hypoplastic and absent in full expression of the malformation.

ANTIMONGOLOID SLANT

- Alport syndrome
- Apert syndrome
- Cri-du-chat syndrome
- Crouzon's syndrome
- Noonan's syndrome
- Treacher Collins syndrome
- Turner's syndrome

Apex Beat, Displaced

It refers the lowest and outermost point of cardiac impulse which gives maximum thrust to the palpating finger. It is located in the intercostal space, distance from the midclavicular line, either medial or lateral. Normal site varies with age. The displacement of the cardiac apex in different age groups is mentioned in **Table 1**.

TABLE 1: Displacement of the cardiac apex in different age groups.

Age	*Location*
Birth to 1 year	Left 3rd ICS lateral to MCL
1–4 years	Left 3rd ICS in the MCL
4–8 years	Left 4th ICS in the MCL
8–12 years	Left 4th ICS medial to MCL
Adolescent	Left 5th ICS medial to MCL

(ICS: intercostal space; MCL: midclavicular line)

CAUSES OF DISPLACED APICAL IMPULSE

- Dextrocardia
- Aortic and mitral valve disease
- Left ventricular hypertrophy
- Right ventricular hypertrophy
- Scoliosis
- Funnel chest
- Pleural effusion
- Pneumothorax
- Ascites
- Abdominal tumor

Apical impulse may be *forcible or diffuse:*

Forcible apical impulse:

- Fever
- Hyperdynamic circulation
- Thyrotoxicosis
- Left ventricular hypertrophy
- Retracted lung

Diffuse apical impulse:

- Thin chest wall
- Hyperkinetic state
- Severe valvular regurgitation
- Complete AV block
- Hypertrophic cardiomyopathy

CHAPTER 32

Aphthous Ulcers

This is the most common form of oral ulceration, and three types are recognized on the size and number of ulcers.

The term minor aphthous ulcer is given to ulcers <5 mm in diameter, which occur intermittently as single ulcers or in crops. The ulcers take from 1 week to 10 days to heal. Larger >1 cm, persistent ulcer on the tongue and palate. These are prone to neoplastic transformation.

Aplasia Cutis Congenita

It is characterized by absence of or failure of formation of a localized of epidermis, dermis, fat, bone, or some combination of these layers. Rarely, they may be associated with limb defects and congenital and genetic anomalies. In majority of cases, only the dermis and epidermis are absent. At birth, the lesion may consist of a sharply circumscribed open and weeping erosion or ulceration. It may be covered by a thin often hemorrhagic membrane or crust. Evaluation should include radiologic studies to assess the depth of lesion to search of associated anomalies. A hair collar sign indicates to rule out underlying neural tube defect.

Apraxia

Praxis refers to carrying out an action. Apraxia is characterized by an inability to perform motor behavior. Specifically, apraxias are acquired disorders of learned movement present, in the absence of disease involving the "motor system" or muscle. To test for apraxia, establish first that the sensory, motor, and musculoskeletal systems are intact.

The patient must be asked to do simple tasks initially and then progress to complex tasks. Each group of muscles must be tested as apraxias may be regional, e.g., buccofacial, limb, truncal, etc.

Apraxias are most frequently seen in patients with lesions involving the parietal lobe on the dominant side, although lesions in other locations of left frontal lobe may also cause apraxic disorders.

Apraxia can be divided into three main types (affecting progressively "higher" elements of the motor system)—kinetic (limb), ideomotor, and ideational—as well as a number of other specific disorders of apraxias.

CLASSIFICATION

Limb Kinetic Apraxia

This is a loss of the components of motor engrams, resulting in coarse or unrefined movements that no longer have the expected appearance of being practiced over time. These apraxias are usually contralateral to a hemisphere lesion.

Ideomotor (Ideokinetic Apraxia)

This is the most common type of apraxia. It involves a loss of the volitional ability to perform learned movements. A lesion in the dominant hemisphere, in the premotor area, anterior corpus callosum, or inferior parietal lobe, can cause ideomotor apraxia.

Ideational Apraxia

Ideational apraxia is an impairment of ideational (conceptual) knowledge resulting in a loss of the links between tools and their actions, as well as the ability to sequence the movements correctly. Movements may be left out, produced in the wrong order, or attempted with incorrect tools. This condition may result from diffuse brain disease or dominant parietal lobe lesions.

Apraxia of Speech

Some patients who have disturbances of motor speech are considered to show an apraxia of buccolingual movements, though this may coexist with—and be difficult to distinguish from—aphasia. The region of damage involves the insula in the dominant frontal lobe.

Dressing and Constructional Apraxia

In patients with lesions of the nondominant parietal lobe, there may be an inability to put on clothes in the correct order, or to identify items that have been turned inside out. Such patients will also show constructional apraxia (i.e., they will have difficulty in copying a diagram, drawing a clock or constructing a figure from matchsticks). This disorder is best considered as a type of visuospatial dysfunction rather than a true apraxia.

Orofacial Apraxia

Orofacial apraxia may be seen with lesions that affect the dominant supramarginal gyrus or motor association cortex. Patients will be unable to lick the lips or pretend to blow out a match, though they will be able to perform these tasks if there is jam on the lips or if a lighted match is held in front of them.

Conduction Apraxia

Conduction apraxia causes selective difficulty in copying movements, so that patients can pantomime a sequence on command better than they can imitate it. This is similar in concept to conduction aphasia. The location of the lesion is not known.

CHAPTER 35

Arteriovenous Malformations

Arteriovenous malformations (AVMs) and fistulas develop from a breakdown in the typical circular pattern by which the arterial blood supply directly connects with the venous system. The bypass occurs via tangled web of ectatic arterial vessels that link with the venous system, whereas the arteriovenous fistula is a single connection between from artery to the vein. Both AVM and fistula lead to a high pressure system joining a low pressure structure, which creates the potential for a point of rupture. The most common locations are the pelvis, extremities, and intracranial circulation.

The extracutaneous lesions typically present with symptoms of pain (deep pelvic pain, headaches, or limb pain), high output failure (pulmonary AVM and hepatic AVM), or bleeding (gastrointestinal or intracranial).

The cutaneous AVMs have insidious presentation as dermal stain at birth followed by swelling that grows with the child. The initial appearance of dermal stain is similar to capillary malformations but differentiated due to warmth and quick refill after blanching the lesions. As these lesions expand with associated swelling, they become pulsatile. Large lesions with fistula formation will often have associated bruits and thrill.

36 CHAPTER

Arthrogryposis

It occurs because of failure of development of or degeneration of muscular structures. This will lead to nonprogressive muscular disorder. The cause is unknown. Anterior horn cells are reduced in number and spinal cord is reduced in size. It involves all the limbs. Joint contractures lead to deformities that include club foot, dislocated hip, and contractures at knee, elbow, and wrists **(Fig. 1)**.

Orthopedic treatment is aimed at providing optimal motor function. Range-of-motion exercises maintain what motion is present. Gradual recurrence of the deformity after surgery is not uncommon, however.

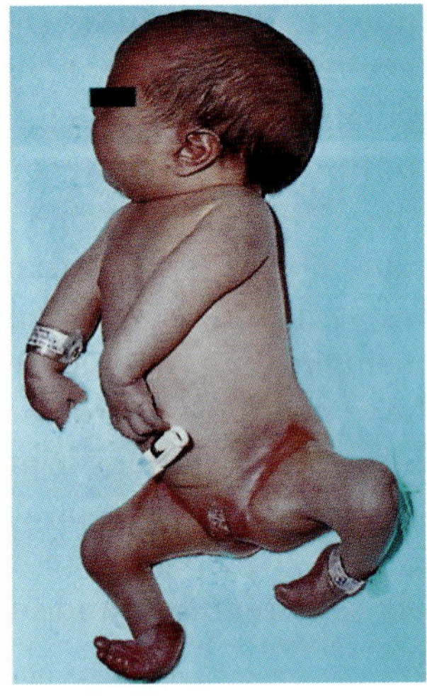

Fig. 1: Arthrogryposis.

CHAPTER 37

Ash-leaf Spots

Congenital, well-demarcated, and hypopigmented macules, termed ash-leaf spots because of their usual lanceolate shape, are often a valuable early marker of tuberous sclerosis. They appear at birth or shortly thereafter as 1–3-cm oval macules on the trunk. Because they are hypopigmented, rather than totally depigmented, they are not as easily appreciated or as bright white as the lesions of vitiligo, and their usual truncal distribution helps distinguish them from the classic location of vitiligo.

The identification of ash-leaf macules may be enhanced (although not as dramatically as is seen in vitiligo) by the use of a Wood lamp, and this method of examination should be part of the assessment of any child, particularly one with a fair complexion, who develops idiopathic seizures in infancy. The visible purple light emitted is absorbed by normal melanin in the skin. Thus in a darkened room, areas of hypopigmentation or depigmentation appear brighter violet, whereas normally melanized skin reflects little visible light and appears dull purple or black. In addition to tuberous sclerosis, Wood lamp examination may also be helpful in delineating the full extent of pigmentary changes in vitiligo and in postinflammatory hypopigmentation.

It is important to recognize that up to 0.5% of otherwise normal newborns will have an isolated hypopigmented macule, which, in the absence of other signs of tuberous sclerosis, is termed a nevus depigmentosus and represents a localized form of pigmentary mosaicism. Nevus depigmentosus is somewhat of a misnomer, because the lesions are not truly depigmented; they are hypopigmented and so do not enhance maximally under Wood lamp.

38 CHAPTER

Asplenia

The spleen plays a particularly important role in preventing invasive infections, especially during the first year of life before specific immunity to certain bacteria has developed. The spleen is able to bind and phagocytose unopsonized encapsulated bacteria, and produces natural antibodies against polysaccharides, demonstrating the critical role of the spleen in preventing sepsis in immunologically immature subjects from encapsulated bacteria. The spleen is also an important location for the phagocytosis of complement and antibody opsonized bacteria, and a key location for the production of antibodies.

Functional asplenia occurs in children with sickle cell disease, initially as a result of vascular occlusion by the sickle cells in the splenic circulation. Congenital absence of the spleen may occur alone or as part of an asplenia syndrome with congenital heart disease. Mutations in NKX2 and ribosomal protein SA have been found in a small number of patients with congenital asplenia. Trauma and surgical splenectomy are also important causes of asplenia.

Individuals without spleens (anatomic or functional) are subject to a severe form of sepsis that is rapid in onset and can lead to sudden death if it is not recognized and treated promptly. Pneumococci are responsible for >50% of such infections; infections with *H. influenzae*, *S. aureus*, group A *streptococci*, gram-negative enteric bacilli, and meningococci also occur.

The diagnosis of anatomic or functional asplenia is suggested by the presence of red blood cell inclusions, particularly Howell-Jolly bodies on peripheral blood smear. Failure of uptake of technetium 99-sulfur colloid, which is normally taken up by the entire reticuloendothelial system or the lack of erythrocyte pitting, is also noted in asplenic patients. Lack of a spleen by ultrasonography of the abdomen is suggestive of asplenia, but accessory splenic tissue may still be present. Functional tests of splenic tissue are a better indicator of asplenia.

The risk of fulminant infection in patients who have undergone splenectomy (from surgery or trauma), or in those with functional asplenia or congenital asplenia, is highest in the first few years. The risk is lower in older children and in adults, probably because they have developed opsonizing antibodies through previous exposure. The management of functional or anatomic asplenia lies mainly in prevention. When splenectomy becomes necessary, partial protection against life-threatening infections can be obtained by immunizing patients with conjugated and polyvalent pneumococcal, *H. influenzae* type b, and meningococcal vaccines. Booster immunization may be needed because of waning immunity with time. Prophylactic antibiotics may be given continuously in a single daily dose for 1–3 years or up to the age of 16 years (some authorities suggest longer periods or even for life) after splenectomy. Parents of older asplenic children are advised to have their children seen by a physician or to administer the antibiotics at the first sign of a febrile illness.

CHAPTER 39

Astigmatism

In the patient with astigmatism, the refractive power differs in various meridians of the eye. In most cases, astigmatism is caused by abnormal curvature of the cornea; in rare cases, lens abnormalities may cause astigmatism. Infants and children with corneal distortion secondary to scarring (trauma or infection) or to external compression (ptosis or hemangioma of eyelid) are at an increased risk for astigmatism. Moderate levels of astigmatism may produce blurring of vision (far and near), leading to squinting, fatigue, headaches, and lack of interest in close-up work in older children and amblyopia in younger children. Cylindric or spherocylindric lenses (usually glasses) are used to improve vision and comfortability.

CHAPTER 40

Ataxia–Telangiectasia

Ataxia-telangiectasia is a multisystem, autosomal recessive degenerative disorder characterized by ataxia, oculocutaneous telangiectasia, immunodeficiency, and a high incidence of neoplasia. The nature of the basic underlying defect is unknown. Affected individuals are extremely sensitive to ionizing radiation and have defective deoxyribonucleic acid (DNA) repair mechanisms. Molecular genetic testing for ATM (ataxia-telangiectasia mutated), the only gene associated with ataxia-telangiectasia, is clinically available. Ataxia is the usual presenting feature, and the course of the neurologic disturbance is rather stereotypic. Tremors of the head may be seen before first year old, and unsteadiness of gait is evident when the child first walks. Progressive global ataxia and slurred, scanning, dysarthric speech are typical during the early school-age years. Loss of deep tendon reflexes and impairment of position and vibratory sensation are evident by the end of the first decade. Adolescence is marked by choreoathetosis, dystonic posturing, gaze apraxia, and progressive dementia. Nonclassic forms of ataxia-telangiectasia have included adult-onset cases and presentations with early dystonia.

The characteristic cutaneous manifestations of this disorder appear by 6 years old. Telangiectasias first appear on the bulbar conjunctivae and develop later over the malar regions, ears, antecubital fossae, neck, and upper chest.

Neuropathologic changes are widespread, with the cerebellum being the site of maximal degeneration. Loss of Purkinje and basket cells, thinning of the granular cell layer, and mild changes in the molecular layer are characteristic findings.

Systemic manifestations include major defects in cellular and humoral immunity. Deficiencies of immunoglobulin A (IgA) and immunoglobulin M (IgM) are characteristic and together with impaired cellular immunity contribute to susceptibility to the recurrent sinus and pulmonary infections that mark this disorder, as well as to the tendency to develop malignancies of the lymphoreticular system (most commonly acute lymphoblastic leukemia or lymphoma) during adolescence or early adulthood. Serum α-fetoprotein levels are elevated, which serve as a nonspecific marker. Adult family members of patients, especially mothers, may also be susceptible to malignancy—breast and lung cancer being the most common.

CHAPTER 41

Athetosis

These are abnormal, nonrepetitive, involuntary slow writhing movements of the periphery. These involve mostly fingers, wrists, face, neck, or trunk. These involve distal part of the limb leading to rotation of limb and spreading toward the proximal part of the limb and trunk. Like chorea, athetosis may occur at rest and is often worsened by voluntary movements. Because athetosis tends to occur with other movement disorders, such as chorea (choreoathetosis) and dystonia, it is often difficult to distinguish as a discreate entity. Choreoathetosis is associated with cerebral palsy, kernicterus, and other forms of basal ganglia injury; therefore, it is often seen in conjunction with rigidity—increased muscle tone that is equal in flexors and extensors in all directions of passive movements regardless of velocity of movement. The site of lesion is basal ganglia especially putamen. The causes are Wilson disease, tuberculosis, kernicterus, birth asphyxia, encephalitis, measles, and diphtheria. It can also be seen with hypoxic-ischemic injury and dopamine-blocking drugs.

CHAPTER 42

Atopic Dermatitis

Atopic dermatitis is one of the most common and stressful of all chronic skin disorders in children. It is now known that mutations in filaggrin, in addition to causing ichthyosis vulgaris, cause the barrier dysfunction, which is characteristic of atopic dermatitis in about 50% of patients. Atopic dermatitis can be divided into three general phases on the basis of the age of the patient, but it is worth noting that these stages may overlap in any given patient.

The infantile phase of atopic dermatitis begins between birth and 6 months old and lasts about 2 or 3 years. Characteristically, the rash is manifested by erythematous, pruritic papules, and plaques that ooze and crust. Lesions are distributed over the cheeks, forehead, scalp, trunk, and extensor surfaces of the extremities and are typically symmetrically distributed. Many infants with atopic dermatitis have overlapping seborrheic dermatitis of the scalp and/or intertriginous areas, such as the neck folds. Several factors that were previously felt to have played a role in atopic dermatitis, including exclusive breastfeeding, the delayed introduction of solid foods, and the use of probiotics and/or fish oils each have been found to have no statistically significant effect on its development.

The childhood phase of atopic dermatitis occurs between ages 4 and 10 years old. The skin lesions are typically dry, papular, and intensely pruritic. Circumscribed scaly patches are distributed on the wrists, ankles, and antecubital and popliteal fossae; these patches frequently become secondarily infected, both as a result of the nonintact skin barrier and from discrete immunologic differences in children with atopic dermatitis, namely a deficiency in two innate antiviral and antibacterial arms of the skin's immune system: β-defensins and cathelicidins. More chronic areas can show lichenification. Cracking, dryness, and scaling of the palmar and plantar surfaces of the hands and feet are also common. The chronic pruritus and sleep disturbance associated with many cases of childhood atopic dermatitis may help to explain the finding that children with atopic dermatitis are more likely to have attention-deficit/hyperactivity disorder (ADHD). It also underscores the importance of comprehensively treating these patients not just for their visible skin findings but also for their systemic and behavioral comorbidities. Remission may occur at any time, or the disorder may evolve into a more chronic type of adult dermatitis. Of children with atopic dermatitis, 75% improve between the ages of 10 and 14; the remaining children may go on to develop chronic dermatitis.

The adult phase of atopic dermatitis begins around age 12 and continues indefinitely. Major areas of involvement include the flexural areas of the arms, neck, and legs. Eruptions are sometimes seen on the dorsal surfaces of the hands and feet and between the fingers and toes. Lichenification may be marked.

Atrial Fibrillation and Atrial Flutter

Atrial fibrillation is uncommon in children and is rare in infants. The atrial excitation is chaotic and more rapid (400–700 beats/min) and produces an irregularly irregular ventricular response and pulse. This rhythm disorder is often associated with atrial enlargement or disease. Atrial fibrillation may be seen in older children with rheumatic mitral valve stenosis. Thyrotoxicosis, pulmonary embolism, pericarditis, or cardiomyopathy may be suspected in previously normal older child or adolescent with atrial fibrillation.

Atrial flutter, also known as intra-atrial reentrant tachycardia, is atrial tachycardia characterized by atrial activity at a rate of 250–300 beats/min in children and adolescents, and 400–600 beats/min in neonates. The mechanism consists of a reentrant rhythm originating in the right atrium circling the tricuspid valve annulus.

CAUSES OF ATRIAL FIBRILLATION

- Rheumatic heart disease—mitral stenosis
- Thyrotoxicosis
  Cardiomyopathy
- Arterial septal defect

Atrial flutter, although usually associated with a regular ventricular rhythm, may produce an irregular pulse if the degree of atrioventricular block is variable.

CHAPTER 44

Auspitz Sign

In psoriasis, there is rapid turnover in epidermal cells produces unknown psoriasis. Although an inherited predisposition is suspected and upper respiratory tract and streptococcal infections may precipitate lesions in children, in guttate psoriasis. Although the increased epidermal growth causes a thickening of skin in the psoriatic, there are also areas between the epidermal ridges where the skin is thin and scale is close to subepidermal vessels. Thus, when it is removed, small bleeding points are often seen. This is called the Auspitz sign. It is hallmark of the psoriasis.

CHAPTER 45

Back Pain

CAUSES OF BACK PAIN

- Vertebral osteomyelitis
- Pancreatitis
- Psoas abscess
- Pelvic inflammatory disease
- Reactive arthritis
- Ankylosing spondylitis
- Sickle cell anemia

SCOLIOSIS

The sideways bending of the spine is scoliosis. Note the site, persistence, or disappearance of scoliosis in forward bending (functional), the number of curvatures, approximate upper and lower limits of the curvatures, the side of the convexity, association with other deformities such as kyphosis. Chest bulges out posteriorly on the convex side of scoliosis known as rib-hump and on the concave side of scoliosis there is crowding of ribs.

Classification of Scoliosis (Cobb's Classification)

- *Postural scoliosis (functional scoliosis):* This type of curve is reversible if the cause is removed, e.g., in pelvic obliquity.
- *Structural scoliosis:*
  - Myopathic scoliosis, e.g., progressive muscular dystrophy.
  - Neuropathic scoliosis, e.g., polio-myelitis and cerebral palsy.
  - Osteopathic scoliosis, e.g., congenital wedge deformity, hemivertebrae, congenital fusion.
  - *Idiopathic scoliosis:*
    - Dorsal type
    - Combined dorsolumbar type
    - Lumbar type
    - Dorsolumbar type

KYPHOSIS

There can be an abnormality in anterior posterior curvature of the spine. If it becomes abnormally prominent posteriorly it is kyphosis.

- Labile kyphosis which may be postural, e.g., myopathy or compensatory, e.g., congenital diaphragmatic hernia (CDH).
- *Fixed kyphosis:*
  - Angular kyphosis (gibbus) due to collapse of one or two vertebrae, e.g., TB
  - Gradual kyphosis (round kyphosis) due to partial or complete collapse of more than two vertebrae, e.g., ankylosing spondylitis.

LORDOSIS

Gradual kyphosis (round kyphosis) due to partial or complete collapse of more than two vertebrae, e.g., ankylosing spondylitis.

An abnormally prominent spinal convexity anteriorly is known as lordosis. Some amount of lordosis is normally present in the lumbar and cervical regions (in tetanus there is posterior curving of whole back-opisthotonus).

In lumbar lordosis due to disease, the abdomen becomes prominent. If the central furrow is deeper, it indicates that the lordosis is exaggerated and if there is no central furrow, there is complete obliteration of the lordosis and flattening of the back. Look for any swelling, sinuses, depression, scar, nevus, tuft of hair (e.g., spina bifida occulta), note any globular swelling, with or without skin cover (spina bifida manifesta and meningomyelocele), compensatory lordosis may be due to bilateral CDH.

CHAPTER 46

Bartholin Gland Abscess

It is a tender mass at the posterior margin of the introitus at the base of the one of the labia majora. It is generally seen in adolescents with gonorrhea and chlamydia. Streptococci and vaginal anaerobes have been documented. Treatment is incision and drainage.

CHAPTER 47 Bleeding

There are two types of bleeding disorders based on the abnormality in either platelets or the coagulation cascade. These include abnormal platelets and abnormal coagulation cascade. Platelet disorders manifest as purpura **(Fig. 1)**, ecchymosis, mucosal bleeds, and epistaxis. Coagulation disorders manifest as hematoma and hemarthrosis. Prolonged bleeding at site of injury will be present.

Bleeding can be classified as:

- *Generalized:*
  - Mucous membrane (petechiae)
    - Platelet disorder
    - Leukemia
    - Aplastic anemia
  - Deep seated bleeding
    - Coagulation disorder
    - Hemophilia
    - Disseminated intravascular coagulation (DIC)
    - Septic shock
- *Localized bleeding:*
  - Nose
    - Pricking the nose
    - Foreign body in nose
    - Hypertension
  - From gums
    - Scurvy
  - From lungs
    - Tuberculosis
    - Bronchiectasis
  - Upper gastrointestinal tract
    - Liver cell failure
    - Drugs
  - From rectum

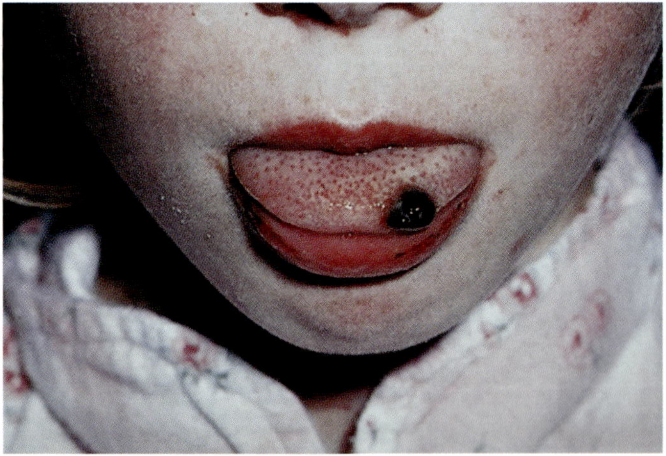

Fig. 1: Idiopathic thrombocytopenic purpura.

TABLE 1: Hematological changes in bleeding-related conditions.

Condition	*Platelet count*	*Bleeding time*	*Activated partial thromboplastin time (APTT)*	*Prothrombin ratio*	*Fibrinogen*	*D-dimer*
• Thrombocytopenia	↓	↑	N	N	N	N
• Von Willebrand's disease	N	↑	↑	N		N
• Hemophilia A or B	N	N	N or ↑	N	N	N
• Warfarin/liver disease	N	N	N	↑	N	N
• Disseminated intra-vascular coagulation	↓	↑	↑	↑	↓	↑

- Fissures
- Polyp
- Hemorrhoids

The various hematological changes in many bleeding-related conditions are mentioned in **Table 1**.

VASCULAR CAUSES OF BLEEDING

- Henoch–Schönlein purpura
- Connective tissue disorder
- Scurvy
- Cushing's disease
- Hereditary hemorrhagic telangiectasia

CHAPTER 48 Blood Pressure

It is the indicator of cardiac output and systemic vascular resistance. Normal blood pressure varies with the age of the child **(Table 1)**.

METHODS OF MEASURING BLOOD PRESSURE

Auscultatory Method

It should be recorded, and the patient should be in comfort. The cuff size is very important. The principle is that it should cover 2/3rd of the length of the arm. Air bag within the cuff should encircle 3/4th of the arm circumference. The children of different ages have different arm sizes. Blood pressure (BP) cuff of appropriate size should be used. The larger cuff gives slightly lower result, and smaller cuff gives false higher result. Hence, it is better to use larger cuff rather than smaller cuff. Cuff should be properly applied. Cuff pressure is raised to obliterate the brachial artery pulsation and slightly more. Now slowly BP cuff pressure is released, and systolic blood pressure is recorded by the appearance of Korotkoff sound by auscultatory method or appearance of radial pulse palpatory method.

Cuff pressure is further released till Korotkoff sound muffles and then disappears. The measurement value between muffling and disappearance of sound is actual diastolic pressure. This cannot be measured by palpation.

TABLE 1: Normal blood pressure.

Age	*Systolic*	*Diastolic*
Birth (3 kg)	50–70	25–45
Neonate	60–90	20–60
Infant (6 months)	85–105	50–60
Toddler (2 years)	95–105	50–60
School age (7 years)	95–110	55–70
Adolescent (15 years)	110–120	65–80

Flush Method

Flush method is used in newborns. The cuff pressure is increased till the forearm appears blanched and slightly above that. Cuff pressure is gradually released, the point when there is sudden flushing, i.e., reappearance of blood supply is the systolic pressure.

Palpatory Method

Radial pulse is felt while cuff is deflated. The point at which radial pulse reappears is systemic pressure.

Doppler Method

Here ultrasound Doppler is used to detect the flow in the radial or brachial artery.

ABNORMALITIES OF BLOOD PRESSURE

Hypertension: If the blood pressure is >95th centile for age and sex. It can be essential or secondary to other systemic illnesses.

Causes

- Acute glomerulonephritis
- Hemolytic uremic syndrome
- Renal artery stenosis
- Neuroblastoma
- Wilms' tumor
- Coarctation of aorta
- Pheochromocytoma
- Cushing's disease

Hypotension: A fall in blood pressure occurs in the following conditions.

- Benign
- Vasovagal syndrome
- Carotid sinus reflex
- Peripheral circulatory failure
- Acute-myocardial failure
- Pericardial effusion

Formulae to calculate expected blood pressure
Systolic blood pressure: 90 + (2 × age in years)
Diastolic blood pressure: 55 + (2 × age in years)

PULSE PRESSURE

It is the difference between the systolic and diastolic pressure.

Increased pulse pressure is seen with:

- Hypertension
- Aortic regurgitation
- Patent ductus arteriosus
- Arteriovenous (AV) fistula
- Complete heart block

Narrow Pulse Pressure

- Shock
- Aortic stenosis
- Cardiac tamponade
- Constrictive pericarditis

49 CHAPTER

Blood Samples

Repeated blood samples for biochemical and microbiological tests are required for very small and ill infants. It is always wise to keep it in mind that infant's blood volume is 80 mL/kg. Prior discussion with laboratory people will often avoid the confusion regarding the volume of the blood to be drawn.

CAPILLARY SAMPLES

Capillary blood is useful for many biochemical investigations. Biochemical investigations include blood gases, blood glucose, serum bilirubin, and blood spots for Guthrie's card test.

The sites used for capillary samples are heel, fingertips, and ear lobe. Disposable lancets are used to prevent infections. Blood samples up to 1 mL can be obtained. It has got limitations. Serum potassium is often high. PCV will be high up to 15% higher than true venous packed cell volume (PCV). This sample cannot be used for blood culture.

Heels must be warmed and made pink. Cotton wool balls soaked in warm water are applied against the heel for a few minutes. Surgical spirit is applied and allowed to dry. Sterile white paraffin is smeared in the surrounding areas. This helps to prevent dispersion of the blood when it begins to flow.

A firm stab into the lateral border of the heel with the lancet deep of 1–2 mm into the skin is given **(Fig. 1)**. Prick should never be in midline as risk of osteomyelitis and os calcis is there. In most infants 1 mL of capillary blood can be easily obtained. It should be collected in small containers. A 5–10 minutes squeezing at the heel may be necessary.

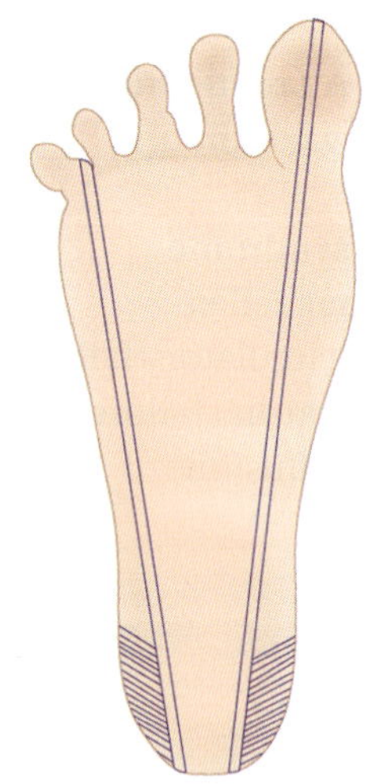

Fig. 1: Sites of heel prick.

Once the blood is collected, pressure is applied with a cotton wool for a few minutes. Ensure that the bleeding is completely stopped. A small protective dressing may be required. A small elastoplast may be used.

VENOUS BLOOD SAMPLES

Blood can be collected in any superficial way. Most commonly proximal veins are used. The superficial vein on the dorsal of the hand, ankle, or feet can be used for the purpose. The other veins usually used are antecubital fossa veins external or internal jugular veins, femoral veins. Use of the femoral vein is discouraged as hip joint is close to it. Prick may induce as well as osteomyelitis.

BROKEN NEEDLE TECHNIQUE

Here the hub of needle no. 21 or 23 is broken off **(Fig. 2)**. Smaller needles are not advised as blood flows slowly. Hence the needle has to be kept for a long time. The needle is inserted into 2 mm in the vein. Blood will flow out quickly. Blood is collected in the tubes. This sample can be used for all investigations except for blood culture. 2 mL of blood can often be obtained.

After collecting blood, needle is removed, by simultaneously applying pressure. This can be done by cotton wool.

Large veins are advised, where specimens are to be withdrawn into a syringe. Cooperation and immobilization of the child is very important. Adequate amount of sample should be obtained in the first attempt especially among sick preterm infants. Apnea may be induced by the procedure. At least two people are required, one to hold the infant and other to collect the sample. The skin should be cleaned by local antiseptics. 21 number needle is used; some may prefer butterfly type needle. Individual doctors have their own particular preference of veins.

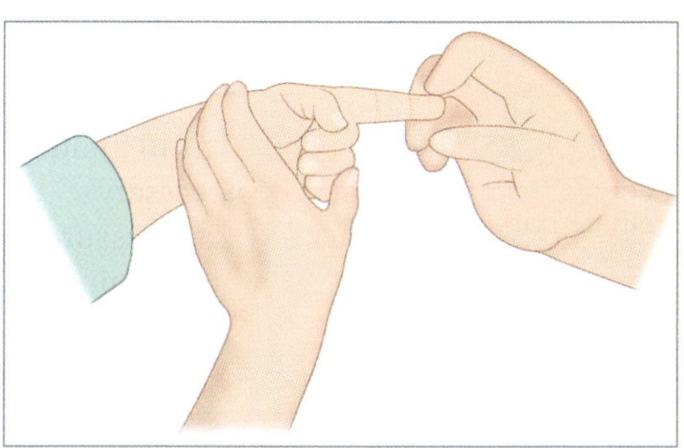

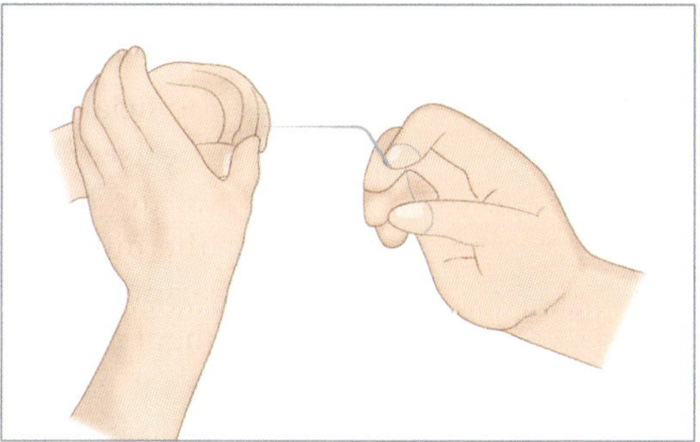

Fig. 2: Broken needle technique.

ANTERIOR CUBITAL FOSSA VEINS

There are two veins in antecubital fossa. They are medial basilic and cephalic veins. The nurse should fix the upper limb by a gentle firm fold of the upper arm below the wrist. Pressure in the upper arm should not be more as it will obstruct the arterial flow.

Needle size of 21 or 23 gauze is used. They will facilitate the easy flow of blood as a result of suctioning by syringe. Gentle local pressure is applied following the removal of the needle. The sample can be used for blood culture.

EXTERNAL AND INTERNAL JUGULAR VEIN

For this purpose, more persons are required to hold head. The neck should be in extension position on the side to be entered. The external jugular can easily be identified by occluding just above the clavicle. Experience is required to locate the jugular vein.

The infant is held supine with its shoulder at the table edge. The needle is inserted in the line of the vein but nearer the angle of the mandible. The needle is then proceeded over the sternomastoid muscle. The size of the needle used is 21. Local pressure is applied, and child is kept under sitting posture **(Fig. 3)**.

FEMORAL VEIN

This vein is avoided as far as possible because of danger of infection into the underlying hip joint. Here the infant is made to sleep on his back. The legs are partially flexed, abducted at hip. Femoral artery is palpated in the midpoint just below the inguinal ligament.

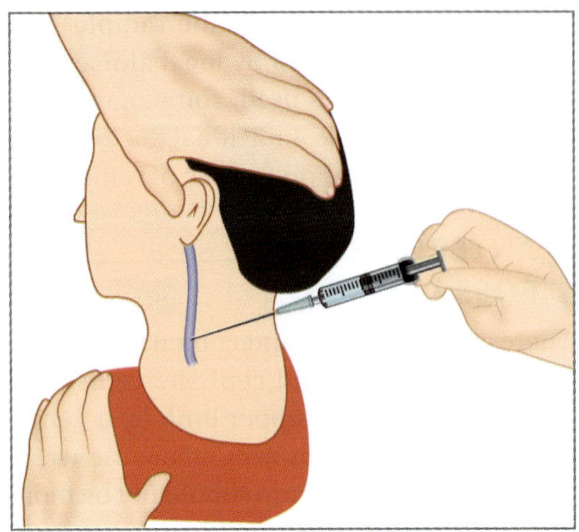

Fig. 3: External jugular vein cannulation.

The femoral vein lies just medial to it. Syringe and needle are held vertically and proceeded further through the skin toward the vein. This should be done with constant gentle suction. Blood will be sucked as soon as it enters the vein **(Fig. 4)**. If the blood is not obtained needle should be withdrawn; no further attempt is made.

Firm pressure should be applied over the vein until bleeding from the vein whether superficial or subcutaneous has stopped. A sterile occlusive dressing should be applied. Risk of entering directly into the artery is alarming.

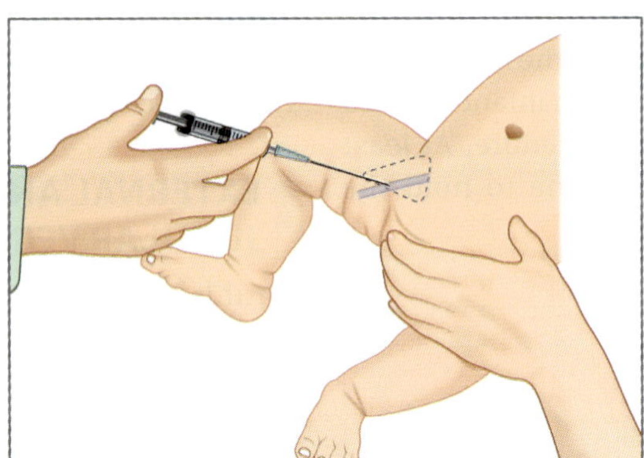

Fig. 4: Femoral vein catheterization.

CHAPTER 50

Blindness

Blindness is very difficult to suspect <3 months of age. Partial loss of vision is called amblyopia and complete blindness is called amaurosis. Blindness in children is caused by damage or lesion of visual pathways bilaterally.

CAUSES OF BLINDNESS

- Optic neuritis
- Retinitis pigmentosa
- Encephalitis
- Tuberculous meningitis
- Brain tumor
- Degenerative brain disease

CHAPTER 51

Blue Dot Sign

It is seen in torsion of testicular appendages. The appendix testis and appendix epididymis are embryologic remnants that are normally undetectable on routine examination. Torsion of appendix, which can occur in the early pubertal age group, may difficult to differentiate from torsion of the spermatic cord. Early after the onset of acute scrotal pain, a small tender mass may be palpable on the upper anterior surface of the testis or epididymis. In light skinned children, the swollen, dark infarcted appendage may be seen through the scrotal skin—"Blue dot sign" of Dresner.

CHAPTER 52

Blue Sclera

The most common cause of the blue appearance to the sclera in an infant is the fact that the normal thinness of the layers of eye allow the darker color underlying tissue to be seen through the white of the eye, thus creating blue hue that is often seen in infant eye.

CAUSES OF BLUE SCLERA

- Prematurity
- Hypophosphatasia
- Osteogenesis imperfecta
- Marshall-Smith syndrome
- Russell-Silver syndrome
- Ehlers-Danlos syndrome
- Marfan syndrome
- Trisomy 18 syndrome

Body Proportion

BODY MASS INDEX

It is calculated as (weight/length^3). It is an important parameter used for the assessment of growth in adolescent especially obesity. The normal body mass index (BMI) lies between 18.5 and 25. BMI between 25 and 30 is called overweight. Obesity is defined as BMI > 30. Adults with BMI <18.5 are termed to have chronic energy deficiency. The BMI <15 is seen among undernutrition. In severe under nutrition BMI is <13.

Body mass index:

$$\text{BMI} = \frac{\text{Weight (kg)}}{\text{Height (M)}}$$

This is like Quetelet's index except that the values are in SI units. BMI values can be used to draw standardized percentile curve in children and adolescents. It is especially useful defining obesity-BMI at or above 95 percentile for age or >30 (whichever is small).

Ponderal index: It is used to define intrauterine growth retardation.

$$\frac{\text{Body weight in grams}}{\text{Length in cm}^3} \times 100$$

In intrauterine growth restriction (IUGR), it is <2, while it is >2.5 in appropriate for gestation (AFG) babies.

PONDERAL INDEX

$$\text{Ponderal index (PI)} = \frac{\text{Height (cm)}}{\text{Cube root of body weight}}$$

Ponderal index	*Comment*
2	Symmetric IUGR
<1.9	Asymmetric IUGR

ARM SPAN

It is the distance measured between the tips of the middle fingers of both arms outstretched at right angles to the body. Abnormal arm span, i.e., more than height are seen in Marfan's syndrome, Homocystinuria, Klinefelter's syndrome. Arm span is less than height in achondroplasia and cretinism.

Normally it will be 1–2 cm less than the body length <5 years. It equals by 10–12 years of age.

UPPER SEGMENT/LOWER SEGMENT RATIO

Lower segment is the measurement made from the symphysis pubis to heel. Upper segment is derived by deducting the lower segment value from the height. Upper segment is measured from the vertex to the upper end of the symphysis pubis.

The ethnic and familial should be kept in mind. Sometimes it may be necessary to measure the parents as well.

Normal ratio	*US*	*LS*
At birth	1.7	1.0
At 10 years	1.0	1.0

Abnormally large and long limbs are seen:

- Chondrodystrophy
- Cretinism
- Dwarfism

Abnormally short trunks and long limbs:
- Rickets
- Chondrodystrophy
- Arachnodactyly

WARNING SIGNS OF DEVELOPMENTAL DELAY FOR FURTHER EVALUATION

4–6 weeks:
- Not responding to nearby voices by 8 weeks
- Absent "startle"
- No social smile by 3 months

At 3 months:
- Not showing interest in people and playthings by 3–4 months
- No head control by 5 months
- No vocalization

At 6 months:
- Persistent Moro's and asymmetric tonic neck reflexes
- Not visually alert
- Not reaching for objects

At 9 months:
- No hand transfer
- Not sitting
- No repetitive babble even by 10 months

At 1 year:
- Not starting a variety of speech sounds
- Not pulling to standing position

At 1.5 years:
- Not moving about to explore
- Not speaking single word by 21 months

At 2 years:
- Avoiding eye contact
- Handedness before 2 years-looks for weakness of opposite hand
- No sentence by 27 months

At 3 years:
- Not following simple directions
- Monotonous play by self

At 4 years:
- No intelligible speech
- Not drawing a human figure

At 5 years: No grammatical speech

SKELETAL MATURITY

Skeletal maturity implies how far the bones of a particular area have progressed toward maturity not in size but in shape and in their relative positions to one another, as seen in a radiograph. The number of centers of ossification present and the stage of development of each gives an estimation of the skeletal maturity.

For a rough estimate of bone age from the left-hand X-ray: Centers of ossification appear as—capitate, hamate (1-year), and lower end of radius (2-year). Triquetral (G-year), lunate (4-year), scaphoid (5-year), lower end of ulna, trapezium, trapezoid (6-year), pisiform (12-year) for the elbow joint, the appearance of centers of ossification of the lower end of the humerus are: Medial epicondyle (5-year), trochlea (1-year), capitulum (1-year), and lateral epicondyle (12-year). The epicondyle for the upper end of radius and ulna appear at 4 years and 8 years respectively.

THUMB RULE

- The number of carpal bones at wrist = age in years plus one.
- There are five ossification centers at birth in term babies—two at knee joint (upper end of tibia and lower end of femur) and three in the foot (talus, cuboid, and calcaneus).

CHAPTER 54

Borborygmi

Borborygmi is the term applied to rumbling noises of varying quality and intensity produced by peristaltic movements of the bowel propelling mixed gaseous and liquid contents.

These sounds, although normally inaudible to the patient or to other persons and detected only by auscultation by means of a stethoscope. They may be due to the powerful peristaltic waves of a bowel that is hypertrophied and dilated above a lowly developing obstruction of the large bowel; here there will usually be accompanying progressive constipation, colicky abdominal pains, and distension.

Bossing: Frontal and Parietal

Frontal bossing is the descriptive term for a prominent forehead.

CAUSES OF FRONTAL BOSSING

- Preterm
- Rickets
- Hemolytic anemia
- Congenital syphilis
- Hydrocephalus
- Achondroplasia
- Mucopolysaccharidosis

Parietal bossing is marked prominence in parietal region.

CAUSES OF PARIETAL BOSSING

- Rickets
- Chronic subdural hemorrhage

56 CHAPTER

Brachial Plexus Injury

The incidence of brachial plexus trauma with current obstetric management is 0.7 per 1,000 live births. The mechanism of injury in most instances is traction on the plexus during delivery. Although lesions have classically been divided into those affecting upper spinal segments (Erb's palsy; **Fig. 1**) and those affecting lower segments (Klumpke palsy), the distinction may not be clearcut in some cases. Injury to the C5 and C6 fibers is most often identified by the child's arm hanging limply adducted and internally rotated at the shoulder and extended and pronated at the elbow. Injury affecting the lower segments of C7 and T1 rarely occurs in isolation, causing weakness of the wrist and hand, and ultimately leads to a claw-hand deformity. There may be sensory loss along the ulnar side of the hand and forearm in the distribution of the T1 dermatome. If the T1 root is affected with interruption of the sympathetic innervation at that level, Horner syndrome (constricted pupil, drooping upper eyelid, and local inability to sweat on one side of the face) may be apparent.

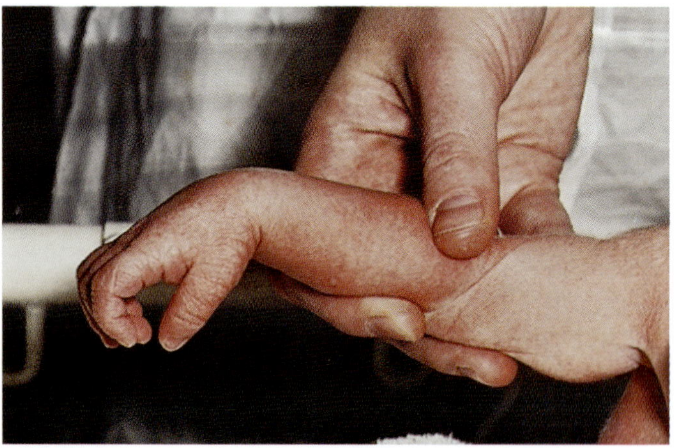

Fig. 1: Erb's palsy.

57 CHAPTER

Breast Lumps

METHOD OF EXAMINATION

Both breasts should first be looked at as a whole to see whether they are symmetrical in size, contour, and level, and whether the two nipples are in the same site and of the same circumference, prominence, and inclination. Skin, areola, nipple, size of the breast, and local swelling in different positions should be inspected. Both the sides are compared for any asymmetry.

If no difference is at first noticed, the patient should be asked to raise both arms slowly above the head and bring them down again to the side, since differences which were previously invisible—particularly dimpling of the skin from attachment of a lump—may come into view as the breast glides over the chest wall.

Each breast is palpated systematically over all quadrants from periphery toward nipple. Presence of any lump and tenderness noted. If any mass is felt, its description such as position, size, consistency, margins, tenderness, and inflammation should be done. Nipple is palpated for any discharge—watery, milky, or bloody is noted. Axilla is palpated for any extension of breast between thumb and finger and presence of nodes. Supraclavicular lymph nodes are palpated.

After the examination, the lump or swelling can be attributed to various factors as mentioned in **Box 1**.

BOX 1: Classification.

Swellings of the whole breast:

- *Bilateral*
  - Pregnancy
  - Lactation
  - ANDI (abnormalities of normal development and involution)
  - Hypertrophy
  - In males from stilboestrol administration
  - Acute mastitis
- *Unilateral*
  - Hypertrophy of the newborn
  - Puberty
  - Unilateral hypertrophy

Discrete lumps in breast:

- *Benign*
  - Fibroadenoma
  - Simple cyst
  - Galactocele
  - Lipoma
  - Plasma cell mastitis (periductal mastitis) (*Rare:* fat necrosis; tuberculous abscess)
  - Phyllodes tumor
- *Malignant*
  - Carcinoma (*Rare:* Sarcoma; lymphoma)

Swellings that are not of the breast:

- *Retromammary abscess:*
  - From disease to rib
  - Chronic empyema
- Chondroma of chest wall
- Deformities of the ribs
- Mondor's disease

BREAST ENGORGEMENT

There will be bilateral fullness of both the breasts. The overlying skin shows no signs of redness, warmth, or local tenderness. There may be milky discharge from the breasts. This is called witch's milk, which is benign phenomenon.

This resolves spontaneously and no intervention is required. It results from the stimulation of breast tissue by high levels of maternal hormones.

SWELLING IN PREGNANCY AND LACTATION

Both breasts are enlarged equally and tense and nodular. The superficial veins are usually prominent and on gentle squeezing a few drops of milk are discharged from the nipple. Montgomery's tubercles will be evident.

CHAPTER 58 Breath Sounds

These are produced by the flow of air through the respiratory tract. They are produced by the vibration of vocal cord caused by turbulent flow of air through the larynx. The sounds are further transmitted through the trachea, bronchi through the lungs to the chest wall. The passage through the lung tissue, the alteration in the intensity and frequency pattern is altered.

TYPES OF BREATH SOUNDS

Types of Normal Breath Sounds

- *Vesicular breathing:* The character of the sound heard over the trachea is hollow tubular sound. This sound gets modified through the passage of air through numerous smaller bronchi, bronchioles, and alveoli. The high-pitched high frequency sound at trachea is changed to low pitched. Low-frequency sound at the peripheral airways and alveoli. This changed sound which we hear normally is called vesicular breath sounds.

  It is characterized by active inspiration due to inflow of air into bronchi and alveoli. This is followed by short expiration due to elastic recoil of alveoli. There is no pause between inspiration and expiration.
- *Bronchial breathing:* The hollow, tubular sounds heard over the laryngotracheal area are usually modified by functioning lung tissue into the low pitched and low frequency vesicular sounds. When the normally aerated lung is replaced by pathological lung, the sound will not be modified and heard as it is to the chest wall without modification.

  It is characterized by active inspiration due to the passage of air in the bronchi. The alveolar phase is absent. Hence there is pause. The expiration is passive.

TYPES OF BRONCHIAL BREATHING

- *Tubular bronchial breathing:* It is high-pitched sound better heard with diaphragm of a stethoscope. They are heard in consolidation.
- *Cavernous bronchial breathing:* It is low-pitched bronchial sound, better heard with bell of the stethoscope. They are heard over the cavities, early pneumonia and bronchopneumonia.
- *Amphoric bronchial breathing:* It is high pitched and has peculiar metallic quality. It resembles the sound produced by blowing through an empty bottle with narrow neck. It is heard over the hydropneumothorax, just above the fluid and in large pulmonary cavity with patent bronchus.

ADVENTITIOUS SOUNDS

Crackles/Crepitations

These are two types:

1. *Fine crepitations:* These are sounds of reopening of peripheral airways, i.e., peripheral bronchioles and alveoli during

inspiration. These peripheral air passages get occluded during expiration due to inflammatory exudate or transudate. It is heard always at the later part of inspiration. These are fine and high-pitched sound. They are more profuse at lower part of the lung. These are seen in pulmonary edema and pneumonia.

2. *Coarse crepitations:* These are also called rales. These are caused by passage of air through secretion of large airways or cavities, bubbling sounds. After coughing, crepitations are diminished or absent because the secretions move out. It is commonly seen in bronchiectasis.

Rhonchi/Wheeze

This is sound produced by narrowed airways. It can be generalized or localized. Generalized wheeze is seen in bronchiolitis and bronchial asthma. Wheezes are usually expiratory and commonly associated with prolonged expiration. Localized wheeze may be seen among localized narrowing of the airway, usually by larger bronchi by some obstruction. Cause of obstruction may be intraluminal, i.e., endobronchial tuberculosis and foreign body or extraluminal, i.e., enlarged lymph nodes due to tuberculosis or lymphoma.

Bronchoscopy and Bronchoalveolar Lavage

Bronchoscopy is the inspection of the airways. Flexible bronchoscopy is commonly in pediatrics. There are several sizes of scopes that enable visualization of the proximal and distal airways. Many fiberoptic bronchoscopes also have a channel that allows for the collection of fluids, or in larger scopes allows for insertion of tools such as forceps, brushes, or baskets.

Bronchoalveolar lavage (BAL) is a method used to obtain a representative specimen of fluid and secretions from the lower respiratory tract, which is useful for the cytologic and microbiologic diagnosis of lung diseases, especially in those who are unable to expectorate sputum. BAL is performed after the general inspection of the airways and before tissue sampling with a brush or biopsy forceps.

Indications for diagnostic bronchoscopy and BAL include recurrent or persistent pneumonia or atelectasis, unexplained, or localized and persistent wheeze, the suspected presence of a foreign body, hemoptysis, suspected congenital anomalies, mass lesions, interstitial disease, and pneumonia in the immunocompromised host. Indications for therapeutic bronchoscopy and BAL include bronchial obstruction by mass lesions, foreign bodies or mucus plugs, and general bronchial toilet and bronchopulmonary lavage.

CHAPTER 60

Brown Syndrome

It is an isolated motility disorder in their inability to elevate the eye when in adduction. This may be caused by a congenital anomaly of the superior oblique tendon, or it may be acquired as in idiopathic inflammation or tenosynovitis of superior oblique tendon. Acquired causes may be persistent, resolve spontaneously and/or respond to anti-inflammatory medicines [nonsteroidal anti-inflammatory drugs (NSAIDs)].

CHAPTER 61

Brushfield Spots

These are found in the patients with Down syndrome. The spots consist of normal iris stroma that are surrounded by rings of mild hypoplasia. These give iris a speckled appearance. They are of no visual or pathological significance.

62 CHAPTER

Bulging Anterior Fontanel

There are six fontanels in the skull as listed below:

1. Anterior fontanel (AF) (located between frontal and parietal bones)
2. Posterior fontanel (located between occipital and parietal bones)
3. Antero lateral fontanel (paired) also called sphenoid fontanel
4. Posterolateral fontanel (paired) also called mastoid fontanel

The AF may vary in size. Persistent delay in closure or unusually large in size indicate increased intracranial pressure or pathological delay in bone growth.

Posterior fontanel is present where the lambdoid and sagittal sutures unite. It is triangular in shape and situated at the junction of occipital and two parietal bone meet. It closes by 2 months. Hypothyroidism should be ruled out when the posterior fontanel persists.

PREMATURE CLOSURE OF ANTERIOR FONTANEL

- Microcephaly
- Craniosynostosis
- Hyperthyroidism

DELAYED CLOSURE OF ANTERIOR FONTANEL

- Rickets
- Hydrocephalus
- Hypothyroidism
- Down syndrome
- Achondroplasia
- Osteogenesis imperfecta
- Hypophosphatasia
- Skeletal dysplasia

Raised intracranial pressure in meningitis is reflected by palpable tension of the fontanel and loss of normal venous pulsation. It is best to assess AF when the child is calm and held upright. The sunken fontanel indicates dehydration.

Bulging AF is seen meningitis, congestive cardiac failure (CCF), vitamin A intoxication, lead poisonings, pseudotumor cerebri, and hypophosphatasia. Although a slight depression of the fontanel is common in normal infants, sunken fontanel is a sign of dehydration.

CHAPTER 63

Butterfly Rash

It appears typically over the nose and cheek. This is seen in systemic lupus erythematosus disease. Anemia, neutropenia, and thrombocytopenia are hematological findings. Associated findings include asthma, splenomegaly, proteinuria, arthritis, and retinal exudates. All these collectively seen in connective tissue disorder.

SECTION 3

CHAPTER 64

Café-Au-Lait Macules

Café-au-lait macules are well-circumscribed tan macules that usually measure <0.5 cm and may be as large as 15–20 cm in diameter. The lesions are found on any cutaneous site and may be present at birth or appear during early childhood. Although café-au-lait spots are seen in 10–20% of normal individuals, the presence of many macules should raise the clinical suspicion of neurofibromatosis **(Fig. 1)**. The presence of six or more café-au-lait spots (>0.5 cm in prepubertal children; >1.5 cm in post-pubertal children) fulfills one of the diagnostic criteria for neurofibromatosis type 1. Although the lesions are not pathognomonic, they are present in most patients with neurofibromatosis and tend to be larger and more numerous. Café-au-lait spots have also been associated with tuberous sclerosis, McCune–Albright syndrome, Turner syndrome, Bloom syndrome, ataxia-telangiectasia, Russell–Silver syndrome, Fanconi anemia, Gaucher disease, and Chediak–Higashi syndrome.

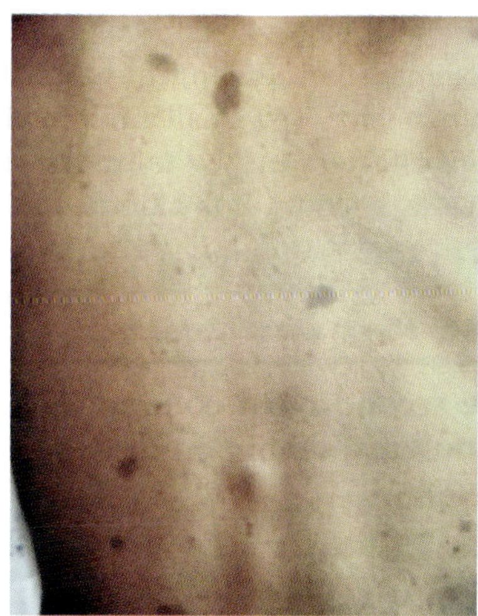

Fig. 1: Café-au-lait macules.

CHAPTER 65

Camptodactyly

It is a nontraumatic flexion contracture of the proximal interphalangeal joint, that is often progressive. The small and ring fingers are often affected. In two-thirds of cases it is bilaterally affected. It is inherited through a dominant gene and is seen in 1.9% of normal population. However, this is also a part of various syndromes such as Down's, Carpenter, and Aarskog syndrome.

66 CHAPTER

Candidiasis

Candidal species, particularly *Candida albicans*, may be considered part of the normal cutaneous flora in most individuals. However, predisposing factors such as endocrinologic disorders, genetic disorders, immunosuppressive conditions, and the administration of systemic corticosteroids or antibiotics may allow for overgrowth of this organism and subsequent infection. Candidiasis refers to an acute or chronic infection of the skin, mucous membranes, or internal organs caused by this pathogenic yeast. Other conditions, such as warmth, moisture, and disruption of the epidermal barrier, further promote invasion and overgrowth. Cutaneous candidiasis can have a variety of clinical manifestations, depending on the site of infection. Some of the most common manifestations include (1) oral candidiasis (thrush), (2) candidal diaper dermatitis, (3) vulvovaginitis, and (4) paronychia.

Oral candidiasis is a common condition of infancy and in immunosuppressed individuals. It is characterized by painful inflammation of the oral cavity with multiple, often confluent, white plaques on an intensely erythematous base. The disorder usually responds to treatment with oral nystatin suspension, which is applied to the oral mucosa four times daily until 2 days after the lesions have completely resolved. Oral fluconazole is another therapeutic option for more extensive or resistant cases. Extensive involvement or failure to respond to treatment may suggest an underlying immunodeficiency disease. Cutaneous lesions in the intertriginous and diaper areas are frequently coexistent with thrush.

CHAPTER 67

Capillary Malformation

Capillary malformations, more commonly called *port-wine stains*, are found all over the body. They can be seen in isolation or as part of a syndrome. Most commonly, they are treated when they are on the face, because they may be obvious and cause social distress for the child. Pulsed dye laser therapy is a common modality used to treat these malformations. Incidence is reported to be about 0.3% of newborns.

Capillary malformations are made up of abnormal collections of capillaries in the skin causing a cutaneous hyperemic appearance. They can be faint to dark in color or appear almost purple. They are present at birth and typically darken with age. Around puberty they can become verrucous in nature. Size can range from as small as a silver dollar to covering half of the entire body from head to toe.

CHAPTER 68

Caput Succedaneum

Normal transit of the fetal head through the birth canal induces molding of the skull and scalp edema, especially if labor is prolonged. The edema, which can be massive, is known as a caput succedaneum. Much of this edema is present at birth and tends to overlie the occipital bones and portions of the parietal bones bilaterally. It is exudation of serous fluid in the soft tissues of the presenting part during delivery **(Fig. 1)**.

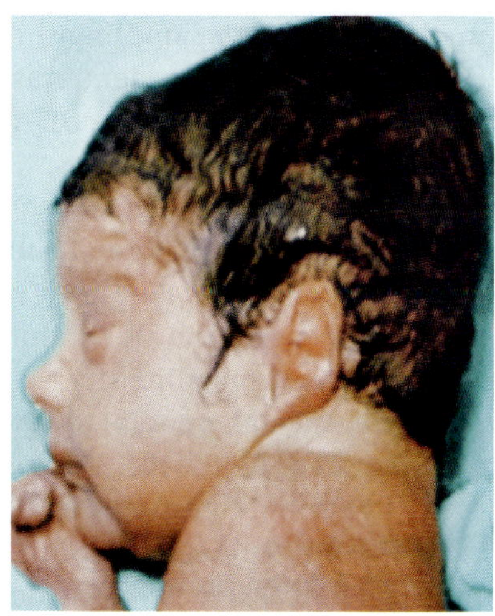

Fig. 1: Caput succedaneum.

It is a diffuse swelling, not limited by suture lines, usually over vertex or face (in case of face presentation). It may disappear anywhere between 24 hours and 3 days and no permanent mark is usually left. In some cases, bruising of the scalp may also be present (especially if a vacuum extractor was used). The presence of a caput requires no therapy, and spontaneous resolution within a few days is the rule. Distinguishing caput from a subgaleal (subaponeurotic) hematoma, a rare but serious complication of delivery, is important. A subgaleal hematoma is a collection of blood within scalp tissues extending beneath the epicranial aponeurosis. Palpation of a large caput succedaneum reveals firm, nonpitting swelling. In contrast, the cranial swelling of subgaleal bleeding is boggy due to the palpation of clotted blood just beneath the epicranial aponeurosis. The collection of blood in this potential space can be quite large, and these infants must be monitored for signs of hypovolemia. Serial examinations, which can include measurement of head circumference and hematocrit, are important to identify ongoing blood loss.

69 CHAPTER Cardiocentesis

It is a method of directly sampling the fetal blood **(Box 1)**. This is done under ultrasound control. This can be carried out after 17 weeks till delivery.

No sedation and preparation are required. It is carried out with full bladder. Umbilical cord is pointed. Place of the placenta is noted. Local anesthesia is given in the abdominal wall at the anticipated puncture site.

A 20-gauze special needle with 9-cm length is attached to 20 mL disposable syringe. Syringe should contain citrated or heparinized saline. Under the continuous ultrasound guidance, needle is introduced into the place of ultrasound sector near the transducer. This is followed by movement toward the insertion of the cord. The cord is punctured at about 1 cm from the placental insertion. According to the stage of gestation 2–4 mL of blood is gently aspirated. It is then collected in the bottle containing culture media and anticoagulant **(Fig. 1)**.

The needle is gently withdrawn and puncture site in cord is watched for the extent of bleeding. Fetus is monitored for the bradycardia. The success and safety of the procedure depends on experience, patience and skill.

BOX 1: Indications.

- Normal hematological values
- Biochemical assay
- Endourological study
- Inborn error of metabolism
- Coagulation profile
- Immunological study
- Endocrinological study

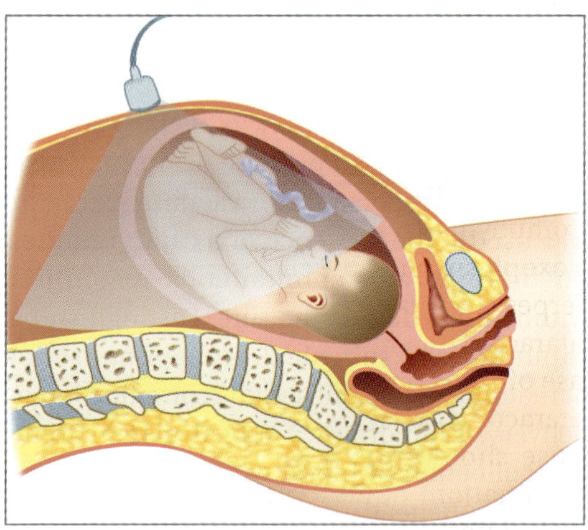

Fig. 1: Cardiocentesis.

CHAPTER 70 Cataract

Most cases of unilateral cataract are idiopathic in origin or associated with other ocular anomalies (persistent hyperplastic primary vitreous and anterior segment dysgenesis). Bilateral cataracts have a known genetic basis in about 60–70% of the cases but this is increasing as novel mutations continue to be described. Cataracts are commonly inherited in an autosomal dominant manner but may be inherited in an autosomal recessive or X-linked pattern. They can be associated with metabolic diseases such as galactosemia or Fabry syndrome. Cataracts found to be a result of a metabolic disease may be reversible by removal of the offending agent; galactosemic cataracts are potentially reversible if lactose is eliminated from the diet promptly. Intrauterine TORCH(S) infections (*T*oxoplasmosis, *R*ubella, *C*ytomegalovirus, *H*erpes simplex, and *S*yphilis) can also cause cataracts. Usually these are bilateral but in the case of congenital rubella infection unilateral cataract may occur. Evaluation for a systemic cause should include a pediatric physical examination, ophthalmologic examination of the infant and family members, urine for reducing substances after lactose-containing milk feeding, labs for TORCH(S) infections, calcium, phosphorus, and glucose. Other metabolic studies, chromosomal evaluation, and genetic consultation may be indicated **(Fig. 1)**.

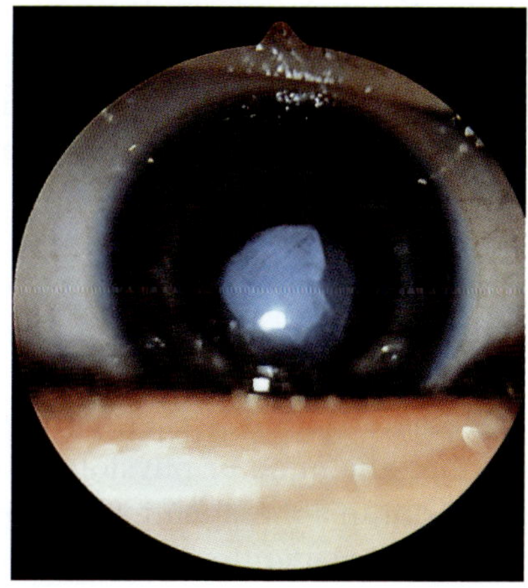

Fig. 1: Cataract.

CAUSES OF CATARACT

- *Prematurity*
- *Hereditary*
- *Genetics:*
  - 13, 18, 21 trisomy
  - Turner syndrome
- *Congenital infection:*
  - Toxoplasmosis
  - Cytomegalovirus (CMV)
  - Syphilis
  - Rubella
  - Herpes simplex
- *Metabolic causes:*
  - Galactosemia
  - Hypocalcemia
  - Hypoparathyroidism
  - Juvenile diabetes mellitus
  - Wilson's disease
  - Mucopolysaccharidoses
- *Drugs:*
  - Steroids
- *Trauma:*
  - Contusion
  - Penetrating injury

Cardiac Catheterization and Angiocardiography

On the basis of the preceding steps of diagnostic evaluation—history, physical examination, ECG, chest X-ray, echocardiogram, and other noninvasive laboratory studies—the pediatric cardiologist has a precise assessment of the anatomic and physiologic abnormalities in simple malformations and considerable useful information about complex malformations. Cardiac catheterization is then performed when further anatomic or physiologic data is needed prior to a therapeutic decision, or when the cardiac condition can be palliated or treated in the catheterization laboratory.

INDICATIONS

In both infants and older children, cardiac catheterization is performed if echocardiography or other noninvasive means cannot provide complete anatomic data. Therapeutic procedures are also performed in the catheterization laboratory such as coil embolization of a patent ductus arteriosus (PDA), balloon aortoplasty in coarctation of the thoracic aorta, balloon atrial septostomy, valvuloplasty of stenotic aortic or pulmonic valves, and placement of atrial septal defect (ASD) devices. In addition, cardiac catheterization is performed to evaluate the efficacy of pharmaceutical therapy. An example of this would be administering nitric oxide or prostacyclin acutely to a child with primary pulmonary hypertension to see its effect on the pulmonary vascular resistance.

The risks of cardiac catheterization (morbidity and mortality) must be explained to the patient's family. Although the risks are very low for elective studies in older children (<0.1%), the risk in distressed infants is in the range of 2%. Interventional procedures such as balloon valvuloplasties will increase these risks.

Carditis

In developing countries, 60–80% cases of rheumatic fever have clinical features of carditis and in 40% is seen during the first attack of rheumatic fever. It is pancarditis involving pericardium, myocardium and endocardium. Carditis occurs within 2 weeks of the onset of the fever.

Pericarditis results in pericardial pain. The pain may be quite severe. Friction rub may be heard on auscultation. ECG shows ST and T wave changes.

A patient of rheumatic pericarditis always has additional mitral or mitral and aortic regurgitation murmur.

Myocarditis presents with cardiac enlargement, soft heart sound and congestive cardiac failure (CCF). Carey Coombs murmur is a delayed diastolic mitral murmur heard during the course of acute rheumatic fever. S3 gallop may be present. Gallop rhythm is an abnormal array of heart sounds in which third and fourth heart sound may also be present and usually indicates active disease of the heart.

Endocarditis is represented by pansystolic murmur of mitral regurgitation. Tricuspid valvulitis results in tricuspid regurgitation.

CLINICAL FEATURES OF CARDITIS

- Murmurs
  - Significant apical systolic murmurs, (musical quality of grade III)
  - Apical mid-diastolic murmur due to edema of valve (Carey–Coombs murmur).
  - Basal diastolic murmur
- Enlarged heart
- Congestive heart failure
- Presence of pericardial rub

Others include:

- Tachycardia (sleeping)
- Heart sounds (decreased or muffled)
- Gallop, arrhythmias, and changing murmurs
- Subcutaneous nodules
- Persistent dry cough, ECG changes laboratory findings raised erythrocyte sedimentation rate (ESR) and presence of C-reactive protein (CRP)
- Valves affected in frequency of occurrence are, mitral 70%, mitral and aortic (7%), tricuspid and pulmonary valves are rarely affected.

CHAPTER 73

Central Venous Pressure Monitoring

INSERTION TECHNIQUE

Internal jugular vein, subclavian vein, and femoral vein are selected for this purpose. Subclavian route is more common for long-term cannulation. Catheter malposition is more common with this. This is very difficult in edematous patient as landmarks are poorly identified. Roller is placed down the back. This allows shoulder to fall back. It helps the needle placement between the first rib and clavicle. The patient should be placed head-down, with the hand turned away from the site of entry.

The sternal notch, angle of the clavicle, subclavian artery and delta pectoral groove are identified before needle insertion. An entry of 0.5 cm lateral and below the mid-third of the clavicle makes it easier to pass between the clavicle and first rib. Needle should be kept parallel to the skin once the needle has entered the skin. This is to avoid the puncture of the lung. The needle should be advanced with the negative pressure on syringe aiming for the triangle. The triangle is formed by clavicular and sternal needs of sternocleidomastoid muscle. Once the needle is located, the syringe should be removed, and flow of the blood is observed. A steady flow indicates that the needle is within the lumen of the vein. Pulsatile flow strongly suggests arterial puncture and needle should be removed. Guide wire should pass easily. The dilator should pass easily and should not be passed >1 cm. Once the catheter has passed, easy aspiration of the blood should be checked. A chest X-ray should be taken to ensure the correct placement.

CHAPTER 74

Cephalhematoma

Well demarcated subperiosteal hemorrhage over parietal bone, restricted by suture line **(Fig. 1)**. It appears 6–12 hours after birth. It is absorbed or calcified in 4–6 weeks.

Causes of cephalhematoma:
- Forceps application
- Vacuum extraction
- Difficult delivery, contribute to its occurrence

Complications that might result from cephalohematoma include:
- Anemia
- Jaundice
- Infection.

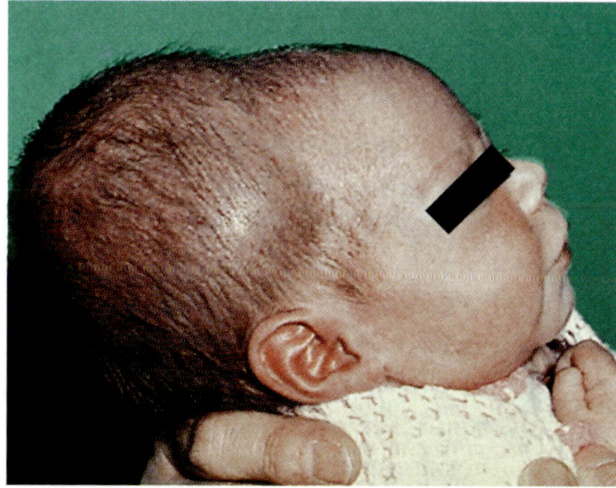

Fig. 1: Cephalhematoma.

Often, confusion arises between the diagnosis of a caput and that of a cephalhematoma. The latter is a localized collection of blood beneath the periosteum of one of the calvarial bones; it may be bilateral but is most often unilateral. It is distinguished from a caput by the fact that its borders are limited by suture lines, usually those surrounding the parietal bones. However, diagnosis can be difficult in the immediate newborn period, when there may be overlying scalp edema. On palpation, the border may feel elevated, and the center depressed. Most patients have an uncomplicated course of slow resolution over one or more months, although calcification may occur. On occasion, these infants may develop jaundice from the breakdown and resorption of the large hematoma. Underlying hairline skull fractures occur with some regularity but are rarely of clinical significance. The exception is the uncommon development of a leptomeningeal cyst. Radiologic investigation for an underlying depressed fracture is indicated in infants whose histories suggest significant trauma and those having depressed levels of consciousness *or* neurologic abnormalities on examination. Infection is another potentially serious but rare complication, which is more likely when the integrity of the overlying skin is broken, such as may occur when a scalp electrode is placed or a scalp abrasion in the normal course of delivery.

Cerebellar Signs

Specific tests used to evaluate cerebellar function include assessment of gait and balance, pronator drift, the finger-to-nose test, rapid alternating action, and heel to shin test. Damage to cerebellum can lead to:

- Loss of coordination of motor movement (asynergia)
- Inability to judge distance and when to stop (dysmetria)
- Inability to perform rapid alternating movements (adiadochokinesia)
- Intention tremors
- Staggering, wide based ataxic gait

- Hypotonia
- Nystagmus
- Scanning speech—words are broken
- Pendular knee jerk
- Truncal ataxia
  - Positive Romberg's sign
- Coordination
  - Dysmetria
  - Dyssynergia
  - Dysdiadochokinesis
- Intention tremor
- Ataxic gait
- Titubation

CHAPTER 76

Cervical Spine Immobilization

Two techniques are described. It is necessary to apply both to achieve adequate spine control.

COLLOR METHOD

Once the collar is in place, the neck is largely obscured. Before placing the collar, tracheal deviation, wounds, laryngeal crepitus, subcutaneous emphysema should be looked for. For successful application correct size collar is important.

Cervical stabilization should be maintained by the assistant. Flat part of the collar is placed under the neck. Shaped part of the collar is placed under the child's chin. Flat part of the collar is folded till it meets shaped part. Fit of the collar is reassessed. If the fit is correct the joining device is secured. In line stabilization is ensured until sandbags, tape, or head bags are in position.

SANDBAG OR TAPE

Sandbag is placed on either side of the head. Tape is applied across the forehead and attached to long spinal board. Tape is attached across the chin piece of the hard collar attached to long spinal board.

Log-rolling

This is to minimize the chances of exacerbating unrecognized spinal cord injury. Non-essential movements of the spine must be avoided until adequate investigation and examination have excluded it. If maneuvered that might cause spinal movements then log rolling should be performed. The aim is to maintain the alignment of the spine during turning of the child. The basic requirements are adequate caretaker and good control.

77

CHAPTER

Chest Circumference

Non-stretchable tapes such as metal tapes, fiber glass tapes are ideal. Tape is passed through nipple line. It is measured at mid respiration at the level of the nipple line. The tape measure is placed at right angles to the vertebral column **(Fig. 1)**. It is measured in recumbent position up to the age of 5 years and with standing thereafter. Measurement is recorded to the nearest 0.1 cm.

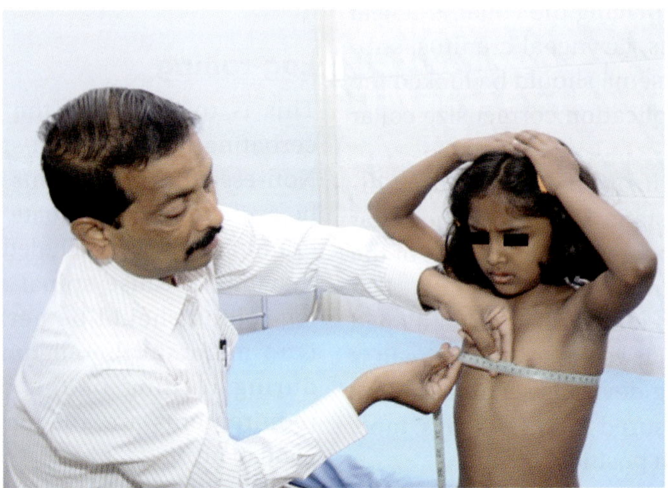

Fig. 1: Chest circumference.

CHAPTER 78

Chest Deformity

SHAPE OF THE CHEST

In infancy and early childhood, the cross-section of the chest is almost circular, the anteroposterior and lateral diameters being about equal. The general shape of the thorax tends to be cylindrical. The shape of the chest in childhood may be greatly modified by hypertrophied adenoids or rickets.

The shape of the chest changes as the age advances.

Abnormal chest: Any abnormality of contour, size, or shape of the chest must be noted carefully, as it may explain the nature of present or past diseases. An abnormal chest may be either symmetrically or asymmetrically abnormal.

Normal contour

Barrel-shaped chest: The anteroposterior diameter is increased relative to lateral diameter. The normal ratio is 5:7. This is seen in emphysema.

Pectus excavatum (funnel-shaped chest): There is a depression in the lower part of the sternum or less commonly depression of the whole length of the body of sternum. Which may be congenital following rickets in childhood or an occupational deformity (in cobblers). Usually asymptomatic, but when there is a very marked degree of depression, the heart may be displaced to the left and the ventilatory capacity of the lungs restricted.

Pectus carinatum: This is a common sequelae to chronic respiratory disease in childhood. It consists of a localized prominence of the sternum and adjacent costal cartilages, often accompanied by indrawing of the ribs to form symmetrical horizontal grooves (Harrison's sulci) above the costal margin, which are themselves usually everted. These deformities are thought to result from lung hyperinflation with repeated strong contractions of the diaphragm while the bony thorax is still in a pliable state. This deformity may also be caused by rickets.

Thoracic kyphoscoliosis: This ranges in degree from the minor changes in spinal curvature to grossly disfiguring and disabling deformities. Severe kyphoscoliosis may have profound effect on pulmonary functions, as the chest deformity reduces the ventilatory capacity of the lungs and increases the work of breathing. Many such patients develop hypoxemia, hypercapnia, and heart failure at an early stage.

Chest Pain

Chest pain can be the presenting complaint for a child feeling chest tightness, burning, pressure, stabbing sensations, palpitations, or heartburn. This can make quickly discerning an etiology difficult, particularly in young children who are not able to verbalize precise symptoms. Chest pain as a symptom affects equal numbers of girls and boys and children under and over 12 years of age.

Due to the rarity of cardiac pathology as the cause for chest pain, it is difficult to develop evidence-based guidelines for evaluation, and the implication of a misdiagnosis of a serious disorder is high. Chest pain caused by noncardiac causes may be the combination of multiple diagnoses, leaving medical providers seeking to "rule out" life-threatening cardiac causes of chest pain.

APPROACH TO THE PATIENT WITH CHEST PAIN

In particular, children and adolescents who have chest pain or syncope that is exertional should be taken seriously, particularly if there is a family history of sudden death.

A complete history and physical examination usually with an electrocardiogram (ECG) used to diagnose chest pain allows medical providers to avoid missing life-threatening cardiac pathology.

HISTORY

One possible approach includes a stepwise, directed history that includes:

- Description of pain
- Assessment for red-flag symptoms, including targeted family history
- Medication review
- Review of known illnesses
- Review of systems including psychosocial evaluation

Eliciting the basics of the chest pain's duration, quality, propensity to radiate, severity, and timing is essential.

Vital signs can indicate the presence of pain by revealing signs of tachycardia and tachypnea, and can provide information regarding potential serious medical illness, including fever, hypoxia, or hypotension. Blood pressures should be obtained in upper and lower extremities, monitoring closely for a gradient between extremities. All vital signs should be evaluated in the context of reference ranges for a child's age and height.

CAUSES OF CHEST PAIN

- Thoracic cause
    - Trauma
    - Costochondritis
- Intrathoracic causes
    - Lungs
        - Pleurisy
        - Pneumothorax
        - Pulmonary embolism
        - Collapse of lung
    - Cardiac
        - Pericarditis
        - Vascular lesion

- Aortic aneurysm
- Aortitis
- Mediastinum
  - Mediastinal emphysema
- Esophagus
  - Esophagitis
  - Achalasia
- Miscellaneous
  - Peptic ulcer
  - Liver abscess
  - Pancreatitis
  - Functional

MUSCULOSKELETAL

Musculoskeletal chest wall pain is perhaps the most identifiable cause of chest pain due to its association with localized tenderness elicited by specific manipulation of the thorax. Pain can involve the ribs, costochondral junctions, costal cartilages, intercostal muscles, sternum, clavicle, or spine. The pain is often worse with movement, coughing, and inspiration.

RESPIRATORY

Respiratory causes of chest pain are often diagnosed through the use of history and general appearance of the patient. Some of these causes can require urgent evaluation and treatment. In a patient with sudden, significant chest pain, medical providers should consider acute pneumothorax or acute pulmonary embolism (along with acute pericarditis, myocarditis, or aortic dissection—discussed in cardiac etiologies of chest pain). Asthma or reactive airway disease is more likely in a patient with audible wheezing and cough.

PSYCHOGENIC/IDIOPATHIC

Psychogenic causes of chest pain are more common in adolescents than in children under the age of 12 years. Patients with psychogenic etiologies of chest pain may also have additional physiologic causes of pain; psychologic risk factors can amplify the clinical presentation of chest pain. Psychologic forms of chest pain are typically recurrent with particular stressors. Children and adolescents may have a history of anxiety and/or stressful life events that are not easily apparent but can have a large impact on their perception of pain. Many psychologic factors, such as anxiety, depression, and psychosomatic features often coexist. Patients with psychogenic causes of chest pain are the most likely to have other somatic symptoms, including breathlessness, fatigue, nervousness, near-syncope, and palpitations. These patients also often demonstrate more bodily worries, more limitations of general activity, and more school absences. The most common etiologies of psychogenic chest pain are hyperventilation and underlying psychiatric illness, such as anxiety, depression, or somatoform disorders (conversion or somatization).

Anxiety, depression, and somatoform disorders can cause episodic chest pain with or without hyperventilation. Within anxiety disorders, chest pain and other symptoms are typically temporally related to stressful situations. Anxiety-related psychogenic chest pain is four times as likely to occur in a patient with a family history of chest pain (often an adult with a history of cardiac ischemia), and the pain is often fleeting and vague in its description.

GASTROINTESTINAL

Esophagitis (reflux, infectious, and eosinophilic) and esophageal motility disorders (diffuse esophageal spasm and achalasia) can cause chest pain in both adults and children. Esophagitis is characterized by symptoms typical of "heartburn," a substernal burning sensation that is exacerbated by eating or position changes, specifically lying supine.

Achalasia classically causes dysphagia, nocturnal regurgitation, and chest pain. It can occur at any age and the chest pain is variably associated with the diagnosis (19–95% of the time). Eosinophilic esophagitis can cause chest pain secondary to esophageal inflammation, dysmotility, and reflux. Other notable gastrointestinal disorders can also cause chest pain including esophageal foreign body, gastric and duodenal ulcers, cholecystitis, pancreatitis, hepatitis, and infections of the subdiaphragmatic space. Esophageal rupture is a rare cause of chest pain; it has been described in patients with bulimia nervosa or after surgical repair of a tracheoesophageal fistula.

OTHER

Breast-related causes of chest pain can occur in both males and females. Females may complain of throbbing or burning chest pain caused by fibrocystic disease, fibroadenoma, swelling with menstruation, mastitis, or pregnancy. Gynecomastia in males can lead to unilateral or bilateral chest pain. Substance abuse of tobacco and/or cocaine in addition to other sympathomimetic substances can also cause chest pain. Foreign bodies in the airways and/or esophagus can be unusual causes of chest discomfort; these diagnoses are typically evident due to other symptoms such as dysphagia, drooling, choking, stridor, or dyspnea. Neoplastic diseases such as mediastinal tumors or lymphomas can also manifest primarily as chest pain.

CARDIAC

Arrhythmias are the most common, whereas patients with myocarditis or myocardial infarction are often the most acutely ill. Heart disease is more commonly found in adolescents than in younger children who complain of chest pain, and adolescents represent the largest group of patients between 1 and 21 years of age who die suddenly of cardiac causes. Supraventricular and ventricular tachyarrhythmias can put adolescents at risk for sudden death. Supraventricular tachycardia (SVT), a narrow complex tachycardia, is the most common arrhythmia in children.

Chest pain that increases during physical exertion or other stress and is relieved by rest, is often poorly localized to the substernal area, and can radiate to the left arm and/or jaw is secondary to a cardiac etiology. This pain is often referred to as anginal and can be secondary to ischemia, although ischemia is not common in children or adolescents **(Box 1)**.

Acute pericarditis causes substernal chest pain that is sharp, stabbing and aggravated by deep inspiration, coughing, or straining. Typical pericarditis pain is improved by being in the sitting position, and patients will avoid lying supine.

Acute myocarditis often is caused by or follows viral infections. Symptoms of acute myocarditis include lethargy, pallor, low-grade fever, anorexia, chest or abdominal pain, and signs of congestive heart failure.

BOX 1: Causes of pediatric anginal chest pain.

- Aortic stenosis
- Hypertrophic cardiomyopathy
- Coronary artery thrombosis
- Anomalous coronary artery location or anatomy
- Coronary vasospasm
- Mitral valve prolapse

CHAPTER 80

Cheyne–Stokes Respiration

It is characterized by rhythmic alteration in the depth of respiration. The gradual increase in respiratory rate is followed by apnea. This happens due to anoxemia. The brain becomes less responsive to carbon dioxide level, as carbon dioxide stimulates respiratory center in brain. During the period of apnea carbon dioxide accumulates and stimulates respiratory center. This results in hyperventilation and hypocapnia. This leads to recurrence of apnea. This cycle repeats until brain recovers. This type of breathing is seen any condition leading with the depression of respiratory center.

CHAPTER 81

Chordee

Chordee (ventral penile curvature) without hypospadias occurs much less frequently than chordee with hypospadias. Chordee may be a minor problem related to skin tethering. It may be a result of abnormal development of urethra and ventral penile structures. It can be due to congenital short urethra in which case surgical correction is required. Surgery includes division of the urethra and interposition of a skin tube. If chordee is suspected neonate circumcision is delayed and justified.

Chorea

Chorea: It is sudden, jerky, and nonrepetitive resembling fragments of normal movements. Most prominent in extremities, however seen in tongue, face. It is exaggerated by emotion and action.

Quasi-purposive movement disappears during sleep.

Common causes:

- Rheumatic chorea
- Drug induced
- TB meningitis encephalitis,
- Chorea gravidarum

Rare causes:

- Wilson's disease
- Huntington's chorea
- Typhoid
- Diphtheria
- Leukodystrophies
- Hallervorden–Spatz syndrome
- Carbon monoxide poisoning

Rheumatic chorea is often associated with:

- Hypotonia
- Pendular jerks
- Flexor plantaris
- Brisk superficial reflexes
- Milkmaid's grip
- Facial grimace
- Bad handwriting
- Dinner fork deformity of hand
- Explosive speech, dysarthria
- Jack in box tongue
- Choreic hand
- Other features of rheumatic disease such as arthritis, carditis, and subcutaneous nodules

SYDENHAM'S CHOREA

Characteristic features of choreiform movements

- Involuntary movements
- Sudden, jerky
- Nonrepetitive
- Occurring at distal joints
- Quasi-purposive
- Disappear during sleep
- Exaggerated by emotions and presence of people are other features seen in Sydenham's chorea
- Associated movements
- Emotional lability
- Muscular hypotonia
- Pendular jerks (depressed or absent deep tendon reflexes)
- Brisk superficial reflexes especially abdominal reflexes

Clinical types of Sydenham's chorea:

- Hemichorea
- *Manic chorea:* Emotional disturbance is more.
- *Paralytic chorea:* Due to excessive hypotonia
- *Chorea gravidarum:* Seen in pregnancy

CHAPTER 83

Chorionic Villus Sampling

This is useful to obtain the fetal tissue. This procedure helps chromosomal, biochemical, and DNA studies. This is indicated in perinatal diagnosis of thalassemia, sickle cell disease, hemophilia, Duchenne's muscular dystrophy, and cystic fibrosis.

This is a relatively safe procedure. Potential complications are listed in **Box 1**. This can be performed at an outpatient basis. This is done with the full bladder, so that the gravid uterus is lifted up into the abdominal cavity. This procedure is done during 9–12 weeks. Twin pregnancy should be excluded. Placental size and position should be noted.

BOX 1: Complications.

- Placental bleeding and fetal death
- Amnionitis
- Increased risk of neonatal respiratory distress
- Fetomaternal hemorrhage
- Premature onset of labor
- Injury to fetal parts
- Postural deformities such as clubfoot

Cervix is prepared with povidone iodine. Polyethylene catheter of the 21–28 is used. Diameter of the catheter is 1–2 mm. This is fitted with a malleable wire obturator. This is then inserted through the cervix under ultrasonographic guidance. Catheter tip is advanced till it lies in chorionic frondosum. Guide wire is gently removed, catheter is advanced through the cervix, so that it stays with chorion **(Fig. 1)**.

A 20-mL syringe filled with 5 mL of tissue culture medium is attached to the catheter, gentle suction of 10 mm is applied, and catheter is slowly withdrawn from the placental site, till the catheter tip lies just above the internal os. Suction should not be applied as the catheter is traversing through the cervical canal. This is to avoid the risk of contamination of mucus and blood. The aspiration of 15–30 mL of trophoblastic tissue is adequate.

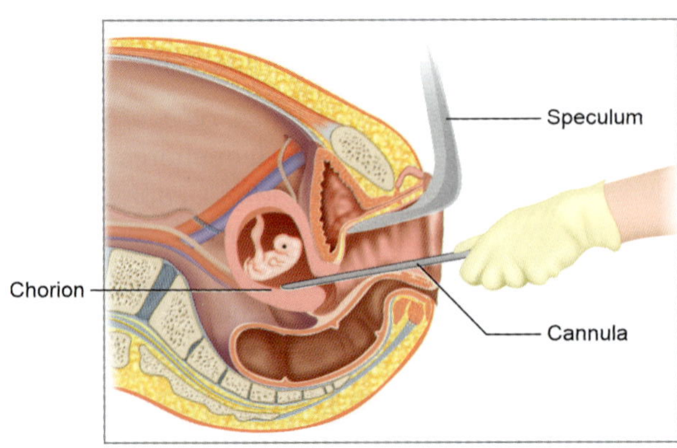

Fig. 1: Chorionic villus biopsy.

CHAPTER 84

Choledochal Cyst

It is a congenital condition, more common in girls. It typically presents within the first several years of life with fusiform to cystic dilatation of the common bile duct. Pain from common bile obstruction or acute pancreatitis may be the initial presenting symptom. Although many lesions are identified on antenatal ultrasound imaging. Surgical excision of the abnormal common duct, with reconstruction with hepaticojejunostomy, is indicated to prevent recurrent episodes of pancreatitis.

85 CHAPTER

Chylothorax

Lymphatic malformations are one of the most common slow-flow lesions seen vascular anomalies. Lesions are made up of small or large cysts or a combination of two. Two special categories include central conducting anomalies and generalized lymphatic malformations. These form clinically chylothorax. Central conducting lymphatic anomalies are malformation of major lymphatic vessels and commonly thoracic duct. This will lead to pooling of chylous fluid within the pleural space. The diagnosis is made by lymphangiogram. This demonstrates abnormal lymphatic flow through the thoracic duct. Magnetic resonance imaging (MRI) demonstrates an obstructed or ectatic thoracic duct. In generalized lymphatic malformation, lymphatic anomalies occur as multiple-sized lymphatic vessels, as well as within various organs of the body.

CHAPTER 86

Clinodactyly

Shortened little fingers, with radial deviation, due to hypoplasia of radial aspect of middle phalanx. The little finger either shows a single crease or its distal crease lies proximal to the proximal crease of ring fingers (normally distal crease of little finger lies distal to the proximal crease of ring finger). Here, the little finger is curved. Hypoplasia of the middle phalanx leads to the congenital deviation of little finger **(Figs. 1 and 2)**. It is seen in Down syndrome, Aarskog's syndrome, and de Lange syndrome.

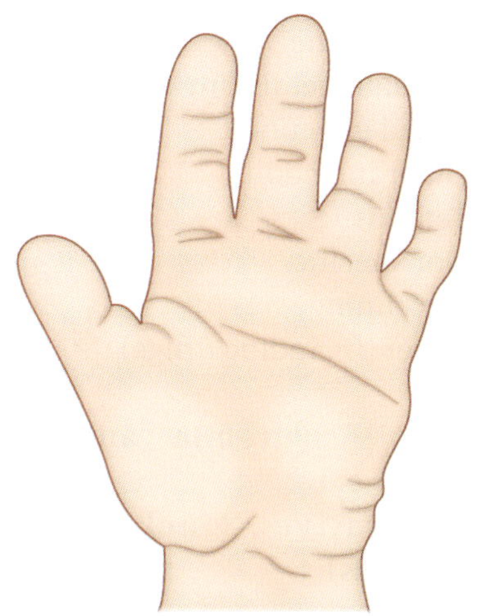

Fig. 1: Clinodactyly—incurving of fifth finger.

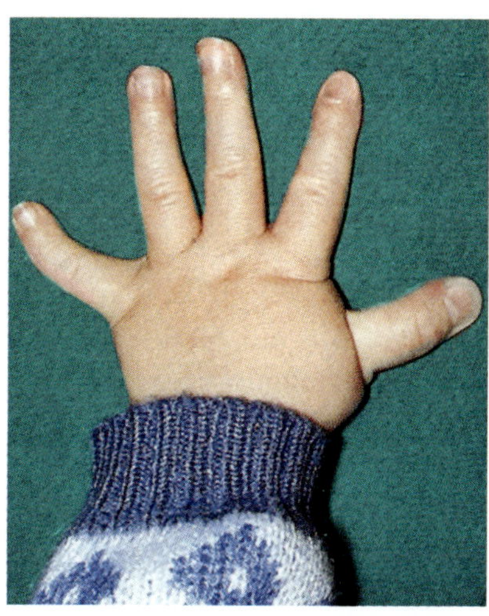

Fig. 2: Clinodactyly.

Clonus

Historic data, including any familial incidence of movement disorders, are essential. Exposure to anoxia, toxins, or trauma should be ascertained. The examination should determine whether myoclonus is focal or generalized.

CLASSIFICATION OF MYOCLONUS

Segmental:

- Brainstem
  - Eye
  - Palate
  - Jaw
  - Face
  - Neck and tongue
- Toxic
  - Limb
  - Trunk
  - Diaphragm
- Etiology
  - Vascular
  - Infections
  - Demyelinating
  - Neoplastic
  - Traumatic
  - Unknown

Generalized (subcortical, brainstem, or spinal cord involvement)

Acute and subacute

- Encephalomyelitis (including polio)
- Toxic and infections
  - Other infection
  - Tetanus
  - Nonspecific
  - Strychnine
  - Other (including drugs)
- Anoxia
- Metabolic (uremia and hepatic insufficiency)
- Degenerative (inclusion body encephalitis)

CHAPTER 88

Cisternal Puncture

It is indicated in neonate, if there is difficulty in lumbar puncture. Nape of the infant neck is shaved. The infant is laid on his side, the pillow is kept under the head to keep the cervical and thoracic spine straight. The lower edge of the occipital bone is palpated. The infant's neck is maximally flexed. Lumbar puncture (LP) needle is inserted in the midline through the atlanto-occipital membrane. It is inserted for 3–4 cm. Aim is to hit the bottom of the occipital bone. The angle of insertion is changed minimally, so that needle passes just through the occipital bone. The direction of the needle should be at the root of the nose. The needle then passes through the dura and enters the cisterns magna at a depth of about 1.5 cm in the term infant.

89 CHAPTER

Clubbing of Fingers

It is thickening of tissues at base of the nail resulting in obliteration of angle between the nail base and adjacent skin of the finger.

Ordinarily, clubbing appears in cyanotic congenital heart disease (CHD), when child is 1 or 2 years old. But in severely cyanotic children, clubbing is seen as early as 2–3 weeks of age.

SIGNS OF CLUBBING

Fluctuation of nail bed and loss of angle between the nail and nail bed are the earliest signs of clubbing.

SCHAMROTH'S SIGN IN CLUBBING

Normally, a diamond-shaped space is formed, when the two thumbs of the child are kept opposed on their dorsal aspect. But in clubbing this shape is obliterated.

PATHOPHYSIOLOGY

- Clubbing occurs due to interstitial edema and dilatation of the arterioles and capillaries.
- Swelling of the subcutaneous tissues over the base of the nail, causes the overlying skin to become tense, shiny, and red with obliteration of skin creases.
- Later on the swelling involves the curvature of the nail especially in its long axis.
- Finally, swelling of the pulp of the finger occurs in all dimensions.
- In a few cases, there may also be hypertrophic pulmonary osteoarthropathy causing pain and swelling of the hands, wrist, knees, feet, and ankles.

MECHANISM

Although the mechanism of clubbing is not clear, it is believed that the stimulus of clubbing is hypoxia. Hypoxia leads to opening up of deep arteriovenous fistula which increases the blood supply of the fingers and toes causing it to undergo hypertrophy.

Another hypothesis is that when reduced ferritin in venous blood escapes oxidation in the lungs and enters systemic circulation, it causes dilatation of arteriovenous anastomosis and hypertrophy of terminal phalanges resulting in clubbing.

SPECIAL FORMS OF CLUBBING

- Unilateral clubbing-aneurysmal dilatation of aorta and its branches, bronchial arteriovenous fistula, pancoast tumor, and erythromelalgia lymphangitis.
- Unidigital—may be hereditary, if bilateral and involving the thumbs. Other causes are median nerve injury, local trauma, tophaceous gout, and sarcoidosis.
- Differential clubbing—only in upper limbs—heroin addicts, due to chronic obstructive phlebitis.
- Only in lower limbs—patent ductus arteriosus with reversal of blood flow.

PSEUDOCLUBBING

In hyperparathyroidism excessive bone resorption may result in disappearance of terminal phalanges with telescoping of soft tissues and drumstick appearance of the fingers resembling clubbing **(Fig. 1)**. However, the curvature of the nail is not present.

CLUBBING

Finger clubbing is an important physical sign and may be the first and only sign of serious organic disease. The relative frequencies of causes are listed in **Box 1**.

BOX 1: Causes of finger clubbing.

- Cyanotic congenital heart disease
- Infective endocarditis
- Bronchiectasis
- Empyema
- Lung abscess
- Cystic fibrosis
- Cirrhosis of liver
- Crohn's disease
- Ulcerative colitis
- Celiac disease

GRADING OF CLUBBING

I: Softening of nail bed
II: Obliteration of angle of nail bed
III: Parrot beak/drumstick appearance
IV: Hypertrophic osteoarthropathy

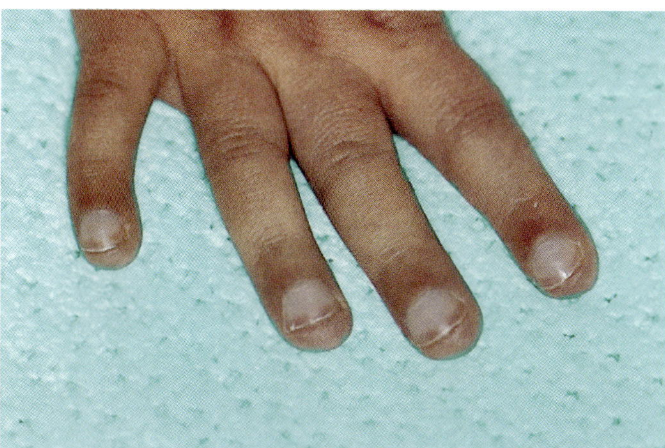

Fig. 1: Clubbing.

CHAPTER

90 Coin Test

It is used test for punctured lung. A punctured lung can cause air or fluid to leak into the pleural cavity, leading to pneumothorax or hydrothorax.

It is done in the case of hydropneumothorax. The coin is placed firmly on the affected side. That coin is percussed with one more coin. The stethoscope is applied directly on the opposite side of the chest. A high pitched, tympanic or metallic sound is heard over the chest. If a tinkling sound is heard, it is likely that air or fluid has found its way into the pleural cavity.

91

CHAPTER

Coloboma of Eyelid

Defects and notches in eyelid margins are seen in coloboma of eyelid. This occurs because of failure of fusion of embryonic fissures in development. This is seen in Goldenhar syndrome. This syndrome consists of vertebral anomalies, dermoids, and preauricular skin tag **(Fig. 1)**.

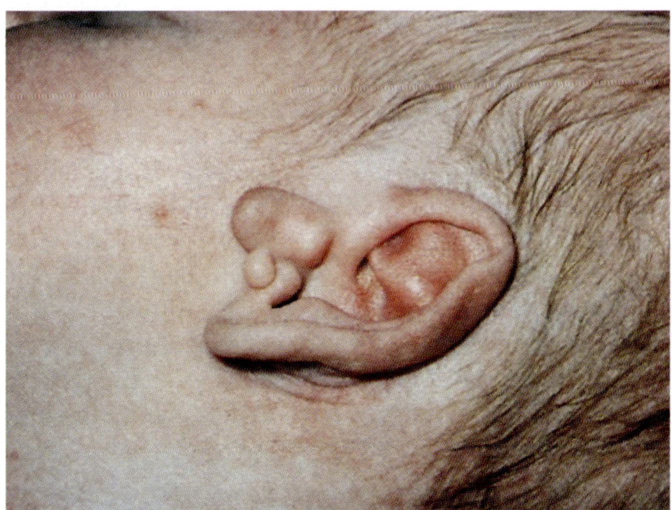

Fig. 1: Preauricular tag.

CHAPTER 92

Coloboma of Fundus

In coloboma of fundus, an extensive well demarcated white area is present which engulfs the optic disc and exposes underlying sclera. Visual acuity is likely to be impaired with large defect. It may occur with other ocular abnormalities, such as microphthalmia. They may also occur in chromosomal abnormalities, e.g., trisomy 13 and 18 **(Figs. 1 and 2)**.

Fundoscopy should be reserved for the end of the examination, right before the child leaves the examining room, unless corneal staining is indicated. Fundoscopy is sometimes a frustrating experience for both the examiner and the child. If you really suspect an abnormality, dilate the pupil to see what you are looking for. Use a short-acting cycloplegic, such as tropicamide 1%, putting one drop in each eye. Pupillary dilation is achieved within at least 20 minutes in most children; it may take a little longer in children with darkly pigmented eyes. The easiest way to put drops in the eyes is to have the patient lie supine with the eye closed. You then put the drop in the inner canthus (corner of the eye) and ask, or wait, for the child to open his or her eyes. Instantly, the drops are in, and nobody has had to fight at least until the next time, when the child may remember your trick. Most young children will not hold their eye still while you try to locate some familiar landmark. Such as the disc or a blood vessel. The solution is for you to stay still, let the child's eye do the moving, and let your

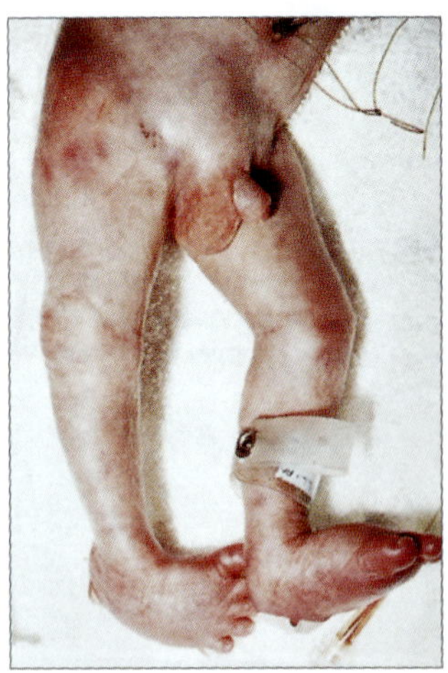

Fig. 1: Edward syndrome.

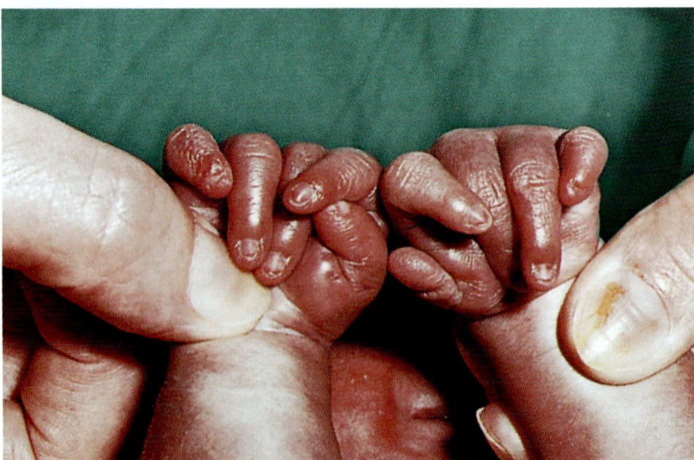

Fig. 2: Trisomy18-Edward syndrome.

eye do the looking. The chances of finding something are far better if you are not moving while you search. Because the other secret of funduscopic success is good old practice (for which there is no reasonable substitute), try to examine the fundi in most infants and children with each complete physical examination. Fundoscopy will become progressively easier for you.

- Evaluate whether the red pupillary reflex is equal in all four fundus quadrants. You can accomplish this goal without having to obtain a perfect focus on the retia; perform the examination at a distance of 25 cm (10–12 inches) from the child.
- Once the fundus is in focus, make sure you can see a normal foveolar reflex. Invite the child to look at your little magic light. Sometimes the child's curiosity prompts him or her to do this anyway when you come close with the direct ophthalmoscopy. One problem is that shining the light on the fovea stimulates the pupillary light response maximally (constriction) and may make viewing of the fundus difficult. Do not despair: The sharp bright foveolar reflection of the ophthalmoscopy is easy to see.
- Visualize at least part of a well demarcated temporal edge of the disc as it passes by.

An even, red pupil indicates an attached retina with no major inflammatory or tumor process. Good fixation plus a sharp foveolar reflex eliminates an organic cause of poor vision, especially if the optic nerve looks normal **(Fig. 3)**. Most optic nerve diseases in the child involve the temporal half early in their evolution.

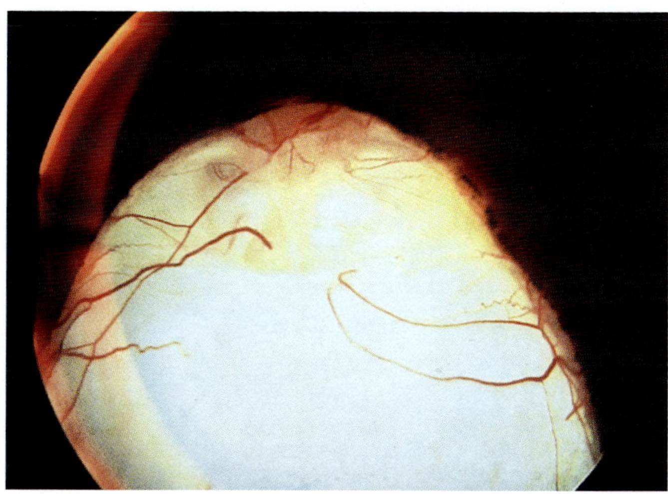

Fig. 3: Coloboma of fundus.

CHAPTER 93

Coloboma of Retina

There is a defect in embryonal fissure closure in optic disc. It manifests as leukocoria. It occurs because of yellow white reflection of underlying sclera. Sometimes there will be red reflex. This is seen as flushing from red to white as eye moves from normal retina to coloboma of retina.

CHAPTER 94 Collodion Body

In several variants of ichthyosis, particularly lamellar ichthyosis or congenital ichthyosiform erythroderma (CIE), the infant can be born encased in a thick, parchment-like scale known as a collodion membrane. This dries and is shed in large sheets within 7–14 days. Affected neonates have ectropion, flattening of the ears and nose, and fixation of the lips in O-shaped configuration. Hair may be absent or may perforate abnormal covering. The membrane cracks with initial efforts.

Significant secondary fluid, electrolyte, and heat losses can occur. Although scaling may only be mild or may even resolve completely in some infants, many go on to develop cutaneous findings typical of the underlying ichthyosis.

Neonatal morbidity and mortality may be due to cutaneous infections, aspiration pneumonia, hypothermia, or hypernatremic dehydration from excessive transcutaneous fluid losses as a result of increased skin permeability. The outcome is uncertain, and accurate prognosis depends on identification of the underlying ichthyosis.

CHAPTER 95

Congenital Hemangioma

The congenital hemangioma is a vascular tumor. The prominent feature to distinguish the congenital hemangioma is that it is fully formed at birth. The classical appearance is of a solitary plaque-like lesion with violaceous appearance. The lesions usually have coarse telangiectasias on their surface and a halo of blanched skin encircling its margins **(Figs. 1 to 7)**.

The congenital hemangioma can then be differentiated into three categories based on its lifecycle. The first category is the non-involuting congenital hemangioma (NICH) that never recedes. The second is the partially involuting congenital hemangioma (PICH) that will flatten in the first year of life but not completely recede. The final category is the rapidly involuting congenital hemangioma (RICH) that will completely recede in the first year of life and typically leaves behind a characteristic atrophied plaque.

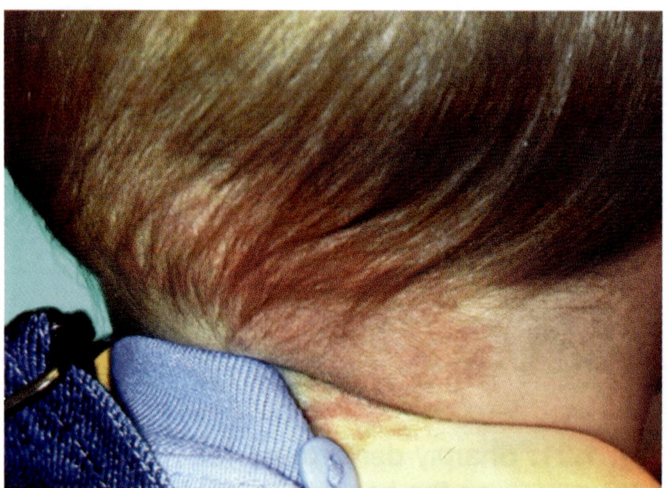

Fig. 1: Salmon patch.

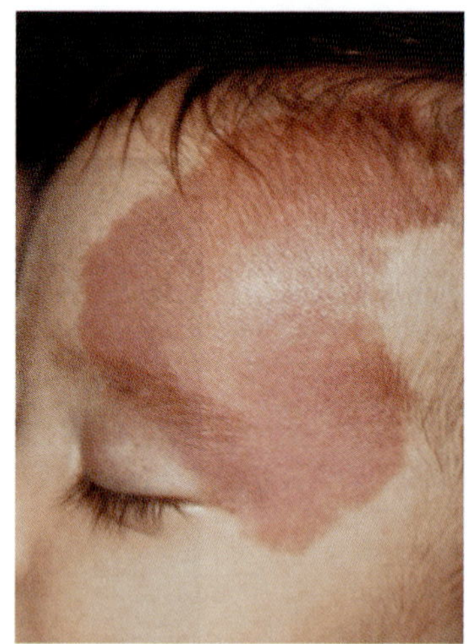

Fig. 2: Port-wine stain.

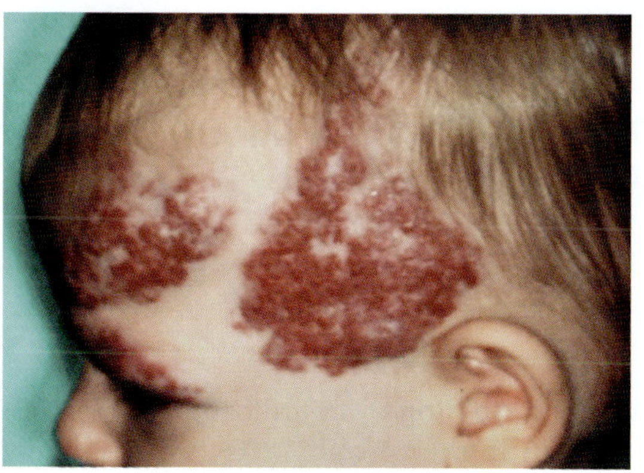

Fig. 3: Multiple hemangiomas.

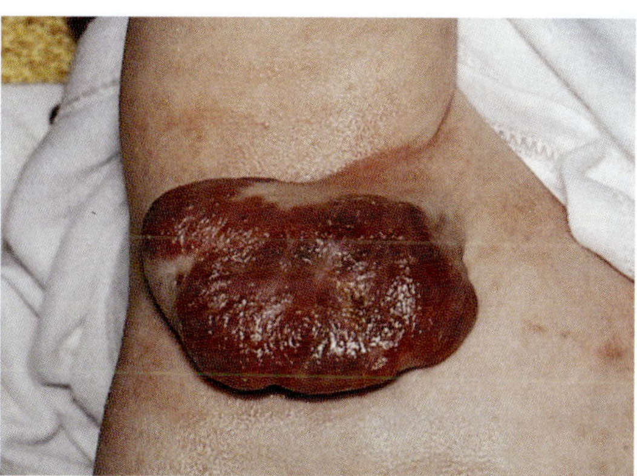

Fig. 4: Cavernous hemangioma.

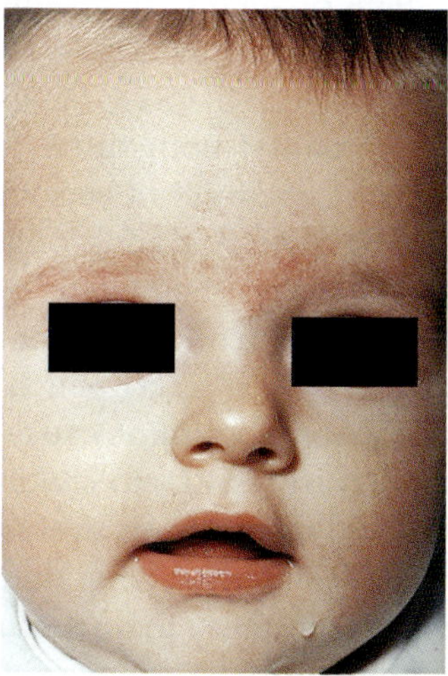

Fig. 5: Salmon patch.

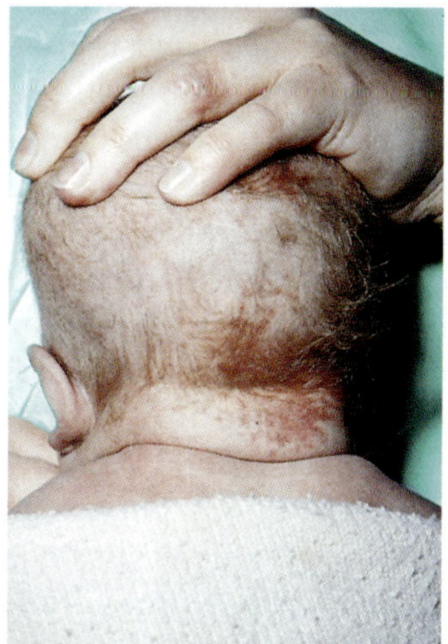

Fig. 6: Salmon patch hemangioma.

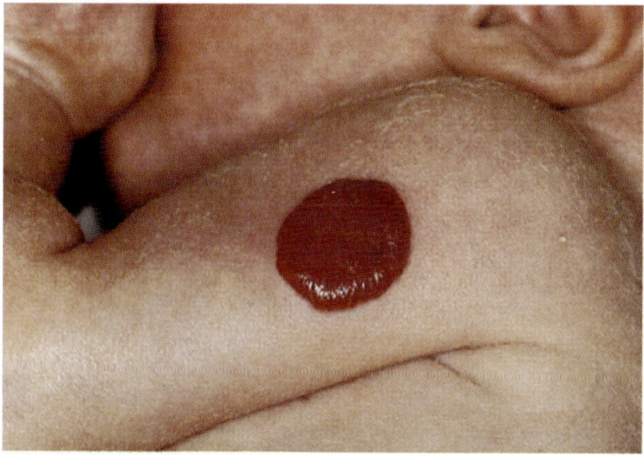

Fig. 7: Strawberry hemangioma.

CHAPTER 96

Congenital Hydronephrosis

Hydronephrosis is the single most common renal abnormality (20%) detected by fetal ultrasonography. It is more reliably assessed by ultrasonographic imaging obtained within 1 week after birth to aid detection of responsible conditions, such as ureteropelvic junction obstruction, high-grade vesicoureteral reflux (VUR), renal dysplasia, or posterior urethral valves in males. Mild-to-moderate isolated hydronephrosis is defined by an anteroposterior diameter between 5 and 15 mm without calyceal dilation, normal renal cortical thickness, and no associated abnormal renal echotexture, hydroureter, or thickened bladder wall on ultrasonography at 1 week after birth. Although urinary tract infection (UTI)/pyelonephritis occurs more commonly in infants with hydronephrosis than in the general population, VUR is uncommon and usually of low grade. Hence, neither voiding cystourethrogram (VCUG) nor antibiotic prophylaxis is definitively required. However, sequential ultrasonography should be done to follow hydronephrosis. Typically, 94% of such cases resolve spontaneously during the first 12–14 months of life.

Severe antenatal congenital hydronephrosis is less common but very important condition that often has additional genitourinary anomalies on imaging suggesting the spectrum of CAKUT (congenital anomalies of the kidney and urinary tract), which together constitute the predominant cause of end-stage renal disease (ESRD) in children. Such children should be promptly evaluated with VCUG and nuclear medicine studies. Any febrile episodes in these infants should lead to prompt and appropriate investigation for UTI and therapy.

CHAPTER 97 Consciousness: Disorders

Consciousness is the state of awareness of the self and the environment when provided with adequate stimuli. Patients who are in normal wakefulness will be fully responsive to stimuli and will display correct behavior and speech in response to these stimuli.

The Glasgow Coma Scale provides a useful measure to assess the level of consciousness. It is based on the observation of level of response to graded stimuli in three modes—eye opening, motor function, and verbal utterance. In the first mode, spontaneous eye opening and blinking score the highest grade, eye opening in response to voice the next highest, eye opening in response to painful stimuli the next, and finally no response of eyes opening to stimuli the lowest.

Several terms are used to define altered states of consciousness, as follows.

CONFUSION

Confusion, or clouding of consciousness, is characterized by an impaired capacity to think clearly and to perceive, respond to, and remember current stimulus. There is usually disorientation.

DELIRIUM

This is a state of severely disturbed consciousness with motor restlessness, disorientation, and delusions. Delirium is associated with a diffusely abnormal EEG and is commonly seen with toxic and metabolic disorder.

STUPOR

Patient responds to strong noxious stimuli. He returns to an unconscious state when stimulus is stopped. When around patient cannot interact with examiner.

COMA

This is a condition of absolute unconsciousness judged by the absence of any psychologically understandable response to external stimulus or internal need. It is the state of total unresponsiveness to even deep painful stimulus reflex motor response may not be tested.

CHAPTER 98

Constipation

Constipation is defined symptomatically as the infrequent passage of hard stools, straining while passing a stool, or pain associated with the passage of a hard stool.

Constipation is classified broadly either as functional or as secondary to underlying conditions, such as anatomic abnormalities, metabolic disorders, neurologic dysfunction, or medication effects. The majority of childhood constipation is functional. The Rome III Criteria for Functional Gastrointestinal Disorders defines functional constipation in two age groups as noted in **Boxes 1 to 3** here.

A rectal motility evaluation may be helpful in the diagnosis and management of chronic constipation. Anorectal manometry can be used to evaluate the integrity of the muscles and the innervation of the defecatory mechanism. Determining the sensory threshold provides valuable diagnostic information—patients who cannot detect a balloon filled with 120 mL of air usually have

BOX 1: Functional constipation—infant/toddler.

Diagnostic criteria—must include 1 month of *at least two* of the following in infants up to 4 years of age:
- Two or fewer defecations per week
- At least one episode/week of incontinence after the acquisition of toileting skills
- History of excessive stool retention
- History of painful or hard bowel movements
- Presence of a large fecal mass in the rectum
- History of large-diameter stools, which may obstruct the toilet

Accompanying symptoms may include irritability, decreased appetite, and/or early satiety. The accompanying symptoms disappear immediately following passage of a large stool

BOX 2: Functional constipation—child/adolescent.

Diagnostic criteria—must include *two or more* of the following in a child with a developmental age of at least 4 years with insufficient criteria for diagnosis of irritable bowel syndrome (IBS):
- Two or fewer defecations in the toilet per week
- At least one episode of fecal incontinence per week
- History of retentive posturing or excessive volitional stool retention
- History of painful or hard bowel movements
- Presence of a large fecal mass in the rectum
- History of large diameter stools, which may obstruct the toilet

BOX 3: Causes of constipation during the neonatal period.

- Meconium plug (rule out cystic fibrosis)
- Meconium ileus (rule out cystic fibrosis)
- Hirschsprung disease
- Intestinal pseudo-obstruction
- Anteriorly displaced anus
- Ectopic anus
- Anal stenosis
- Imperforate anus
- Spina bifida
- Hypothyroidism
- Hypercalcemia
- Neuronal intestinal dysplasia types A and B
- Medications (opioids, paralytic agents, and magnesium)

encopresis. Hirschsprung disease is unlikely if reflexive relaxation of the internal anal sphincter occurs in the presence of rectal distention.

CAUSES OF CONSTIPATION

Functional:

- Habitual
- Psychological

Organic:

- Imbalanced diet
- Recent acute illness
- Surgical causes
  - Hirschsprung's disease
  - Rectal stenosis
  - Anal stenosis/fissure
  - Stricture
  - Volvulus
- Metabolic
  - Dehydration
  - Hypokalemia
  - Hypercalcemia
  - Pan hypopituitarism
- Endocrinal
  - Hypothyroidism
  - Cystic fibrosis
- Drugs
  - Narcotics
  - Antidepressants
- Central nervous system
  - Cerebral palsy
  - Spinal cord lesion
  - Myotonic dystrophia

CHAPTER 99 Continuous Murmurs

Of the many causes of continuous murmurs, only two are of major importance. The most common continuous murmur is a normal finding known as the venous hum. In children whose circulation in hyperkinetic, continuous turbulence is audible over the jugular veins and usually is loudest in the right supraclavicular fossa. This murmur, usually heard only in the sitting or upright position, varies considerably in intensity with movement of the child's head, and its intensity may be influenced by light pressure on either jugular vein. The turbulence also may be palpated with light pressure on the jugular vein. With light finger pressure, a thrill may be palpable.

The other important continuous murmur is that of a patent ductus arteriosus (PDA). It is heard maximally on the left side of the thorax, usually just below the clavicle or between the left sternal border and the midclavicular line in the second interspace. In contrast to the venous hum, it is heard clearly in the supine position. Flow through a PDA of average size increases aortic runoff and left ventricular (LV) stroke volume.

CHAPTER 100

Coombs Test

This will evaluate the patient's blood for the presence of anti-RBC antibody and complement on RBCs or in the serum, respectively, identify immune-mediated hemolytic anemia. Antibody and complement-mediated RBC destruction produces spherocytes on peripheral blood smear. Coombs-positive hemolytic anemia in the newborn most often represents an alloimmune hemolytic anemia. This is caused by maternal antibody that crossed placenta into the neonate, hemolyzing the newborn RBCs. Maternal antibodies form fetal RBC antigens when the fetal blood gains entry into the maternal circulation via break in the placental integrity. Maternal antibodies then cross the placenta and cause fetal RBC hemolysis. In the majority of cases of severe hemolytic anemia, the maternal antibody is directed at Rh RBC antigens. ABO-mediated disease is less severe due to the decreased number of these antigens on fetal RBCs.

CHAPTER 101

Contact Dermatitis

Contact dermatitis refers to a group of conditions in which an inflammatory reaction in the skin is triggered by direct contact with environmental agents. In the most common form, irritant contact dermatitis, changes in the skin are induced by caustic agents, such as acids and alkalis, hydrocarbons, and other primary irritants. Anyone exposed to these agents in a high enough concentration for a long enough period will ultimately develop dermatitis. The rash is usually acute, with well-demarcated erythema, crusting, and/or blister formation.

In contrast, allergic contact dermatitis is a T-lymphocyte-mediated immune reaction to an antigen coming into contact with the skin. Although patients typically present with acute onset of erythema, vesiculation, and pruritus, in some cases they delay seeking care until after the rash has become chronic with scaling, lichenification, and pigmentary changes. Often, the allergen is obvious, as is the case with poison ivy or nickel jewelry. However, in other cases, careful questioning or more formal patch testing may be required to detect the inciting agent.

The initial reaction occurs after a 7- to 14-day period of sensitization in susceptible individuals. Once sensitization has occurred, re-exposure to the allergen provokes a more immediate reaction, sometimes within hours. This is a classic example of type IV (delayed) hypersensitivity.

CHAPTER 102 Coordination

Coordination will give an assessment of cerebellar function. Cerebellar function includes integration of sensory feedback and motor output. Fine coordination is not fully developed until 4–6 years of life. Hence methods of testing coordination depends on the level of neuromuscular maturation.

FINGER-NOSE TEST

Here the examiner's finger is held at an arm's length in front of the patient. Patent is asked to touch the examiner's finger and his nose alternately. Gradually the patient is asked to do it progressively faster. In cerebellar lesion, the patient develops the intestine tremor as his finger approaches the target. Over shooting of the target occurs.

Patient is asked to perform some repetitive movements such as supination and pronation rapidly. Unable to do this is called dysdiadokokinesia. This is seen is cerebellar lesion. Here, there is incoordination and patient is unable to do so. He has irregularity and slowness of movements.

HEEL-SHIN TEST

Patient is asked to touch the heel of the leg along the shin of the other leg repeatedly. Patient with the cerebellar lesion cannot do it.

TANDEM WALKING

Here the patient is asked to walk on a straight line. It is the most sensitive test. It detects even the latent ataxia especially truncal ataxia.

ROMBERG SIGN

This tests both for coordination and posture. It assesses the cerebellar and sensory system. The patient is asked to stand with eyes open for some time. If the patient is unable to stand, it indicates Romberg sign positive with the cerebellar defect. It can stand with eyes open, but he cannot sustain when the eyes are closed. This means Romberg positive with sensory defect. The defect is in the ascending tract of Gall and Burdach.

CHAPTER 103

Corneal Reflex

This is the most sensitive test of sensory trigeminal nerve function.

Patient is asked to direct his gaze to one side keeping the eyes open. The examiner then approaches the adducted eye from the lateral side with a wisp of cotton that has been twisted to a point. The examiner touches the corner over the iris just lateral to the pupil (avoid contact with conjunctiva, sclera, or pupil).

The normal response is immediate blinking of both eyes, occasionally with movement of the head away from the stimulus.

Afferent limb: Ophthalmic division of trigeminal nerve

Efferent limb: Facial nerve-corneal reflex pathway.

- If there is damage to the ophthalmic nerve, no response will be seen in either eye if the corner of the involved side is touched. Blink response both eyes will be observed when the cornea of the normal side is touched.
- In lesions of the facial nerve, no response is present on the involved side when either cornea is touched. Blink response on the normal side will present regardless of which cornea is touched.

MOTOR COMPONENT

To test the muscles of mastication, i.e., masseter, temporalis and medial pterygoid, patient is asked to close his mouth and clench his teeth.

The examiner palpates the contraction of the muscle on both sides. Muscle contraction should be equal and symmetrical.

The temporalis muscle can be palpated in the temporal fossa during the same maneuver.

To test the lateral pterygoid muscle, ask the patient to open his mouth and rude the lower jaw. Deviation of the jaw to one side suggests weakness or paralysis on the ipsilateral side.

It is the sensitive test for the sensory function of trigeminal nerve. The afferent pathway is from ophthalmic division of trigeminal nerve and afferent pathway is from fascial nerve.

Here the child is asked to look at one side keeping the eye open. The examiner touches the cornea over the iris just lateral to the pupil with the help of the wisp of cotton.

The normal response is immediate blinking of both eyes. Sometimes head moves away from the stimulus.

If there is damage to the ophthalmic nerve, no response is seen in either eye. Blink response in both the eyes will be observed when the cornea of the normal side is touched. If there is lesion in fascial nerve, no response is present on the involved side, when either cornea is touched.

Motor component is tested by asking the patient to close the mouth and clench his teeth. The examiner palpates the contraction of muscle on both the sides. Muscle contraction should be equal and symmetrical.

104 CHAPTER

Cortical Sensory Function

Cortical or discriminatory sensory function tests cognitive ability to interpret sensations associated with coordination abilities. Inability to perform these should make you suspect a lesion in the sensory cortex or the posterior column of spinal cord. The patient's eyes are closed during these procedures.

STEREOGNOSIS

The common objects used daily are given to the patient such as keys and coin. Ask the patient to close the eyes. Patient is asked to identify by touch and manipulation. Tactile agnosia, i.e., unable to identify by touch is seen in parietal lobe lesion.

TWO-POINT DISCRIMINATION

Here the two sterile needles are used. These needles are touched alternatively with one or two points simultaneously at various locations. The distance should be noted at which the patient can longer distinguish two points. The minimal distance of discriminating two points should be tested.

GRAPHESTHESIA

With the blunt object, a letter or a number is drawn on any part of the body. The letter or number should be easily recognized.

Point localization: An area of the patient skin is touched and withdrawn. The patient should localize the point of touch.

EXTINCTION PHENOMENON

Simultaneously touch the cheek, hand or other area on each side of the body with a sterile needle. Ask the patient how many stimuli there are and where they are. Both the sensations must be felt.

POINT LOCALIZATION

Touch an area on the patient's skin and withdraw the stimulus. Ask the patient to point to the area touched. There should be no difficulty in localizing the stimulus. Usually tested simultaneously with superficial tactile sensation.

Cough

Cough is a complex physiological event that protects the lungs from mechanical, chemical, and thermal injury. It is a normal reflex and therefore helps humans adapt to an ever-changing environment. It is a common and normal response in all healthy people following the inhalation or aspiration of foreign material. Cough can also be a pathologic reflex in that it may be of biologically negative significance. It may be an important and often the only sign of serious disease and may significantly contribute to the spread of airborne infection, and in some instances, may result in severe functional or structural damage to the organism. Cough may be an exhausting and debilitating experience that greatly contributes to the morbidity of acute self-limiting and chronic incurable diseases.

MECHANISM

The afferent pathway includes the sensory end organs within the pharynx, larynx, trachea and bronchi, and sensory fibers within the ninth and tenth cranial nerves. The act of coughing usually comprises a sudden and severe or violent expiration after a deep inspiration and closure of the vocal cords and may be associated in severe case with bronchospasm or glottic spasm, resulting in dyspnea, cyanosis, anoxia, and death.

The cough reflex has five components: (1) Cough receptors, (2) afferent nerves, (3) a poorly defined medullary cough center, (4) efferent nerves, and (5) effectors (diaphragm and intercostal and other muscles). Cough begins with stimulation of cough receptors or, less commonly, the afferent nerve pathways.

DIFFERENTIAL DIAGNOSIS

Infection

Infections in infants: Viral upper respiratory infections (common cold); croup (laryngotracheobronchitis); viral bronchiolitis, particularly with respiratory syncytial virus (RSV) or human metapneumovirus; and viral pneumonia are the most frequently encountered respiratory tract infections and hence the most common causes of cough in infancy.

Viral upper respiratory infections (URI): Viral URI symptoms and signs usually include stuffy nose with nasal discharge, sore throat, and sneezing. There may be fever, constitutional signs (irritability, myalgias, and headache), or both. Cough is common and may persist for 5–7 days.

Croup (laryngotracheobronchitis): Infectious croup is most common in the first 2 years of life. Its most dramatic components are the barking ("croupy") cough and inspiratory stridor, which appear a few days after the onset of a cold. In most cases, the patient has a low-grade fever, and the disease resolves within a day or two. In severe cases, the child can be extremely ill and is at risk for complete laryngeal obstruction. There may be marked intercostal and suprasternal retractions and cyanosis. Stridor at rest signifies significant obstruction.

Bronchiolitis: Bronchiolitis is a common and potentially serious lower respiratory tract disorder in infants. It is caused usually by RSV but on occasion by parainfluenza, influenza, human metapneumovirus, adenovirus, enterovirus, and human rhinovirus. It mostly occurs in the winter months, often in epidemics. RSV bronchiolitis is seen uncommonly in children >4 years. Typically, "cold-like" symptoms of rhinorrhea precede the harsh cough, increased respiratory rate, and retractions. Respiratory distress and cyanosis can be severe. The child's temperature is seldom elevated above 38°C.

The chest is hyperinflated, widespread crackles are audible on inspiration, and wheezing marks expiration.

The diagnosis is confirmed with demonstration of RSV by polymerase chain reaction (PCR) of nasopharyngeal secretions.

Pertussis (whooping cough): Pertussis is a relatively common cause of lower respiratory tract infection in infants, children, adolescents, and adults, especially in those who are underimmunized or not immunized. The causative organism, *Bordetella pertussis*, has a tropism for tracheal and bronchial ciliated epithelial cells; thus, the disease is primarily bronchitis, but spread of the organism to alveoli, or secondary invasion by other bacteria, can cause pneumonia.

Pneumonia: The features discussed for viral pneumonia in infants are relevant for viral pneumonia in older children. Adenovirus and influenza pneumonia may present similar to bacterial pneumonia in severity and acuteness.

Bacterial pneumonia is more common in toddlers and older children than in infants. The most common pathogen is *Streptococcus pneumoniae (S. pneumoniae)*. Cough may not be as prominent a presenting symptom or sign as tachypnea and grunting. Raised respiratory rates (>50 in infants 2–12 months old, >40 in children 1–5 years old) plus retractions and grunting with or without hypoxia (oxygen saturation <90%) have a high specificity and sensitivity for pneumonia.

Chest pain, abdominal pain, headache, or any combination of these symptoms may occur. Upper lobe pneumonia may produce meningeal signs, and lower lobe involvement may cause abdominal pain and an ileus.

Examination of the chest shows tachypnea but may be otherwise surprisingly normal. In older children, there may be localized dullness to percussion, with crackles or amphoric (bronchial) breath sounds over a consolidated lobe.

Aspiration

Inhaling food, mouth or gastric secretions, or foreign bodies into the tracheobronchial tree causes acute, recurrent, or chronic cough. Interference with normal swallowing disrupts the coordination of swallowing and breathing that prevents aspiration. Structural causes of disordered swallowing include esophageal atresia (in neonates), strictures, webs, or congenital stenoses. Mediastinal lesions (tumors and lymph nodes), including vascular rings, may compromise the esophageal lumen and esophageal peristalsis, increasing the likelihood of aspiration.

Functional disorders include central nervous system dysfunction or immaturity, dysautonomia, achalasia, and diffuse esophageal spasm. Prior neck surgery, including tracheostomy, may alter normal swallowing. Tracheoesophageal fistula and laryngeal clefts are congenital malformations with direct physical connections between the tracheobronchial tree and the upper gastrointestinal tract; thus, oral contents enter the lungs directly.

Foreign Body

Any child with cough of an abrupt onset should be suspected of having inhaled a foreign body into the airway. Toddlers, who by nature put all types of things into their mouths and who have incompletely matured swallowing and airway protective mechanisms, are at high risk. Infants with toddlers or young children in the household who may "feed" the baby are also at risk. In older children, it is usually possible to obtain an accurate history of the aspiration event. These events are described as choking, gagging, and coughing while something (e.g., peanuts, popcorn, small toys, sunflower seeds) is in the mouth. The child may come to the physician with cough and wheeze immediately after the event, with a clear history and a straightforward diagnosis. In many children with a tracheobronchial foreign body, however, the initial episode is not recognized; these children may not come to medical attention for days, weeks, or even months. The initial episode may be followed by a relatively symptom-free period lasting days or even weeks, until infection develops behind an obstructed segmental or lobar bronchus. At this point, cough, perhaps with hemoptysis, with or without wheeze, recurs.

Gastroesophageal Reflux

Gastroesophageal reflux (GER) is a common cause of cough in all age groups. The typical patient is an infant in the first 6 months of life who spits up small amounts of milk frequently after feedings. This "regurgitant reflux" most commonly resolves by 1 year of age. However, many toddlers and children continue to have reflux, although it may be "silent" or non-regurgitant (without spitting up).

A major mechanism for gastroesophageal reflux disease (GERD) with cough is mediated by vagal esophagobronchial reflexes (bronchoconstriction), stimulated by acid in the esophagus. Whether acid in the esophagus is sufficient stimulus to cause bronchoconstriction by itself or whether it merely heightens bronchial reactivity to other stimuli is not yet clear.

The diagnosis of GERD must also be considered in the child with chronic or recurrent cough with no other obvious explanation. The child who coughs after meals or at night, when the supine position may provoke GER, should be evaluated for GER. If GER is confirmed, the next step is a therapeutic trial of anti-reflux therapy.

Asthma

Cough is frequently the sole or most prominent manifestation of asthma; wheezing may be entirely absent. In fact, asthma is almost certainly the most common cause of recurrent and chronic cough in childhood. Treatment for asthma manifesting as cough is the same as the treatment for asthma.

Habit (Psychogenic) Cough

On occasion, a school-aged child may develop a cough that lasts for weeks, often after a fairly typical cold. This cough occurs only during wakefulness, never during sleep. In many cases, the cough is harsh and foghorn-like. It often disrupts the classroom, and the child is asked to leave. The child is otherwise well and may seem rather unbothered by the spectacle created. There is no response to medications. It seems that this type of cough, previously termed "psychogenic," or "psychogenic cough tic," but now called habit cough, has given the child valuable attention. This attention then serves as the sustaining force, and the cough persists beyond the original airway inflammation. In the small minority of cases, there may be deep-seated emotional problems of which the cough is the physical expression.

BOX 1: Red flags for cough.

- *If associated with severe, acute:*
  - Hemoptysis
  - Dyspnea
  - Hypoxemia
- *If associated with chronic:*
  - Failure to thrive
  - Steatorrhea
  - Decreased exercise tolerance
  - Digital clubbing
- *Persistence of:*
  - Cough for 6 weeks or more
  - Radiographic abnormality, especially if asymmetric
- *Failure to respond to empirical therapy:*
  - Antibiotics for presumed infection
  - Bronchodilators for presumed reactive airways

Common red flags for cough are mentioned below in **Box 1**.

CAUSES OF COUGH

- Upper respiratory tract infection
- Nasobronchial allergy
- Bronchial asthma
- Bronchiolitis
- Pneumonia
- Pulmonary suppuration
- Measles
- Whooping cough
- Empyema
- Foreign body in air passage

CAUSES OF CHRONIC/ RECURRENT COUGH

- Inflammatory disorder of airway
  - Bronchial asthma
  - Infection
  - Inhalation of irritants
- Suppurative lung disease
  - Bronchiectasis
  - Cystic fibrosis
  - Foreign body retained in bronchi
  - Congenital malformation
    - Sequestrated lobe
    - Broncho malaria
    - H-type tracheoesophageal fistula
  - GERD
  - Intestinal lung disease

CAUSES OF CHRONIC COUGH

- *From the birth:*
  - Laryngeal webs
  - Vascular rings
  - H-type tracheoesophageal fistula
- *Early infancy:*
  - Congenital infections—rubella, cytomegalovirus (CMV)
  - Gastroesophageal reflux
- *Late infancy:*
  - Bronchitis
  - Asthma
  - Cystic fibrosis
  - Whooping cough
- *Preschool age:*
  - Recurrent bronchitis
  - Allergic bronchitis
  - Asthma
  - Foreign body
  - Chronic suppurative lung disease
  - Pulmonary eosinophilia
- *At all ages*
  - Bronchial asthma
  - Whooping cough
  - Viral bronchitis
  - Foreign body aspiration

CAUSES OF RECURRENT OF PERSISTENT COUGH

- Recurrent respiratory infection
- Asthma
- Suppurative lung disease
- Recurrent aspiration—gastroesophageal reflux
- Persistent endobronchial infection
- Inhaled foreign bodies
- Tuberculosis
- Tracheobronchomalacia
- Tracheoesophageal fistula

106 CHAPTER

Costochondral Beading

In active childhood rickets, the costochondral junction enlarges producing the so-called "rickety rosary". The soft plastic ribs are readily molded. A depression is produced above the costal margins with a flaring outward of the costal margin itself. This deformity may remain and is known as Harrison's sulcus.

107 CHAPTER

Craniosynostosis

Abnormal shape or dimension of the skull is caused by premature closure of one or more skull sutures **(Fig. 1)**.

PATHOGENESIS

Although suture lines are not normally palpable after 5th or 6th month, final fusion occurs only by fourth decade of life. The metopic suture closes in early infancy in 90% of the people. In the remaining 10% it never closes.

Premature fusion of sutures leads to growth of the skull in the areas of unfused sutures and growth is arrested in the area of fused sutures. This leads to various cranial distortions seen.

Premature fusion is clinically made out by loss of mobility, prominent bony ridges, and absent fontanelle.

Cephalic index (CI): It describes the relationship between

$$\frac{\text{(Maximum breadth) biparietal diameter}}{\text{(Maximum length) occipitofrontal diameter}}$$

Normal range 75–85% when outer to inner biparietal diameter and mid frontal to midoccipital, occipitofrontal diameter (OFD) are used. Cranial sutures can be imaged by ultrasonography (USG).

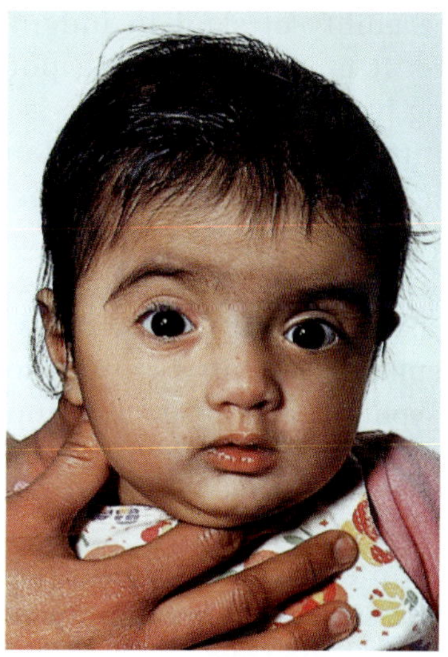

Fig. 1: Craniosynostosis.

Dolichocephaly diagnosed when cephalic index decreased to 75%. Here the anteroposterior diameter is increased and is often due to premature fusion of sagittal suture.

Brachycephaly cephalic index increased to 85%. Here, the skull is flattened anteroposteriorly.

Other types of craniostenoses are:

- Trigonocephaly
- Oxycephaly
- Turricephaly

108 CHAPTER

Craniotabes

It is the ability of skull to indent under pressure. It is just like a ping pong ball, to spring back into shape. This is normal in infants, especially among lambdoid sutures. Persistence of craniotabes more than few months indicates inadequate bone mineralization. This is seen among rickets. This is physiological till 3 months of age, hydrocephalus, vitamin A intoxication, congenital syphilis, and osteogenesis imperfecta.

Craniotabes means soft and compressible skull bones:

- Refers to the occurrence of thin parchment such as soft mushy areas in the skull that can be indented like a ping-pong ball.
- Most commonly present along the suture lines and in the parietal bones at the vertex.

METHOD OF PALPATION

- Hold the head with the left hand.
- Press the skull, one above and one behind the ear, over parietal bone and appreciate the "ping-pong ball" feel and the degree of softness.
- *Caution:* Remember to do this, at the end of the examination as it is a very painful procedure.

CAUSES OF CRANIOTABES

- Rickets
- Hydrocephalus
- Hypervitaminosis A
- Osteogenesis imperfecta
- Congenital syphilis

Auscultation is done for soft bruit over vertex, temples, and eyeballs. Loud harsh bruit suggests arteriovenous malformation or transmission of abnormal sounds from the heart or vessels. The causes of bruit are fever, thyrotoxicosis, anemia, cardiac murmur, patent ductus arteriosus (PDA), arteriovenous (A-V) malformation, and intracranial tumors.

Crepitus (Subcutaneous Emphysema)

Subcutaneous emphysema is due to air trapped under the skin, though uncommon if present can be recognized by crackling sensation produced by lightly compressing the part affected. It starts in and is usually confined to, the neighborhood of the air passages, on rare occasions it may result from the clostridial infection of soft tissues after injury (gas-gangrene). The most common situation is the subcutaneous emphysema over chest, neck due to post-measles bronchopneumonia causing mediastinal emphysema and consequent leak of air into subcostal plane.

The presence of subcutaneous air over the chest wall or up into the neck, which is felt as a crackling under the skin on palpation of the neck or chest, indicates an air leak and is usually associated with pneumomediastinum, which can be confirmed by chest radiograph. Pneumothorax may or may not be present but should be investigated because of its potential seriousness.

CAUSES

- Fractured rib
- Ruptured pneumothorax
- Ruptured alveoli in post-measles bronchopneumonia

CHAPTER 110 Cryptorchidism

During embryogenesis, the testes migrate from their original location near the kidney through the abdomen and descend into the scrotum. Cryptorchidism or failure of the testes to descend into the scrotum, occurs in approximately 3% of infant males. Treatment of cryptorchidism is usually delayed until 6–12 months old to allow the testicle to descend spontaneously. If there is failure of descent, an orchiopexy is performed. A cryptorchid testicle may be intrinsically abnormal and is more likely to undergo malignant transformation. Although surgical intervention may not completely alter the risk of malignancy, placing the testicle in its proper location allows for earlier detection of a suspicious mass.

CHAPTER 111 Cutis Marmorata

Cutis marmorata is characterized by symmetric reticulated cyanosis involving the trunk and extremities. This marbled appearance usually appears when the skin is cool and resolves upon rewarming of the infant. This benign condition typically improves with age. When this vascular pattern is seen in older infants or children, it may be associated with Down syndrome, Cornelia de Lange syndrome, or hypothyroidism.

Cutis marmorata should be differentiated from cutis marmorata telangiectasia congenita (CMTC). The persistent cutis marmorata of CMTC is characteristically asymmetric, often segmental, mottled, or marble-like, and more localized than physiologic cutis marmorata. In addition, the reticulated mottling of CMTC is darker in color and does not resolve with rewarming. Although CMTC improves with age, the abnormal vascular pattern is more persistent than that seen in physiologic cutis marmorata. It may be an isolated entity or may have distinct associations, including atrophy or hypertrophy of the affected extremity, ulcerations, or coexistent vascular malformations and tumors, and other extracutaneous anomalies.

Cutis marmorata is characterized by a transient, netlike, reddish blue mottling of the skin caused by variable vascular constriction and dilation. It is a normal response to chilling, and on rewarming, normal skin color returns. The discoloration occurs symmetrically over the trunk and extremities in infants. In neonates the condition usually abates by 6 months, but it may persist longer in fair-skinned individuals. When cutis marmorata is fixed, asymmetrical, and does not fade with warming, the clinician should consider the diagnosis, cutis marmorata telangiectatica congenita, which is a type of vascular malformation present at birth that can be accompanied by atrophy and other systemic findings when it is extensive.

Cyanosis

Cyanosis is a bluish color of skin and mucous membrane due to presence of reduced hemoglobin in blood: Cyanosis is clinically apparent when approximately 5 g desaturated hemoglobin is present per deciliter of blood. Minimum cyanosis appears as a dusky hue when PO_2 is in between the range of 80–85, and it is easily visible when PO, is below 80%.

There are two physiological types of cyanosis—central and peripheral cyanosis. The difference between the two are described in **Table 1**.

ACROCYANOSIS

It is a clinical manifestation characterized by blue lower extremities and pink upper extremities. For demonstration of differential cyanosis, the patient is asked to sit and keep prewarmed hands on the dorsum of feet. Then a comparison of color is made between the two. This clinical sign is typically seen with right to left shunting across a ductus arteriosus in the presence of a coarctation or interrupted aortic arch.

CAUSES OF CENTRAL CYANOSIS

- *Cardiac causes:*
  - Fallot's tetralogy
  - Pulmonary atresia
  - Transposition of great arteries
  - Pulmonary A-V malformation
  - Congestive cardiac failure (CCF)
  - Atrial septal defect (ASD)/ventricular septal defect (VSD)/patent ductus arteriosus (PDA) with reversal of shunt (Eisenmenger's physiology)
- *Pulmonary causes:*
  - Severe pneumonia
  - Bronchopneumonia
  - Collapse of lung

CAUSES OF PERIPHERAL CYANOSIS

- Shock
- Local vasoconstriction
- Polycythemia

TABLE 1: Characteristic difference between central and peripheral cyanosis.

Characteristics	*Central*	*Peripheral*
1. Visible in	Warm areas (lips and tongue) Skin (nose, conjunctivae and skin)	Skin (nose, cheek, and fingers)
2. Cause	Venous admixture and defective ventilation perfusion	Vasoconstriction and low cardiac output diffusion
3. Pathophysiology	Diminished arterial O_2 saturation	Increased arteriovenous O_2
4. Deoxygenated hemoglobin	Increased	Normal
5. Clubbing of finger	Present	Absent
6. Relief	O_2 useful in cyanosis of pulmonary	Warmth and cardiovascular system (CVS) support

Cystic Hygroma

It is the lymphatic malformation of the floor of the mouth and neck. These lesions may cause significant macroglossia that obstructs the airway requiring tracheostomy. Large neck lesions can cause airway compromise. Imaging is important in defining the extent and nature of the lesion, and in guiding the treatment of the malformation. Lesions that are composed of large cysts (macrocystic) respond better to drainage and sclerosis than lesions made up of tiny cysts (microcystic). The microcystic often acts as solid mass and makes treatment especially challenging. The goals of treatment are to preserve function and cosmesis as much as possible. A combination of drainage, sclerosis, and surgical excision is often necessary in a multispecialty team.

CHAPTER 114 Dandy–Walker Malformation

The Dandy–Walker malformation is a primary developmental abnormality characterized by progressive cystic enlargement of the fourth ventricle beginning early in fetal life. This is accompanied by enlargement of the posterior fossa and upward displacement of the tentorium, torcula, and transverse sinuses. Associated hydrocephalus is almost universal and may be present at birth or may develop later, during infancy or childhood. Of affected individuals, 60% show signs of hydrocephalus and increased intracranial pressure by 2 years old.

Clinical manifestations of Dandy–Walker malformation are variable and depend on the severity and rate of progression of the associated hydrocephalus. A child with a symptomatic condition often has an unusually prominent bulging occiput in addition to the usual findings of hydrocephalus. In children younger than 1 year old, transillumination of the skull effectively demonstrates the posterior fossa cyst. Ataxia, nystagmus, and cranial nerve deficits may also be prominent features.

Plain skull radiographs demonstrate posteroinferior enlargement of the cranial vault, thinning and ballooning of the occipital squama, and upward displacement of the torcula. CT or MRI scans confirm the presence of a large posterior fossa cyst, a small cerebellar remnant, and associated hydrocephalus.

Deafness

TUNING FORK

A 512-Hz tuning fork is used. Basically in these tests, air conduction (AC) and bone conduction (BC) are assessed.

Rinne Test

First keep the vibrating tuning fork on the mastoid process (bone conduction) and ask the child to inform you when he stops hearing the sound. Then, move it besides the ear for air conduction, and is impaired ask him if he can still hear it. It should still be audible.

- Normally, air conduction is better than bone conduction—Rinne positive.
- In conduction hearing loss, bone conduction is better than air conduction and is impaired while retaining their normal relationship of air conduction better than bone conduction—Rinne positive.

Weber Test

The base of the vibratory tuning fork is placed over center of the forehead. The child is asked to indicate the side the tone is heard louder.

Normally, the tone is heard equally on both sides. In patients with unilateral sensorineural deafness, the tone is better heard, i.e., the lateralized to normal ear (positive). In patients with unilateral conductive deafness, the tone is heard louder as diseased side lateralized to affected ear (negative).

Absolute Bone Conduction Test

In infants, startle response is assessed. The response may be blinking of the eyes, sudden change in bodily movements, turning of the head toward the sound. The sound stimulus should not be visible to the infant.

In infants, lack of response to sound may be due to general developmental retardation. If the hearing problem is suspected, it should be examined to clarify between middle ear disease and nerve deafness. Normally, air conduction is better than bone conduction. In middle ear disease, bone conduction is unaffected, air conduction is diminished. In nerve deafness, both are affected. This can be evaluated clinically by tuning fork of 256 Hz.

Caloric Testing for Vestibular Function

The patient is made to lie with the head tilted at 30°. This is to bring the lateral semicircular canal in the vertical plane. The patient is asked to gaze at a fixed point.

The external ear canal is irrigated with the water at 30°C and 44°C for 30–40 seconds. This causes thermal gradient across the bone.

Cold water produces nystagmus away from the ear being irrigated and warm water induces nystagmus toward the ear being irrigated.

Each ear is irrigated with water at both temperatures with suitable gap between each test. There should be suitable time gap between induced nystagmus. The evoked nystagmus is analyzed using electronystagmography.

In patient with nonfunctioning vestibular apparatus, i.e., in canal paresis, there will not be any response to caloric stimulus on that side.

In pontine lesion, there is asymmetric response in two eyes. Here, the disease involves medial longitudinal fasciculus or lesions of extraocular nerves.

In bilateral cerebral disease, both the eyes are tonically deviated to the side of the cold water irrigated.

CAUSES OF ACQUIRED DEAFNESS

- Extreme prematurity
- Hypoxic-ischemic disease of newborn
- Neonatal jaundice
- Recurrent otitis media
- Glue ear
- Severe adenoids
- Trauma
- *Drugs:*
    - Aminophylline
    - Furosemide

CAUSES OF CONGENITAL DEAFNESS

- Familial
- Mental retardation
- Cerebral palsy
- Down syndrome
- Hypothyroidism
- Albinism
- Cleft palate
- Osteogenesis imperfecta
- *Maternal disease:*
    - Rubella
    - Syphilis
    - Chickenpox
- *Maternal drugs:*
    - Aminoglycoside
    - Quinine

CHAPTER 116

Decerebrate Rigidity

It is also known as extensor posturing, describing involuntary extensor positioning of the arms, flexion of the hands, with knee extension and plantar flexion when stimulated as a result of a midbrain lesion.

All limbs are extended, arms pronated, fists closed, and feet plantar flexed. Lesion is in brainstem at midbrain at the level of superior colliculus.

Decorticate Rigidity

It is seen lesion at intercollicular level and at the level of basal nuclei and cortex. Disinhibition of red nucleus results in facilitation of rubrospinal tract. There is disruption of lateral cortical tract. There is flexion posture of upper limb and extension of lower limb. Arms are flexed and bent inward over the chest. Elbows, wrists, and fingers are flexed. Hands clinched in the wrist. Legs are extended and feet are turned inward.

CHAPTER 118

Defibrillation

It is a treatment for life-threatening cardiac dysrhythmias specifically ventricular fibrillation and nonperfusing ventricular tachycardia. A defibrillator delivers a dose of transthoracic electric current to the heart, often called as counter shock. Defibrillators can also restore hearts beating if the heart suddenly stops.

Most defibrillators are attached to adult paddles, i.e., 13-cm diameter. Paddles of 4.5 cm diameter are suitable for use in infants. Paddles of 8-cm diameter should be used for small children. The usual placement is anterolateral. One paddle is put over the apex in the midaxillary line and other is placed just to the right of the sternum immediately below the clavicle. If the anteroposterior placement is used, one paddle is placed just to the left side of the lower part of the sternum and other just below the tip of the left scapula. Gel pads or electrode gel is used for good contact.

Delayed Puberty

Delayed puberty is the failure of development of any pubertal feature by 13 years of age in females or by 14 years of age in males. A lower cutoff may be appropriate in a child with a strong familial pattern of early puberty.

SEXUAL MATURITY RATING

Introduction: The Tanner staging is widely used for assessing sexual maturity rating (SMR). Five stages are described separately for boys and girls in different secondary sexual characters **(Box 1 and Table 1)**. Pubic hair and breast development for girls and pubic hair, penis, and testis development for boys.

CONSTITUTIONAL DELAYED PUBERTY

In the classic case, the affected child had a normal length at birth, a slowdown in height velocity between 6 months and 2 years of age that resulted in short stature, and a normal or near-normal height velocity thereafter along the child's current height percentile.

BOX 1: Sexual maturity rating (SMR) in girls.

SMR public hair:
- Preadolescent
- Sparse, lightly pigmented, straight, medial border of labia
- Darker, beginning to curl, increased amount
- Coarse, curly, abundant but less amount than adult
- Adult feminine triangle, spread to medial surface of thighs

SMR breast:
- Preadolescent
- Breast and papilla elevated as small mound, areolar diameter increased
- Breast and areola enlarged, no contour separation
- Areola and papilla form secondary mound
- Mature; nipple projects, areola part of general breast contour

TABLE 1: Sexual maturity rating (SMR) in boys.

SMR public hair	***Penis***	***Testes***
• None • Scanty, long slightly pigmented • Darker, starts to curl, small amount • Resemble adult, the amount less; larger, glans and breadth; larger, scrotum dark coarse, curly • Adult distribution spreads to medial surface of thighs	• (Preadolescent) • Slight enlargement • Longer • Larger, glans and breadth • Increase in size • Adult size	• (Preadolescent) • Enlarged scrotum, pink, texture altered • Larger • Larger, scrotum dark • Adult size

The physical examination findings are unremarkable, and, depending on the age, the child may have delayed puberty. The cardinal diagnostic result is a bone age that is moderately delayed in comparison with chronologic age. There may also be a history of delayed dentition.

CAUSES OF DELAYED PUBERTY

- *Central:*
  - Physiological delay
  - Hypothalamic and pituitary (Kallmann syndrome):
    - Developmental
    - Destructive:
      - Surgical
      - Radiotherapy
      - Tumor
    - *Drugs:* Cyproterone acetate, leukotropin-releasing hormone agonist
- *Gonadal:*
  - *Developmental:*
    - "Vanishing testes" caused by antenatal testicular torsion
    - Anatomical abnormalities of female genital tract
  - *Chromosomal:*
    - XXY—Klinefelter syndrome
    - XO—Turner syndrome
  - *Immunologic:*
    - Autoimmune endocrinopathy
  - *Destructive*:
    - Surgical removal gonads
    - Radiation/chemotherapy

GONADAL ABNORMALITIES

Hypogonadotropic Hypogonadism

A variety of central nervous system insults may disrupt production of gonadotropins. The gonadotropin-releasing hormone (GnRH) pulse generator may be disrupted by an interfering substance, such as excess prolactin (with or without hypothyroidism), or by stress, chronic illness, malnutrition, or excessive physical activity. The hypothalamic arcuate nucleus may be damaged by trauma, radiation, infection, infiltration, increased intracranial pressure, or surgery. The most common mass lesions are craniopharyngiomas, gliomas, and cysts. Congenital conditions or malformations may have allowed enough GnRH for infantile development but not enough for pubertal needs.

Hypergonadotropic Hypogonadism: Males

If the testes are small, they may have been damaged by torsion, sickle cell disease, infection, autoimmune disease, chemotherapy, or radiation and may not be able to respond to luteinizing hormone (LH) and follicle-stimulating hormone (FSH) stimulation. If the bone age is greater than 10 years and the hypothalamus has probably matured, the serum LH and FSH may then be high.

Klinefelter syndrome: This occurs in 1:500 males and is often associated with a 47,XXY karyotype; common features include reduced intelligence, adolescent gynecomastia (often pronounced), and small, firm testes. The testes rarely exceed 5 mL in volume (approximately 25% of the average adult volume). Patients, often tall and thin with an eunuchoid habitus, may have delayed puberty. Virilization may be incomplete, the phallus is often smaller than average, and infertility nears 100%.

Hypergonadotropic Hypogonadism: Females

In this condition, the ovary may be unable to synthesize estrogen (an inherited metabolic defect, possibly associated with excess adrenal mineralocorticoid and hypertension), the ovary may not be formed normally (dysgenesis), or the ovary may have been damaged by any of the factors listed for testicular damage and by galactosemia.

Turner syndrome: The two most common features of Turner syndrome are short stature (involving the limbs to a greater degree than the trunk) and ovarian insufficiency **(Figs. 1A and B)**. Lymph edema and a webbed neck are diagnostic features present in a neonate. Additional features include a shield chest, increased carrying angle (cubitus valgus), short 4th metacarpal, hypoplastic nails, renal anomalies, and left-sided heart defects (coarctation of the aorta, bicuspid mitral valve, etc.).

Kallmann syndrome: This is the combination of an impaired or absent sense of smell and gonadotropin deficiency. Other features include color blindness, atrial septal defects, and renal structural anomalies (unilateral renal agenesis). The X-linked form is caused by a mutation of the *KAL* gene; there are autosomal recessive and autosomal dominant forms.

Females with Delayed or Absent Adrenarche

If a female has advanced breast development but no androgen signs, she may have a deficiency of androgen receptors, as occurs in androgen insensitivity syndrome (testicular feminization). In females, the androgens come predominantly from the adrenal glands (adrenarche).

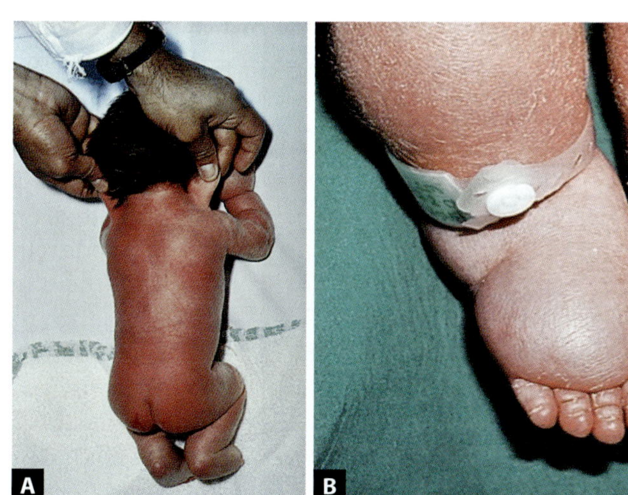

Figs. 1A and B: Turner syndrome.

CHAPTER 120

Dennie Sign

Ocular manifestations of allergic manifestation include cobblestoning of the conjunctiva, the allergic shiner, and Dennie sign. Dennie sign refers to prominent folds or creases on the lower eyelid running parallel to the margin. Although these lines were originally thought to indicate a predisposition to allergy, data suggest that they may be present in any conditions associated with periocular pruritus and scratching of any nasal congestion.

121 CHAPTER

Depressed Nasal Bridge

A low nasal bridge is when the bridge of the nose is flatter or lower than usual. It can be caused by genetic condition, an accident, or an infection. It can cause chronic sinus problem. The underlying causes are present at birth and are diagnosed at or shortly after birth.

Flat nasal bridge is seen among Carpenter syndrome, Williams syndrome. Depressed nasal bridge is seen among thalassemia **(Fig. 1)**, Down syndrome, ectodermal dysplasia, Hurlers syndrome, hypothyroidism, and congenital syphilis.

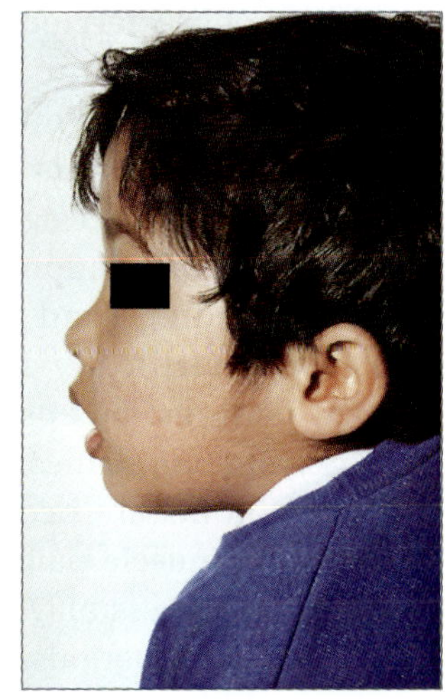

Fig. 1: Thalassemia.

122 CHAPTER

Dermatomyositis

Dermatomyositis is characterized by perivascular inflammation in muscles and skin, occasionally with gut and other organ involvement. Dermatomyositis is more common in girls and the average age at onset is 8 years. The main manifestations include characteristic skin findings and proximal muscle weakness, specifically involving the neck flexors, deltoids, biceps, triceps, quadriceps, psoas, and hamstrings **(Figs. 1A and B)**. These symptoms are occasionally accompanied by mild muscle pain, fatigue, or poor endurance. Weakness may be subtle and not recognized for long periods. Frequent early symptoms include difficulties rising from the floor, climbing stairs, climbing in and out of a minivan, and combing the hair.

Skin manifestations include Gottron papules, which are scaly, erythematous plaques or papules that appear over the metacarpophalangeal (MCP) and proximal interphalangeal (PIP) joints on the hands. Similar lesions are seen on the extensor surfaces of the elbows and knees and over the medial malleoli. The distribution of the rash, which may be misdiagnosed as eczema or psoriasis, is an early clue to the diagnosis. The periungual capillaries may become grossly dilated and may develop thromboses that can be visualized either with the naked eye or with mild magnification. Heliotrope rash is a violaceous discoloration of the upper eyelids that is often accompanied by mild edema and is pathognomonic for dermatomyositis.

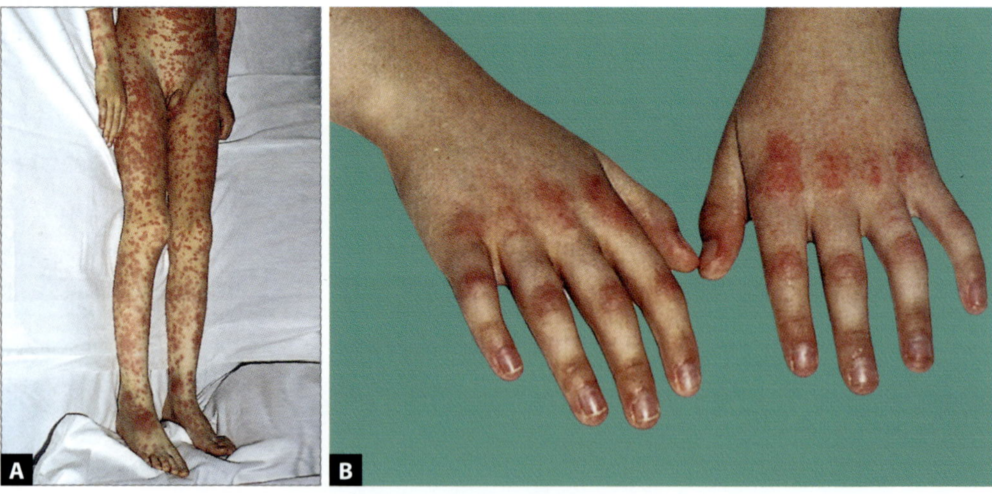

Figs. 1A and B: Dermatomyositis.

Some children develop more extensive erythroderma that may appear over the shoulders, termed the shawl sign, or in a V-neck distribution on the chest. With severe disease, some patients may also develop vasculopathic skin ulcerations.

The diagnosis is suggested by the rash and proximal muscle weakness detected on physical examination. Muscle enzymes are elevated in most, but not all, children with dermatomyositis. There may be elevations in only one or a few enzymes and, therefore, testing for aspartate aminotransferase, alanine aminotransferase, lactate dehydrogenase, creatine kinase, and aldolase should be performed. The child with a characteristic rash, definite proximal muscle weakness, and elevated muscle enzyme levels may not require additional testing for diagnosis. If weakness is questionable, or if the rash is not characteristic, an EMG can confirm the presence of muscle inflammation.

CHAPTER 123

Diaper Dermatitis

It occurs over the groin and upper thigh. The eruption is sharply marginated, usually bilaterally symmetrical involves intertriginous fold and occasionally the perianal regions and buttocks. The margins are abrupt, erythematous and scaly, red to brown in color, and central clearing with an active border.

Previous exposure to substance concerned with 48–96 hours between contact and the development of cutaneous changes. Activation of previously sensitized skin by contact with the same allergen elsewhere on the body. Persistent of the allergy for many years. Allergic dermatitis tends to produce erythema, edema, and vesicles in acute allergic reaction. The lesions are lichenified in more chronic form.

Irritant contact dermatitis: It is caused by wide varieties of substances with no predictable time in interval between contact and appearance of the rash. Dermatitis occurs soon after exposure and the severity varies with quantity, concentration, and length of exposure to substance concerned. Previous sensitization is not necessary. It presents as slightly scaling, itching, or extensive epidermal damage resembling a superficial burn with inflammation.

- Friction dermatitis occurs where the friction is more pronounced (the inner surface of the thigh, genitalia, buttocks, and abdomen).

  It consists of shiny glazed surface and occasional papules with mild erythema.
- Irritant (contact) dermatitis usually confined to convex surface of the buttocks perineal area, lower abdomen, and proximal thigh sparing intertriginous creases.
- Allergic dermatitis frequently localized to convex areas and the skin is diffusely redden with papules, vesicles, edema, and scaling. The lesions may be shiny, wrinkled, and parchment paper like during resolution stage.
- Intertrigo is a common type of skin eruption in the diaper area with well demarcated lesions associated with maceration and oozing, generally involving inguinal region, the intergluteal area, and the fleshy folding of the thigh.

Diarrhea

The term diarrhea refers to the passage of three or more loose stools per day. Diarrhea is a symptom and it is preferable to consider diarrhea if there is increased frequency, volume, and fluidity. Diarrhea is also a sign when the loss of water is >15 g/kg/day in children <3 years of age and >200 g/kg/day in children >3 years of age.

ACUTE DIARRHEA

The term acute diarrhea refers to a condition where the child passes loose stools lasting for 3–7 days.

INTERMEDIATE DIARRHEA

The term intermediate diarrhea includes children with acute onset of diarrhea lasting for 8–14 days.

DYSENTERY

It is the term used for diarrhea with visible blood and mucus, often associated with fever and tenesmus.

Diarrheal disease is an important problem of children <5 years of age, and in this age group, the primary target is children between 6 months and 2 years of age. As the child grows older, the incidence decreases.

Breastfeeding has a definite impact on the occurrence of diarrheal diseases. Infants who are breastfed have a lower incidence of infective diarrhea. The protective factors in breast milk prevent diarrhea. The early introduction of cow's milk and commercial formulae increase the incidence of diarrhea.

The early introduction of weaning foods will not only be a source of infection but also result in macromolecular absorption of allergens and predispose to the onset and perpetuation of diarrhea. This is more evident if breast milk is discontinued at the time of weaning. Exclusive breastfeeding is, therefore, recommended till the age of 6 months.

The incidence of diarrhea is more in bottle-fed infants than in breastfed infants. When top milk is essential, the child should be given teaspoon feeding or "paladai" feeding. This form of feeding is much superior to bottle feeding as the utensils can be cleansed properly.

Diarrhea and malnutrition form a vicious cycle and the nutritional status may worsen after an episode of diarrhea. Malnutrition is also a precipitating factor in predisposing to persistent diarrhea.

The presence of associated infections such as urinary tract infections, acute suppurative otitis media, bronchopneumonia, and sepsis in a child with acute diarrhea is well recognized precipitating factor for progression to persistent diarrhea if not treated promptly.

There are certain factors which are peculiar to children and infants which can aggravate the effects of diarrhea. They are:

- The greater body content of water in infants
- The larger turnover of water in the infant as compared to adults
- The greater insensible loss of water, since the surface area is two to three times that of an adult
- The greater metabolic requirements
- The immaturity of the kidney in handling solutes and the poor concentrating capacity
- The inability of the infant to quench his thirst by drinking water

TYPES OF ACUTE DIARRHEA

Acute diarrhea can present as:

- Acute watery diarrhea
- Acute dysentery

The term "parenteral diarrhea" refers to a clinical state in many children who present with diarrhea where the primary disease may be outside the gastrointestinal tract, e.g., otitis media, respiratory or urinary tract infection.

PATHOPHYSIOLOGY

Malabsorption Diarrhea

There is decrease in absorptive surface area, intestinal resection (short bowel syndrome) or with intestinal villous atrophy are the causes of malabsorption diarrhea. This is seen in celiac disease.

Secretory Diarrhea

Bacterial toxins, gut regulatory peptides, short-chain fatty acids, and bile salts cause secretary diarrhea. These induce intestinal water secretion. Secretory diarrhea does not alter with eating and the osmolality of the stool can be accounted for by normal ionic constituents. Therefore, doubling the sum of sodium and potassium concentrations in stool should equal the fecal osmolality.

Intestinal Pathogens Causing Diarrhea and/or Vomiting

- *Viruses:* Rotavirus, adenovirus, and others
- *Bacteria: Escherichia coli, Shigella, Salmonella, Campylobacter jejuni, Yersinia enterocolitica, Aeromonas*, and others
- *Parasites: Entamoeba histolytica, Giardia lamblia*, and *Cryptosporidium*

Protozoal Diarrhea

Illnesses due to intestinal protozoa tend to be more prolonged, sometimes for 2 week or more, but usually self-limited in the otherwise healthy host. In general, the duration and severity of *Cryptosporidium* diarrhea is strongly influenced by the immune and nutritional status of the host. A protozoal etiology should be suspected when there is a prolonged diarrheal illness characterized by episodes of sometimes explosive diarrhea with nausea, abdominal cramps, and abdominal bloating.

CHAPTER 125 Diastasis Recti

Diastasis recti is not a pathological entity. The broad angles of the subcostal margins in infants are such that the rectus muscles in infants can be widely separated in the upper abdomen, creating linea that can be relatively thin, allowing a ventral ovoid bulge between the umbilicus and xiphisternum with straining. This bulge is of no clinical significance; in time, with growth, gradual approximation of the rectus muscles occurs and it disappears.

Diastasis of the rectus muscle may be noted as a protrusion in the midline, usually from the xiphoid to the umbilicus but occasionally down to the symphysis pubis. Ordinarily, the protrusion is ½–2 inches size; it is usually common normal variant but may be caused by a congenital weakness of the musculature in a chronically distended abdomen. Diastasis of rectus abdominis ordinarily resolves by 6 years of age.

CHAPTER 126

Diastrophic Dysplasia

It is one of the skeletal dysplasias inherited in an autosomal recessive manner. It results from the mutation in the diastrophic dysplasia sulfate transporter gene (DTDST) located on the chromosome 5. The mutation results in deficient uptake of sulfur by chondrocytes, resulting in abnormal cartilage. It is characterized by short limb dwarfism, severs joint deformities, kyphoscoliosis, clubbed feet, an adducted thumb, and characteristic malformed pinnae of the ears.

CHAPTER 127

Diplopia

Ocular muscle weakness produces diplopia. Here, light will fall on retina of both the eyes.

False image is pallor and less distinct. Images are separated and is more in the direction in which weakness has its poorest action. Weak muscle will displace the false image furthest. Displacement of the false image may be horizontal, vertical, or both.

METHOD OF EXAMINATION

Cover one of the patient's eye with a transparent red shield. A point of light is used to move the object to right and left horizontally, upward and downward in the midline, and vertically when the eyes are deviated to one side. In each position, ask the child:

- Whether he sees one object or two.
- If double, do the two images lie side by side, or one above the other.
- In which position are they farthest apart.
- Which is the red image.

Interpretation of Results

If the images are exactly side by side, it will be only the external or internal recti that are involved. If they are one above the other, either of the obliques, or the superior and inferior recti, may be defective.

CHAPTER 128

Dysmorphology

Anatomical defect that is present at birth is called as congenital malformation. Malformation is a morphological defect of an organ, part of an organ resulting in abnormal development.

A *disruption* is a morphological defect of an organ, part of an organ, or a larger region of the body resulting from the extrinsic breakdown of or an interference with an originally normal development process, e.g., amniotic band syndrome.

A *deformation* is an abnormal form, shape, or position of a part of the body caused by mechanical forces. These forces may be extrinsic (as a result of intrauterine constraint) or intrinsic (fetal hypomobility caused by nervous system defect).

A *dysplasia* is an abnormal organization of cells into tissue and its morphological structure. It is a process and consequence of dishistogenesis.

A *polytopic* defect is pattern of anomalies derived from the disturbances of a single developmental field.

A *sequence* is a pattern of multiple anomalies derived from single known or presumed prior anomaly or mechanical factor. A malformation, a disruption, or a mechanical factor may rise to a cascade of secondary problems in subsequent morphogenesis.

An *association* is nonrandom occurrence in two or more individuals of multiple anomalies not known to be a polytopic field defect, sequence, or syndrome.

CHAPTER 129

Dysphagia

Dysphagia is a symptom that describes difficulty swallowing. Patients with dysphagia report the feeling of the inability to pass esophageal contents into the stomach. When the sensation is in the posterior pharynx or upper esophagus, it can be considered a globus sensation. When it is present, one must consider esophageal inflammation or a primary dysmotility disorder. More common pediatric disorders associated with dysphagia or the globus sensation include reflux esophagitis with or without stricture, achalasia, eosinophilic esophagitis, and esophageal strictures.

Eosinophilic esophagitis is an inflammatory disorder of the esophagus that is a common cause of dysphagia in children. The etiology of eosinophilic esophagitis is not known, although it is generally thought to be the result of an aberrant antigenic immunologic response. Although food antigens are most often suspected, any environmental antigen that traverses the esophagus can lead to its presentation. Similar to other atopic diseases, it is believed that the incidence of eosinophilic esophagitis is increasing. Symptoms include dysphagia, feeding refusal, epigastric abdominal pain, early satiety, and even food impaction. Symptoms of reflux or esophagitis can complicate the diagnosis.

130 CHAPTER

Dysuria

Dysuria is defined as painful urination and can be related to uncomfortable contraction of the muscles of the bladder or when urine comes into contact with the inflamed genitourinary mucosa. The cause of dysuria varies based on age of the child or adolescent; therefore, specific elements of the patient history, potential causes, and diagnostic evaluation will vary with age.

Urethritis caused by herpes simplex virus may occur in both males and females of this age group from autoinoculation from herpes stomatitis; however, presence of genital ulcers should always elicit questioning about sexual activity and/or assault.

Other etiologic factors that may lead to urethritis and resultant dysuria include infection (fungi, pinworms, and scabies), irritation (soap, shampoo, detergent, and bubble bath), systemic illness (Stevens-Johnson syndrome), and trauma (abuse, play, tight clothing, and masturbation).

Urinary tract infections (UTIs) are much more common in adolescent females than adolescent males. Risk factors for recurrent UTIs in females include frequency of sexual intercourse (higher frequency leads to higher risk), maternal history of recurrent UTI, a new sexual partner in the past year, and spermicide use in the past year. Common pathogens in this age group include *Escherichia coli*, *Proteus* species, *Klebsiella* species, *Staphylococcus saprophyticus*, and enterococcus. Although often recommended by clinicians, no evidence supports the thought that postcoital urination leads to a reduction in the frequency of UTIs.

One of the most common causes of dysuria in adolescent males and females is sexually transmitted infections (STIs). Adolescents represent an age group at high risk for acquisition and transmission of STIs. Although many STIs are asymptomatic and are diagnosed by screening asymptomatic sexually active individuals, STIs can present with dysuria, vaginal discharge, penile discharge, and genital lesions. The most likely time for this to happen is within 1 month of beginning a relationship with a new sexual partner.

Chlamydial genital infection is the most frequently reported bacterial STI. Infections with *Chlamydia trachomatis* may be asymptomatic or may present with dysuria, discharge, intermenstrual bleeding, or dyspareunia.

Gonorrhea, caused by *Neisseria gonorrhoeae*, is the second most frequently reported bacterial STI. Infections with *N. gonorrhoeae* may be asymptomatic or may present with dysuria, discharge, intermenstrual bleeding, or dyspareunia. *N. gonorrhoeae* infection may lead to pelvic inflammatory disease (PID); late complications include ectopic pregnancy and infertility. *N. gonorrhoeae* urogenital infection can be detected in women by testing urine or collecting swab specimens from the endocervix or vagina; in men, the diagnosis can be made through urine or urethral swab.

Vaginitis due to various causes can cause dysuria in adolescent females. Vulvovaginal candidiasis, bacterial vaginosis, and trichomoniasis are common causes of vulvovaginitis in adolescents. Other causes are local chemical or allergic irritants, bacterial infections caused by *Streptococcus* or *Staphylococcus* species, trauma, and secondary infections from foreign bodies.

Phimosis is a narrowing of the preputial opening and manifests as failure to retract the foreskin. Paraphimosis is an incarceration of the prepuce behind the glans. Balanitis is an infection of the prepuce.

Dystonia

These are prolonged slow alternating contraction and relaxation of agonists and antagonists. This frequently occurs in proximal joints. This causes abnormal posturing of limbs. This includes twisting for a prolonged period of time. This may affect one or more parts of the body and sometimes the entire body. This condition can be mild or severe.

Some causes of acquired dystonia include birth injury (hypoxia—a lack of oxygen to the brain, and neonatal brain damage) and infections.

The causes include benign dystonia of infancy, cerebral palsy, ataxia-telangiectasia, encephalitis, medications, metabolic disorders, and perinatal asphyxia. Dystonias can be divided into three groups—idiopathic, genetic, and acquired. Idiopathic refers to dystonia that does not have any cause. Many are idiopathic.

Genetic forms of dystonia include:

- DYT1 dystonia is caused by a mutation in the *DYT1* gene. It begins in childhood, and progresses causing significant disability. Because the gene's effects are so variable, some people who carry a mutation may not develop dystonia.
- Dopa-responsive dystonia, also known as Segawa's disease. Onset is during childhood and has progressive difficulty with walking. Symptoms characteristically fluctuate and are worse late in the day and after exercise. Some are due to mutations in the *DYT5* gene.

Acquired dystonia results from damage to the brain by the medication, heavy metal and carbon monoxide poisoning, trauma, or stroke. Acquired dystonia does not spread to the other parts of the body.

Earache

Earache (otalgia) is pain that arises from a pathologic process in the external, middle, or inner ear or that is referred to the ear from another structure. Acute otitis media (AOM) is the most common cause of otalgia in children.

Examination of an infant's ears is a two-person procedure. The infant's head must be immobilized and his or her hands kept out of the ways. Many new parents are reluctant to restrain their baby. Explain carefully that appropriate positioning and restraint actually reduces discomfort and facilitates a shorter and more accurate examination. A variety of effective positions and techniques may be used. At each encounter, you will need to choose a combination of techniques to match the child's age, variation of mood, level of anxiety, and ability to cooperate.

It often is easier to examine infants placed supine on a table with the parent or your assistant holding the arms at the sides and immobilizing both the arms and the body. The examiner then uses one hand to hold the infant head against the table and the other to hold the otoscope. If the examiner needs both hands to manipulate the external ear for successful completion of the examination (or to remove wax), a second person must immobilize the baby's head. Many older infants and young children can be held by the parent against their shoulder or chest with one hand while holding the head steady with the order hand.

Earache is a common presentation enquire about:

- *Site:*
  - Deep in the ear
  - Pain felt on moving/touching pinna suggest otitis externa
  - Over the jaw point
- *Onset:* Should be linked if possible to any known causative factors

RECENT UPPER RESPIRATORY TRACT INFECTION—INDICATING MIDDLE EAR DISEASE

The otoscope is held with the right hand, using the left thumb and forefinger to grasp apply traction away from the head and slightly posteriorly. This position straightens the normally curved external auditory canal, enabling you to see better. Depending on your level of manual dexterity, it also may be helpful to use the third finger of the left hand to gently push the tragus anteriorly, thereby opening the auditory canal further.

Inspect the external auditory meatus and gently place the tip of the otoscope there. Your head will be away from the otoscope as you are not yet looking thought it. Once the otoscope tip is in position at the meatus, move your head up close to the otoscope and look through it; gently aim at the otoscope to see the ear canal beyond. Your head should move with the otoscope as it is aimed in different directions.

Once the lumen is clearly visualized, gently advance the instrument. The external auditory canal is exquisitely sensitive even in the absence otitis externa or a furuncle. Observe carefully for the presence of a foreign body or signs of inflammation. You may be able to work around small amounts of wax. If your view is obstructed, the wax will have to be removed. Never rest the instrument's weight against the auditory canal or you may cause bleeding in addition to pain. The ability to guide the otoscope through the canal without touching the walls only comes with practice.

TYMPANIC MEMBRANE

Because you usually have only a few seconds in which to inspect the eardrum, you must know what you are looking for. The most easily recognized landmark is the long process (handle) of the malleus. The light source is reflected from the umbo as a narrowed cone starting at the center and expanding in an inferior-anterior direction. The normal tympanic membrane (TM) is most concave at the umbo. Changes in middle ear pressure result in alterations to the concavity of the membrane and the diffusion of the light cone. The TM is thinner in the anterosuperior quadrant, the pars flaccida, because of the absence of the fibrous membrane present in the pars tensa. Early signs of inflammation may be observed in the pars flaccida.

Color changes in the TM are notoriously unreliable. Particularly in infants, the vascular changes seen on the cheeks with fever or crying are also observed in the TMs. There is a real risk of over diagnosis of otitis media. It is essential to focus on the TM shape and landmarks; if they are normal, the infant does not have otitis media. Other causes of fever and crying then must be considered, especially serious bacterial infections such as pyelonephritis and meningitis.

DIAGNOSIS

Bacterial Cultures

In selected instances (e.g., persistent treatment failure, severe pain, an immunocompromised host, and a neonate), culture of otorrhea from the external auditory canal or cultures of middle ear fluid by tympanocentesis may guide therapy. In a child with AOM, the offending pathogen is usually present in the nasopharynx.

Tympanometry

Tympanometry is an objective, painless method for detecting the presence of middle ear effusion by providing information about TM compliance. A soft plastic probe is inserted into the external auditory canal in order to obtain an airtight seal. The tympanometer measures the flow of sound energy into the middle ear under conditions of changing air pressure. When the air pressure is equal on both sides of an intact eardrum, with the drum in neutral position, the transmission of sound energy through the TM is at its maximum. The peak on the tympanogram represents the pressure at which the flow of sound energy is maximal.

Acoustic Reflectometry

Acoustic reflectometers are used to detect middle ear effusion. The device directs sonar-like sound waves of varying frequency toward the TM and measures the intensity of reflected sound. Middle ear effusion is detected not by the frequency but by the magnitude of maximal reflected sound. When middle ear effusion is present, reflectance is increased in comparison with that in the air-filled middle ear.

CHAPTER 133 Ear Discharge

OTITIS EXTERNA

The external canal can become vulnerable to infection from excessive moisture from warm humid weather, moisture in the canal, or swimming. The moisture may cause small abrasions in the protective lipid layer of skin in the ear canal. These abrasions become infected on exposure to pathogenic bacteria. Dryness or presence of underlying skin conditions (such as eczema) and trauma (including cotton ear swabs) can also predispose the external canal to infection.

The presenting symptoms are often intense pain (especially with manipulation of the pinna, pressure on the tragus, or jaw movement), erythema, and otorrhea. On physical examination, the ear canal is red, edematous, and tender. Otorrhea may be present in the external canal.

Chondritis is a potential complication of severe otitis externa. It occurs when the infection progresses into the cartilaginous structures of the ear canal. This complication is rare without a history of previous trauma or surgery.

MALIGNANT OTITIS EXTERNA

Malignant otitis externa, also known as necrotizing otitis externa, is an extension of infection to the temporal bone and skull base causing extensive tissue destruction. The illness may result in chondritis and osteitis of both the middle and inner ears. Presenting symptoms include a markedly swollen and laterally displaced pinna associated with fever, malaise, and persistent, deep-seated otalgia out of proportion to findings on examination. Occasionally, facial nerve paralysis may be noted.

ACUTE OTITIS MEDIA

Acute otitis media is most commonly a bacterial complication of a preceding or concurrent viral upper respiratory tract infection (URTI), usually several days after the onset of URTI. The viral infection enables pathogenic bacteria in the nasopharynx to ascend through the eustachian tube into the middle ear either by impairing local host defenses or by eustachian tube dysfunction. The bacterial pathogens then cause a secondary infection.

RECURRENT ACUTE OTITIS MEDIA

Recurrent otitis media is defined as three episodes of AOM in a 6-month period or four episodes in a 12-month period with at least one episode in the preceding 6 months.

Risk factors for recurrent AOM include:

- Onset of AOM in the first year of life, especially if the first episode is before the patient is 6 months of age
- Male gender
- A sibling's history of recurrent AOM
- Cleft palate

- Craniofacial anomalies
- Trisomy 21
- Daycare attendance
- Household cigarette smoke exposure
- Human immunodeficiency virus infection
- Lack of breastfeeding
- History of atopy/allergies

Children with recurrent otitis media present a particular challenge with regard to treatment options. Long-term, low-dose antibacterial agents have been used as a method of prophylaxis in children with recurrent AOM in attempts to prevent additional episodes. While there is some evidence of decreased episodes of AOM, this only occurred while receiving the prophylactic antibacterial, without benefits after discontinuation of the antibacterial.

OTITIS MEDIA WITH EFFUSION

Otitis media with effusion, also known as "glue ear," may occur after an acute episode of otitis media or because of eustachian tube obstruction resulting from another cause [most commonly, upper respiratory tract infection (URTI)]. Otitis media with effusion (OME) differs from AOM in that there is middle ear effusion present without signs or symptoms of acute infection. The most common presenting complaint with OME is decreased hearing. A middle ear fluid can persist for weeks after AOM. 2 weeks after AOM, approximately 75% of children will have persistent effusion. If effusion persists for 3 months or longer or any time language delay, learning difficulties, or significant hearing loss is suspected, hearing testing should be performed.

Based on the guidelines, the following children are candidates for surgical intervention:

- Children with OME persisting for >4 months with associated persistent hearing loss
- At-risk children with persistent OME regardless of hearing status
- Children with structural damage to the middle ear or tympanic membrane secondary to OME

MASTOIDITIS

Mastoiditis is a potentially serious acute or chronic suppurative complication of otitis media. Life-threatening complications of mastoiditis are related to intracranial extension of the suppurative process. Mastoiditis begins with the development of hyperemia and edema of the mastoid process. This progresses to a suppurative process that may produce demineralization and necrosis of bone, abscess formation, and contiguous spread to intracranial or other head and neck areas. Mastoiditis with periosteitis indicates that the infection has spread to the periosteum of the mastoid process and manifests most commonly in children <2 years, although children of any age may be affected. Otalgia, posterior ear pain, fever, and otorrhea are frequent symptoms. Posterior auricular tenderness and erythema, anterior-inferior pinna protrusion, loss of the posterior auricular crease, middle ear effusion, a bulging or perforated tympanic membrane, and sagging of the posterior auditory canal wall are observable signs. Acute mastoid osteitis designates further spread of infection causing bony trabeculae destruction. Mastoiditis may result in transverse sinus thrombosis.

CHOLESTEATOMA

Cholesteatomas are cyst-like growths of the middle ear or mastoid formed by keratinizing squamous epithelial cells. They can be either congenital or acquired. Congenital cholesteatomas likely result from epithelial cells implanted during otologic development in utero. Acquired cholesteatomas are potential complications from chronic otitis media or secondary to a deep retraction pocket (or invagination) in the tympanic membrane. Cholesteatomas can cause bony resorption by expansion, often to the mastoid, but occasionally intracranially with potentially life-threatening consequences. This condition should be suspected in children with history of chronic OM, persistent otorrhea, and a tympanic membrane with a retraction pocket or perforation with white debris overlying the area.

The clinician must be aware of the following red flags associated with these conditions:

- Laterally displaced pinna (malignant otitis externa and mastoid osteitis)
- Mastoid tenderness (mastoid osteitis)
- Perforated tympanic membrane
- A pearl-like tumor in the tympanic membrane (cholesteatoma)
- Subacute headache, meningismus, and altered mental status (brain abscess, subdural or epidural empyema)

CHAPTER 134

Ectopia Lentis

Displacement of lens may be complete or partial, referred to as luxation or subluxation, respectively. The signs and symptoms include blurring, diplopia, anterior chamber may appear deeper, iridodonesis, edge of lens visible in pupillary aperture. Displacement may be seen in condition such as Marfan's syndrome and homocystinuria wherein the lens is displaced upward and laterally, downward and medially respectively. The other conditions are Weill-Marchesani syndrome and sulfite oxidase deficiency.

Edema, Dependent

CAUSES OF LOCALIZED EDEMA

- *In newborn:*
    - Caput succedaneum
    - Cephalhematoma
    - Milroy's disease
    - Abdominal edema—peritonitis, appendicitis, and necrotizing enterocolitis
- *In infancy and childhood* **(*Fig. 1*)**:
    - Angioneurotic edema
    - Boils
    - Dental abscess
    - Lymphangitis
    - Mumps

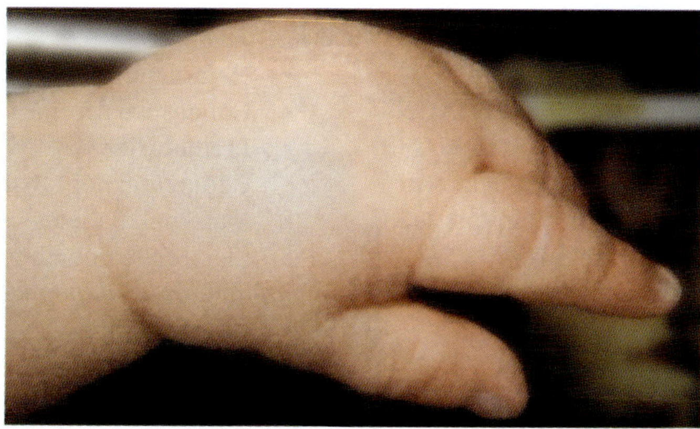

Fig. 1: Edema.

136 CHAPTER

Edema, Generalized

It is the presence of excess fluid in the interstitial space. Systemic disease will produce generalized edema. It usually occurs due to any one of these mechanisms.

- Reduced oncotic pressure
- Increase blood volume
- Increase capillary permeability

MECHANISM OF EDEMA IN VARIOUS CONDITIONS

- In angioneurotic edema—vasculitis.
- In acute glomerulonephritis (AGN)-decreased glomerular filtration rate (GFR) causes hypervolemia
- In nephrotic syndrome protein loss leads to decreased oncotic pressure
- Cardiac-increased systemic venous congestion.
- *Hepatic:*
  - Decreased protein synthesis
  - Lymphatic obstruction causes portal hypertension.

TYPE AND DISTRIBUTION OF EDEMA

- *Lip, tongue:* Angioneurotic edema
- *Waxy edema:* Nephrotic syndrome
- *Painful:* Cellulitis and venous thrombosis
- *Non pitting:* Cretin and Turner's syndrome

CAUSES OF GENERALIZED EDEMA

- *In newborn:*
  - Hemolytic anemia
  - Congestive cardiac failure
  - Prematurity
  - Congenital nephrosis
  - Maternal diabetes
  - Electrolyte imbalance
- *Infancy and childhood:*
  - Kwashiorkor
  - Nephrotic syndrome
  - Acute nephritis
  - Congestive cardiac failure
  - Indian childhood cirrhosis

137 CHAPTER Electrocardiogram

The electrocardiogram (ECG) is for the diagnosis of dysrhythmias and may offer the best clue to the specific diagnosis of congenital lesions (e.g., left axis deviation in a blue baby, suggesting tricuspid atresia).

INTERPRETATION

The sequence of recording the findings of the ECG **(Fig. 1)** is usually as follows:

- *Rate:* The paper speed at which ECGs are normally obtained is 25 mm/s. Each small square is 1 mm, and each large square, 5 mm. Therefore, five large squares represent 1 s, one large square 0.2 s, and one small square 0.04 s. A common method of estimating the ventricular rate is to count the number of small squares between two QRS complexes and to divide this number into 1,500. If QRS complexes appear at a rate of one per five small squares, the ventricular rate is 300; if QRS complexes appear every 12 small squares, the ventricular rate is 125, and so on.
- *Rhythm:* Sinus rhythm is always present in normal children. In contrast to adults, premature atrial and ventricular contractions are uncommon during childhood.
- *P wave:* In the pediatric patient, the P wave is normally not taller than 2.5 mm or more than 0.08 s in duration. The P wave is usually best seen in leads II and V_1.
- *PR interval:* This interval is measured from the beginning of the P wave to the beginning of the QRS complex. It increases with age and with slower rates. The PR interval ranges from a minimum of 0.11 s in infants to a maximum of 0.18 s in older children with slow rates. The PR interval is commonly prolonged in patients who have rheumatic heart disease and by digitalis.
- *QRS complex:* This represents ventricular depolarization, and its amplitude and direction of force (axis) reveal the relative size of (viable) ventricular mass in hypertrophy, hypoplasia, and infarction. Abnormal ventricular conduction (e.g., right bundle branch block, anterior fascicular block) is also revealed. Interpretation of the QRS complex is one of the most important aspects of cardiologic diagnosis.
- *QT interval:* This interval is measured from the beginning of the QRS complex to the end of the T wave. The QT duration is affected by drugs such as digitalis and electrolyte imbalances such as hypocalcemia and hypokalemia (really QU interval prolongation). The normal duration is rate-related and must be corrected using Bazett's formula:

$$QTc = \frac{\text{QT interval(s)}}{\sqrt{\text{R - R interval(s)}}}$$

The normal QTc is <0.44 s or <0.46 s in post-pubertal females.

- *ST segment:* This short segment lying between the end of the QRS complex and the beginning of the T wave is affected by drugs and electrolyte imbalances and reflects myocardial injury.
- *T wave:* The T wave represents myocardial repolarization and is altered by electrolytes, myocardial hypertrophy, and ischemia.

The placement of the lead electrodes on the chest are depicted in **Figure 2**.

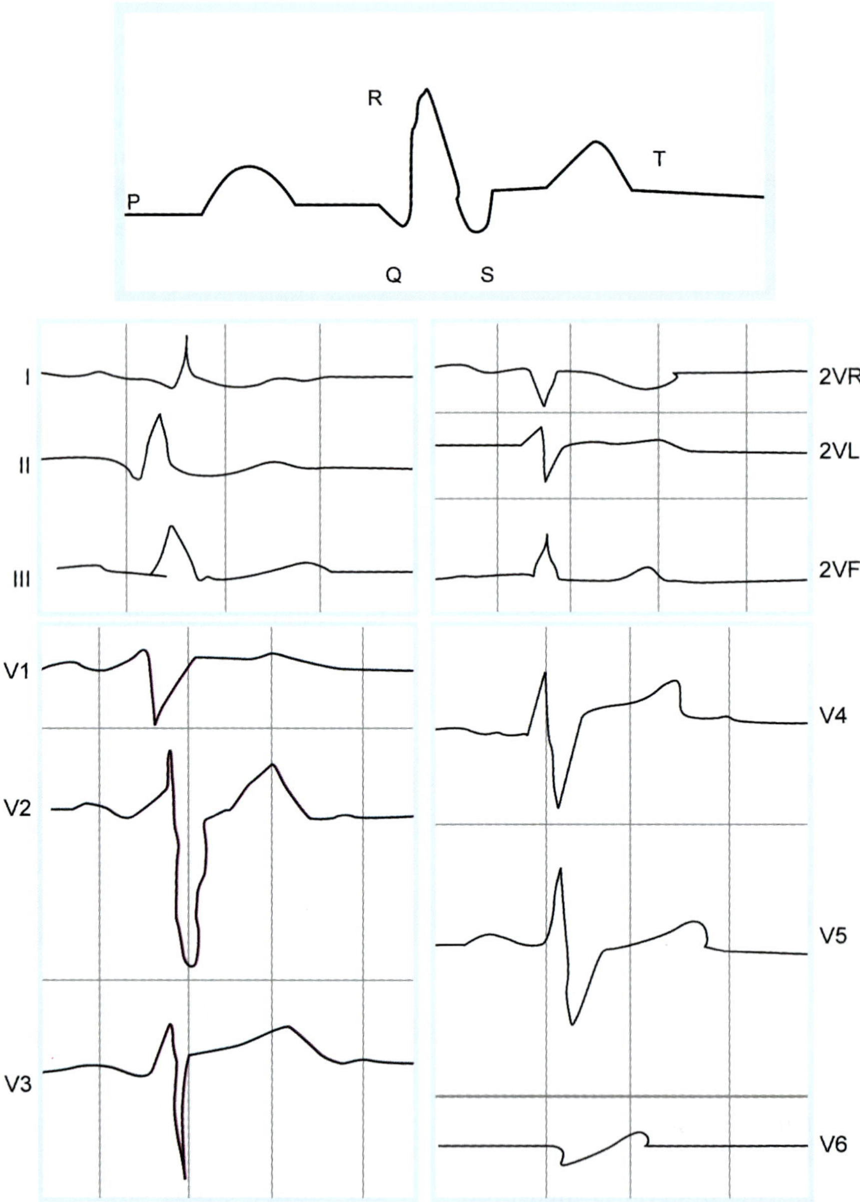

Fig. 1: Normal electrocardiography.

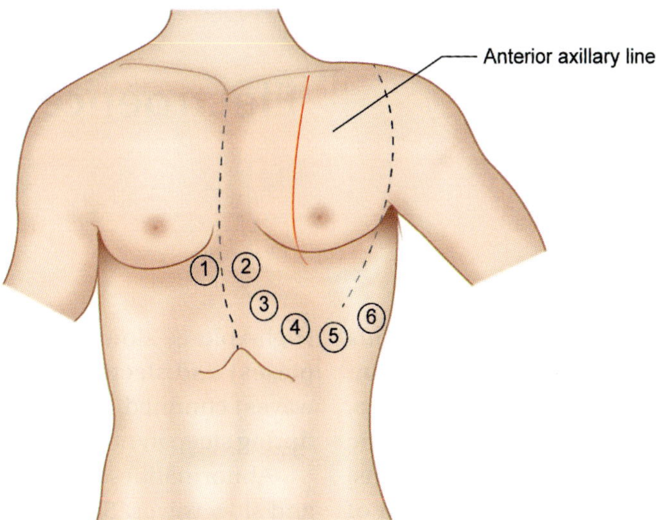

Fig. 2: Position of electrodes in the chest lead recordings.
V1: Right sternal edge in fourth intercostal space
V2: Left sternal edge in fourth intercostal space
V3: Halfway between V2 and V4
V4: Midclavicular line fifth intercostals space
V5: Anterior axillary line horizontal to V4
V6: Midaxillary line horizontal to V4 and V5

CHAPTER 138

Electroencephalogram

An electroencephalogram is a continuous recording of electrical activity of the brain. The electrodes are placed on the scalp. Electrical activity originates from postsynaptic potentials in the dendrites of cortical neurons. Not all potentials are recorded because of buffering effect of the scalp, muscle bone, vessels, and subarachnoid fluid.

The EEG waves are classified according to their frequency as delta (1–3/s), theta (4–7/s), alpha (8–12/s), and beta (13–20/s). These waves are altered by age, state of alertness, closure, drugs, and disease states. High-voltage slow and sharp waves (K complexes) and sleep spindles (regular 12–14/s waves) confined to the central regions occur during sleep in normal EEG.

Abnormalities of waveform include spikes and slow waves. Spikes are characteristically paroxysmal, sharp, and high voltage followed by a slow wave. Spikes and slow waves are associated with epilepsy. Focal spikes are often associated with irritating lesions, including cysts, slow-growing tumors, and glial scar tissue.

CHAPTER 139

Encephalocele

It is a midline usually occipital, defect through which meninges and brain have herniated **(Fig. 1)**. Frontal or nasopharyngeal encephalocele also occur but are less common. Neurological problems such as mental retardation, visual impairment and seizures are common, and hydrocephalus may occur.

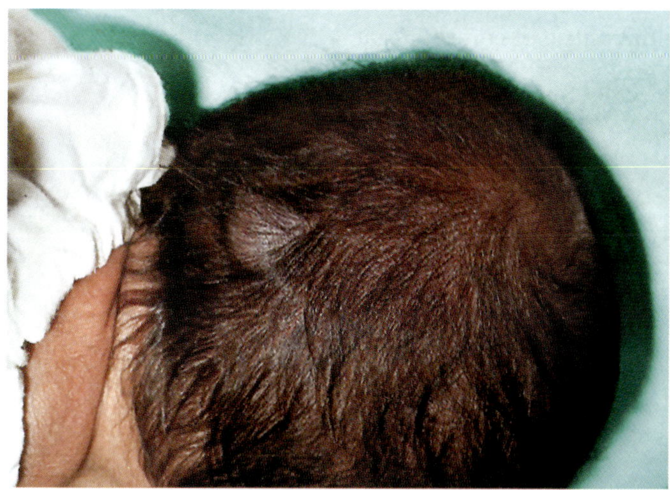

Fig. 1: Encephalocele.

CHAPTER 140

Encopresis

Encopresis is defined as passage of stools in clothes beyond an age when bowel control should have been achieved (usually 4 years). It may be retentive (associated with constipation) or non-retentive primary (never achieved bowel control) or secondary loss of control after an initial phase of control for at least 6 months) primary encopresis is usually associated with constipation while secondary is associated with significant psychological stressors. Behavioral therapy with positive reinforcement and treatment of constipation are necessary.

Enophthalmos (Retraction of the Eyeball)

Enophthalmus suspects enophthalmus, if the eye appears sunken or small. The usual causes are as follows:

Enophthalmus is suspected, if the eye appears sunken or small.

The usual causes **(Box 1)** are as follows:

- Damage to cervical sympathetic nerve
- Microphthalmus
- Apparent retraction in children with chronic malnutrition or acute dehydration

BOX 1: Causes of enophthalmos.

- Congenital (e.g., microphthalmus; also known as nanophthalmus)
- Phthisis bulbi
- Fracture of the orbital floor
- Atrophy of the orbital contents
- *Wasting diseases:* Human immunodeficiency virus (HIV) infection, malignancy
- Horner's syndrome, cicatrizing orbital lesions

Entropion and Ectropion

Entropion is an inversion of the eyelid. Eyelids with the lashes are rolled inward. Eyelashes rub against the conjunctiva or cornea. This may be present at birth, severe blepharospasm, inflammation, or trauma.

Ectropion is an outward rotation of the eyelid margin. Ectropion can lead to problems of corneal exposure. There will be spasm of orbicularis oris muscle and cicatricial contraction of the palpebral conjunctiva. Ectropion may be congenital. It may be caused by any condition (trauma and scleroderma), causing the eyelid skin to contract and evert the eyelid. Ectropion may occur after seventh cranial nerve palsy.

Enuresis

Enuresis means incontinence of urine in children, and is usually nocturnal, though it can also be diurnal. Involuntary discharge of urine after the age at which bladder control should have been established.

The following questions should be asked in history while dealing with a case of enuresis.

- History of bed wetting
- Family problems
- History of emotional disturbances
- Behavior abnormalities

COMMON CAUSES OF ENURESIS

- *Developmental delay*
- *Psychogenic enuresis:*
  - Toilet training difficulties
  - Emotional stress
- *Organic causes:*
  - Obstructive lesions:
    - Chronic constipation
    - Urethral valve
    - Ectopic ureters
    - Urethral strictures
    - Meatal stenosis
    - Contraction of bladder neck
    - Bladder diverticulum
    - Hydrocolopos and hematocolpos
    - Marked phimosis, prostatic tumor, and abscess
  - Neurogenic disorders:
    - Myelomeningocele
    - Sacral neuropathic bladder
    - Occult neuropathic bladder
    - Seizures and spinal cord injury
    - Spinal cord tumors
    - Diastematomyelia and spinal dysraphism
  - Infections:
    - Urinary tract infections
    - Osteomyelitis of vertebral body
    - Spinal epidural abscess
  - Disorders associated with polyuria and polydipsia
    - Diabetes mellitus
    - Sickle cell disease
    - Renal disorders
  - Miscellaneous causes
    - Allergy-chocolate, eggs
    - Obesity
    - Jiggle micturition
    - Global retardation

CHAPTER 144 Epicanthic Fold

Epicanthic fold is a vertical fold of skin which projects from upper eyelid over the medial epicanthus **(Fig. 1)**. These are normally seen in some newborns till 3 months of age. This is seen in Down syndrome, Turner syndrome, Smith Lemli-Opitz syndrome, and Noonan syndrome.

UPWARD AND DOWNWARD SLANTING OF EYEBALL

It is a line connecting the lateral and medial angles in oblique. If the lateral margin is >2 mm higher than medial margin, that is upward slant. If the medial margin is higher, that is downward slant.

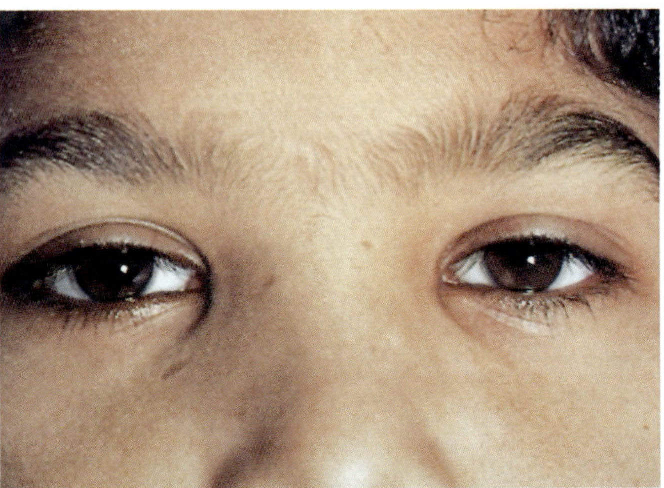

Fig. 1: Epicanthic fold.

CHAPTER 145

Epidermolysis Bullae

Epidermolysis bullae (EB) is a group of inherited mechanobullous disorders characterized by the development of blisters after the skin is subjected to mild friction or trauma. The three general types are EB simplex, junctional EB, and dystrophic EB. These types are classified according to the level at which blister formation occurs. Modes of inheritance vary with subtypes in each group, and blistering, with few exceptions, begins in the newborn period. Other systemic associations may include pyloric stenosis or atresia, muscular dystrophy, and cutaneous localized absence of the skin, especially on the shins.

CHAPTER 146

Epididymis

Epididymal inflammation may be bacterial or nonbacterial in etiology. True bacterial epididymitis is rare in children. Nonbacterial inflammation may be caused by reflux of sterile urine into the ejaculatory ducts or ectopic insertion of a ureter into the seminal vesicle or vas deferens. In many cases of nonbacterial epididymitis, anatomy is normal, and no obvious etiology is evident. Nonbacterial epididymitis would appear to be more common than bacterial inflammation or at least is named as a diagnosis related to scrotal swelling in more instances. The clinical presentation of epididymitis may be indolent or acute, as with torsion. Fever often accompanies bacterial epididymitis, and the urinary sediment may reflect infection. Examination of the scrotum in early stages demonstrates a tender, slightly swollen epididymis, but later the entire scrotal contents are replaced by an inflammatory mass. The cremasteric reflex is present, and elevation of the testis on the pubis may relieve pain (Prehn sign). A color Doppler examination demonstrates increased blood flow. Ultrasound may show an enlarged epididymis. If torsion of the spermatic cord cannot be excluded, surgical exploration must be carried out promptly. All children with bacterial epididymitis should undergo complete upper and lower urinary tract radiographic evaluation after resolution of the acute process [renal ultrasound and voiding cystourethrogram (VCUG)]. Scrotal abscess formation may result from bacterial epididymitis. Nonbacterial epididymitis is treated expectantly. Administration of nonsteroidal anti-inflammatory drugs (NSAIDs) and limitation of activity to bed rest for 48 hours in cases with severe scrotal swelling usually result in rapid improvement of clinical symptoms.

CHAPTER 147

Epigastric Hernia

Epigastric hernia is a congenital defect of the linea alba along the line between the umbilicus and the xiphoid, usually in the lower third of the linea alba (above the umbilicus). These hernias typically present as a recurrent lump with a palpable tiny defect or as a small lump of preperitoneal fat protruding through and trapped by a tiny midline defect. There is little change in size over time and rarely any associated discomfort.

These defects do not resolve spontaneously. Surgical intervention is not urgent, although time may lead to the accumulation of more fat in the tiny defect, leading to a significant subcutaneous lump. Surgical repair is usually advised for the sole reason of minimizing progression to a cosmetically more significant lesion.

CHAPTER 148

Epispadias

Epispadias represents the less severe end of the spectrum of exstrophic anomalies and has a spectrum of severity. Approximately 55% of patients are boys with penopubic epispadias and urinary incontinence. These boys have a palpably and radiographically widened pubic symphysis and a broad, spade-like penis with the urethra opened fully on its dorsal surface up to the level of the bladder neck. The penis is usually tethered dorsally, and the patient is usually incontinent. A smaller percentage of boys demonstrate only penile or balanitic (glandular) epispadias. These boys have normal urinary continence. In girls with epispadias (the rarest cases of epispadias), incontinence is usually accompanied by a wide urethra and a bifid clitoris. The cosmetic appearance of the genitalia in both genders can be improved by genitoplasty, but the larger problem is incontinence, which is accentuated by small bladder capacity. Surgical correction is the rule and may be performed in stages. Renal ultrasonography and voiding cystourethrogram (VCUG) should be performed in all cases.

Epistaxis

It is important to realize that epistaxis (bleeding from the nose) is a sign, not a disease. Possible causes of the condition are shown in **Box 1**.

BOX 1: Causes of epistaxis.

- Trauma to Little's area
- Ulceration and excoriation
- Nasal fracture
- Nasal infections
- Tumors of the nose and sinuses (e.g., juvenile angiofibroma and squamous cell carcinoma)
- Septal granulomas and perforations
- Foreign bodies
- Drugs, anticoagulants, nonsteroidal anti-inflammatory drugs (NSAIDs), and cytotoxic drugs
- Hypertension
- *Coagulopathies:* Hemophilia, Christmas disease, and von Willebrand's disease
- *Dyscrasias:* Purpura and leukemia
- Hereditary hemorrhagic telangiectasia
- Vitamin deficiency—vitamin C and vitamin K

Chapter 150: Epulis

Congenital epulis is a benign soft tissue tumor. It is seen on alveolar mucosa at birth. It is pedunculated swelling found on anterior maxilla but may on the mandible and on both jaws. The mass is firm on palpation. Histologically, sheets of larger granular cells are seen.

CHAPTER 151 Erb's Palsy

It is generally described as the upper trunk or C5-6 palsy. It is the most common injury seen, and together with C5-7, it is called extended Erb's palsy. These two groups have a greater recovery rate resulting in functional arm **(Figs. 1A and B)**.

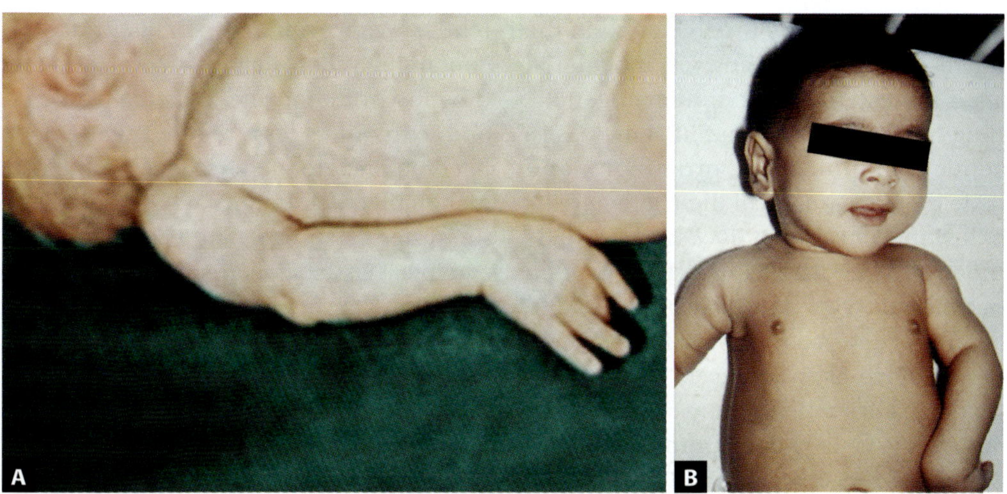

Figs. 1A and B: Erb's palsy.

CHAPTER 152 Erysipelas

Streptococcus pyogenes (*S. pyogenes*) and other pyogenic β-hemolytic streptococci are the cause of erysipelas, an unusual and distinctive infection involving a localized area of the dermis and superficial lymphatics. The causative organisms are usually found in the upper respiratory tracts and are inoculated through a break in the skin; hematogenous seeding has been postulated in some cases. Systemic symptoms are prominent and precede the appearance of the characteristic skin lesion. The onset is abrupt and is heralded by fever and chills, which is often in association with nausea, vomiting, and headache. This prodrome is followed by the appearance of an intensely painful skin lesion that consists of a circumscribed, raised plaque that is usually deep purplish-red but that may be red or even pink. The raised border, although irregular, is well demarcated and spreads centrifugally. Red lymphatic streaks may advance ahead of it toward the regional nodes. On close inspection, the skin is edematous and may have a thickened peau d'orange character. Palpation demonstrates the skin to be indurated, hot, and exquisitely tender. With evolution, small surface blebs containing yellow fluid may form. The face is the most common site, with the trunk, neck, and extremities less frequent. Patients may become bacteremic and develop metastatic foci of infection. Infants are at particular risk for systemic spread. The clinical picture of erysipelas is so characteristic that streptococcal infection can be presumed, and parenteral antimicrobial treatment initiated. Cultures of tissue aspirate from the advancing border of the lesion are typically positive for *S. pyogenes*, as are blood cultures in septic patients. However other β-hemolytic streptococci and, less commonly, *Staphylococcus aureus (S. aureus)* may be isolated.

153 CHAPTER Erythema Toxicum

Erythema toxicum neonatorum is a benign, self-limited, asymptomatic disorder of unknown etiology that is most often seen in otherwise healthy newborns. It occurs in up to 50% of full-term infants and has no racial or sexual predisposition. Lesions usually begin 24–48 hours after birth but may appear up to the 10th day of life. The disorder has been described as a "flea-bitten" dermatosis of the newborn, owing to the intense erythema with a central papule or pustule that resembles a flea bite **(Fig. 1)**. The central papule or pustule is typically 2–3 mm in diameter and is surrounded by a much larger area of erythema. There may be a few to several hundred lesions on the back, face, chest, and extremities. The palms and soles are usually spared. A smear of material from a central pustule reveals numerous eosinophils, and concomitant circulating eosinophilia is present in up to 20% of patients. The eruption fades spontaneously within 5–7 days. No treatment is necessary.

Differential diagnosis includes transient neonatal pustular melanosis, staphylococcal folliculitis, milia neonatorum, miliaria rubra, and herpes simplex. Infections often can be excluded clinically or with a Gram stain, Tzanck smear, and viral and bacterial cultures, when necessary.

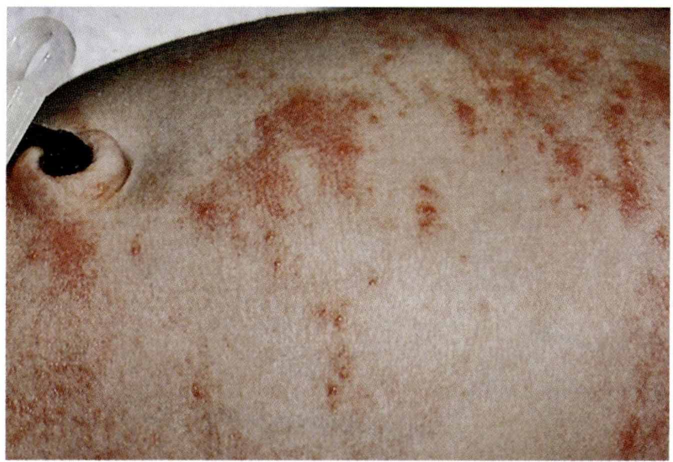

Fig. 1: Erythema toxicum.

Exophthalmos

Exophthalmos is suspected if the eyes appear large or protruding. It occurs in the following conditions:

- Hyperthyroidism (due to retraction)
- Glaucoma (due to enlarged eyes)
- Retro-orbital tumors
- Hemorrhage or metastasis
- Xanthomas of Hand-Schüller-Christian disease
- Neurofibromatosis
- Lymphangioma
- Hemangioma and optic gliomas
- Orbital abscess
- Sinus and cerebral thrombosis

In children with exophthalmos the distance from the angle of the eye to the front of the cornea is >1.5 mm.

This condition may be either bilateral or unilateral.

155 CHAPTER Eye Inflammation (Red Eye)

The term *red eye* usually refers to inflammation of the conjunctiva that causes the eye to appear red. Much less commonly (and much more seriously), the sclera is injected. The causes of red eye include infection of the ocular surface (cornea, conjunctiva, and sclera), allergy, intraocular inflammation, glaucoma, foreign body, and trauma. Evaluation must be directed toward discerning whether a child's red eye is caused by a benign condition that will spontaneously resolve (viral conjunctivitis) or easily be treated with topical medication (bacterial conjunctivitis) or whether the cause is potentially vision threatening (iritis, corneal ulceration, and glaucoma) and requires urgent ophthalmologic evaluation. Signs that should raise concerns for a serious etiology of red eye are in an immunocompromised host, severe pain, proptosis, limitation of eye movements, opacified cornea, abnormal pupil response, or lack of response to therapy.

CONJUNCTIVITIS

Conjunctivitis may be associated with a mucopurulent ocular discharge. The lids may be stuck together after sleep; the pain is generally slight and allayed by closing the eyes. Mucopurulent conjunctivitis is characterized by more profuse discharge and is frequently due to infection by *Staphylococcus* or *Streptococcus* and *Haemophilus* species.

Conjunctival allergies are characterized particularly by edema of the conjunctiva (conjunctival chemosis) and of the skin of the lids, epiphora, and itch. They include non-specific responses to a wide miscellany of drugs, cosmetics, and other irritants. Three specific clinical forms are recognized.

1. Hay fever, from exogenous pollens, etc.
2. Phlyctenular conjunctivitis (due to an allergic reaction, e.g., to a *Staphylococcus* organism), featuring marked photophobia and one or more round yellowish, raised masses at the corneoscleral junction surrounded by a localized area of vascular conjunctiva. In some cases, the phlycten encroach on the corneal surface, being followed by a trail or leash of conjunctival vessels.
3. Spring catarrh, which exists in palpebral and bulbar forms, the former showing polygonal flat-topped conjunctival nodules resembling cobblestones, the latter showing focal gelatinous limbal thickening.

Face, Abnormalities of Appearance and Movements

CRETINOID FACIES

The face is broad, and remarkable for thick eyelids, broad flat nose, thick lips, and widely spaced eyes. The mouth is usually open, the tongue may be more or less constantly protruded, and the chin is poorly developed. The hair is scanty and brittle, the skin coarse, dry or muddy, and often almost yellow.

CONGENITAL SYPHILITIC FACIES

The facies which is unmistakable—an overhanging forehead, perhaps frontal bosses, a depressed nasal bridge, striated scars radiating from the corners and other parts of the lips, which a sallow, earthy complexion.

MYASTHENIC FACIES

It includes lid lag with tired face. There will be characteristic sneer smile patients suffering from myasthenia gravis **(Fig. 1)**.

DOWN SYNDROME

There will be upward slanting of eyes, epicanthic folds, hypertelorism, flattened nasal bridge, and protuberant tongue. Head is brachycephalic.

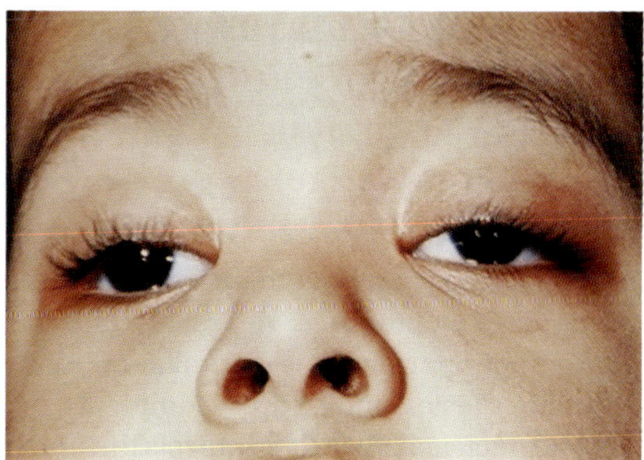

Fig. 1: Myasthenia gravis.

ADENOID FACIES

This is used to be described in the sufferer with a wide-open mouth resulting in the oral breathing demanded by nasal obstruction, and the over-slung lower jaw and dental occlusion with consequent incomplete musculature of the mouth and receding cheeks.

TETANUS

Risus sardonicus due to the spasm of the platysma muscle, the corners of mouth move downward and outward, the lip is stretched across the teeth.

CHAPTER 157 Face Paralysis

TYPES OF FACIAL NERVE PARALYSIS

Facial Nerve Paralysis of Central Origin [Supranuclear or Upper Motor Neuron (UMN) Type]

In central facial paralysis, there is paresis of the lower portion of the face with relative sparing of the upper portion. It is contralateral to the pathologic lesion and is rarely complete.

The nuclear center that controls the upper portion of the face has both contralateral and ipsilateral supranuclear connections whereas the nuclear center which supplies the lower portion of the face has only contralateral supranuclear innervation.

The extent of involvement in a supranuclear palsy may vary from the lower 1st to 2/3rd of the face as there is a great deal of individual variation in facial innervation.

Supranuclear lesions do not produce atrophy of the facial muscles.

Supranuclear facial palsy is of two types.:

1. *Volitional palsy:* In this, involvement is most marked on voluntary contraction. Paresis is apparent when the patient attempts to retract the angle of the mouth. However, on involuntary contractions such as spontaneous smiling or crying, there is preservation of function with little or no evidence of paresis.

   Volitional type of central facial paresis results from involvement of:
   - Cortical center in the lower third of the precentral convolution that control facial movements
   - In the pathway between this center and motor nucleus.
2. *Emotional type of central facial palsy:* In this type of central facial palsy, impairment is marked on smiling or crying however, patient can voluntarily retract his mouth without any difficulty. It results from extrapyramidal, basal ganglion, thalamic, or hypothalamic involvement.

PERIPHERAL FACIAL PALSY (NUCLEAR, INFRANUCLEAR/ LOWER MOTOR NEURON TYPE)

In the peripheral or lower motor neuron (LMN) type of facial paralysis (Bell's palsy) there is:

- Flaccid paralysis of all muscles of facial expression on the involved side (ipsilateral) and paralysis is complete. In LMN type of paralysis—there is atrophy of the facial muscles.
- Affected side of face is smooth, no wrinkles on forehead.
- Eyebrow droops, eye is open, inferior lid lags.
- Nose is flattened or deviated to the opposite side.
- Patient is unable to raise eyebrows, frown, close the eyes, smile, cough, show his

teeth, whistle, or retract the chin on the affected side.

- One attempted movement, mouth is deviated to normal side.
- Food accumulates between teeth and affected cheek.
- Saliva may drip from the paretic side.
- There is difficulty in articulation, especially vowels which require pursing of lips.
- Nasolabial folds are shallow/absent; alae nasi are sunken and do not move with respiration.
- Palpebral fissure is wider than normal due to lagophthalmos (inability to close the eye).
- There are epiphora-excessive tears.
- The stapedius may be paralyzed—hyperacusis for low tones which appear louder and higher.

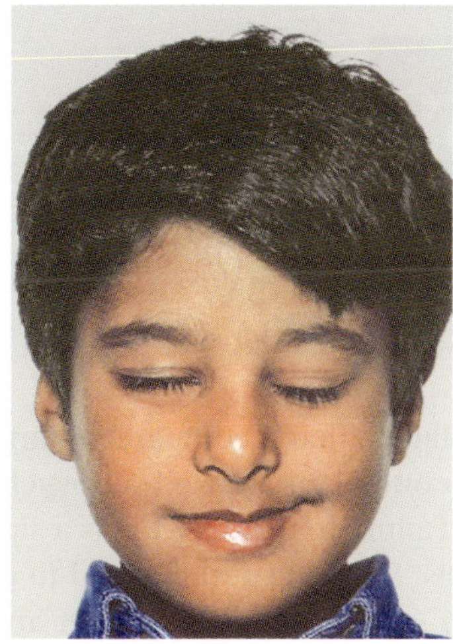

Fig. 1: Bell's palsy.

- In comatose patient—function of facial nerve is elicited by nothing response to painful pressure over the supraorbital ridge **(Fig. 1)**.

CHAPTER 158

Failure to Thrive

Growth failure that accompanies many pathological conditions as well as psychosocial causes. Failure to thrive (FTT) is a sign, not a diagnosis. FTT is generally used to describe children <2 or 3 years who meet any of the following criteria:

- Growth under the third percentile on World Health Organization (WHO) weight for age growth charts (<3% = <3 standard deviations below mean)
- Weight for height or body mass index (BMI) less than the 5th percentile
- Growth patterns that have crossed two major percentiles downward on the weight for age charts within 6 months
- Growth velocity less than normal for age

Infants who are born small for gestational age and are *symmetrically* small are believed to have a reduced number of somatic cells in relation to their normal-sized peers as a result of an early intrauterine event. Infants who are *asymmetrically* small for gestational age, with sparing of the head circumference and possibly length, suffered a late intrauterine event, such as poor maternal nutrition or placental insufficiency. These infants often eat voraciously and experience catch-up growth early in life. Children with genetic short stature have short height for age with appropriate low weight.

Children with FTT caused by calorie insufficiency typically have decreased weight gain, at first with sparing of height and head circumference (wasting). Long-standing calorie insufficiency results in height deceleration (stunting). Height or length is the best predictor of chronic malnutrition. Only in the worst, long-standing cases is head growth decreased. This typical pattern suggests calorie insufficiency and informs the clinician of the chronicity of the problem.

MEDICAL HISTORY

The perinatal history includes problems with labor, method of delivery, and the newborn's growth parameters at birth [i.e., appropriate (AGA), small (SGA), or large (LGA) for gestational age].

The child's medical history should be reviewed for chronic conditions and recurrent, acute conditions, such as recurrent emesis, diarrhea, constipation, neurologic symptoms, or recurrent infections. Hospitalizations, surgical procedures, medications, and allergies should be explored. Immunization status should be ascertained.

FAMILY HISTORY

Is there any history of heart, renal, or gastrointestinal disease in the family? Have there been any early childhood deaths? Is there any sickle cell disease or other anemic condition? Are there any family members with genetic or metabolic conditions? Is there a family history of mental illness that might affect the child or the caretakers? Is there a consanguinity?

SOCIAL HISTORY

Many cases of FTT do not have a primary medical etiology, and thus the social history is vital. Is the child in group daycare, or has the family traveled to an area where a chronic infection such as a parasite might have been acquired? Although the social history can be the most revealing part of the history, it can be the most difficult to elicit. Often the clinician must establish trust with the family before they can reveal the source of their inability to meet their child's nutritional needs.

Constitutional: The examiner should ask whether there are any fevers, night sweats, or changes in activity. Assess sleep hygiene, amount of sleep, and whether sleep is disrupted by snoring or awakenings.

Gastrointestinal: The examiner should inquire about choking, swallowing, dysphagia, vomiting, and spitting up. Night waking and coughing may indicate reflux. Diarrhea, constipation, abdominal pain, distention, or discomfort may indicate organic disease. Pocketing food, or retaining food in the mouth, may indicate oral-motor dysfunction that impedes adequate intake.

Cardiopulmonary: The examiner should ask about coughing, wheezing, night waking, shortness of breath, exercise intolerance, and early tiring during feeding.

Renal: The examiner should inquire about dysuria, hematuria, increased urinary frequency or volume, secondary enuresis, and urine that seems unusually diluted.

EVALUATION

When the history and physical in an infant or child with failure to thrive do not suggest a specific underlying organic disease, unfocused protocols of laboratory investigations and imaging studies almost never provide the answer.

When there are no clear-cut signs suggesting organic disease, a complete psychosocial history and direct observation of the child and family (as described in Chapter 1) usually allow a diagnosis of deprivational growth failure and malnutrition to be made on distinct positive grounds rather than by exclusion.

ENERGY INTAKE AND REQUIREMENTS

Once the history, family observation, and physical examination are complete, the most useful subsequent clinical observation is quantitation of the youngster's daily energy intake, a process that often is best accomplished with the help of a therapeutic nutritionist **(Table 1)**. Quantitation is essential.

Two bits of knowledge are essential for proper clinical evaluation and for a successful plan of management.

- Knowledge of the normal (average) intake for a child of this age (or of this height-age)

TABLE 1: Daily energy requirements at different ages.

Age	*Sex*	*Units (kcal/kg/day)*
0–2 months	Both sexes	100–120
3–5 months	Both sexes	95–100
6–8 months	Both sexes	95–97
9–11 months	Both sexes	97–99
1 year	Both sexes	101
2–3 years	Both sexes	94
4–6 years	Both sexes	100
7–9 years	• Male • Female	88 76
10–12 years	• Male • Female	73 61
13–15 years	• Male • Female	57 46
16–18 years	• Male • Female	51 40

- Appreciation of the facts that achieving growth recovery (i.e., "catch-up growth") requires a daily energy intake that averages 50% more than the normal daily intake of a well-nourished child of the same height.
- The combination of anorexia and a greatly increased energy requirement for recovery makes for a major challenge, which explains why hyperalimentation methods (enteral or parenteral) are so often required at the outset to induce nutritional and growth recovery in these children.

PHYSICAL EXAMINATION

The examination should start with accurate measurements of height or length, weight, and head circumference; these parameters should be plotted on a standard growth curve. Weight for height or BMI (if >2 years of age) should also be plotted. Historical events should be obtained and plotted to identify patterns of growth. As part of a complete physical examination, the following signs should be sought:

- *General:* Degree of emaciation, state of fat distribution and muscle mass, dysmorphic features, vital signs (including blood pressure)
- *Head, eyes, ears, nose, and throat:* Fontanel size, evidence of chronic ear infections, allergic stigmata, patency of upper airway
- *Cardiorespiratory:* Respiratory effort, lower airway sounds, cardiac sounds, pulses, and edema
- *Gastrointestinal:* Organomegaly, abdominal distention, rectal fissures, or prolapse
- *Genitourinary:* Renal masses, Tanner staging
- *Musculoskeletal:* Joint swelling, bone deformities
- *Skin:* Hydration, evidence of chronic inflammation, bruising or scarring, rashes, hair quality and distribution, nails
- *Lymph nodes:* Local versus generalized.
- *Neurologic:* Muscle volume, tone (hypo or hypertonic), strength, coordination, swallowing and drooling, assessment of development and interaction with the examiner.

LABORATORY EVALUATION

The choice of the appropriate initial laboratory tests may include several general screening tests (complete blood count, urinalysis, serum electrolyte levels, and blood urea nitrogen level) to detect treatable conditions. A complete blood cell count can reveal clinically inapparent anemia, which, although usually secondary to the poor nutritional state, can sometimes contribute to the poor dietary intake or suggest anemia of chronic disease. A urinalysis and urine culture can reveal evidence of an occult urinary tract infection or renal tubular acidosis. An erythrocyte sedimentation rate or C-reactive protein may provide evidence of chronic inflammation or infection. The examiner may need to test for celiac disease, in which poor weight gain may be the only symptom for many years. Other specific tests are directed by the history and physical examination as mentioned in **Box 1**.

BOX 1: Investigation.

- Complete blood count
- Serum creatinine urea
- Electrolytes, acid–base status
- Calcium, phosphate
- Liver function tests
- Thyroid function tests
- Acute phase reactant, e.g., C-reactive protein
- Immunoglobulins
- IgA tissue transglutaminase antibodies
- Urine microscopy, culture, and dipsticks
- Stool microscopy, culture and elastase
- Karyotype in girls
- Chest X-ray and sweat test

CHAPTER 159

Faints or Syncope

It is a "transient loss of consciousness due to a reduction in the cerebral blood flow". Syncope is a common phenomenon among children and adolescents.

PATHOPHYSIOLOGY

The pathophysiologic mechanism of syncope includes decrease cerebral perfusion. Vasomotor changes, decreasing venous return, and primary dysrhythmia causes decrease in cardiac output. Clinical features include blurred vision and constriction of visual fields before losing consciousness, as well as nausea, pallor, sweating, and dizziness, which are accompanied by hypotension (systolic blood pressure <60 mm Hg) and by bradycardia (heart rate <40 beats/min).

The common causes of syncope are summarized in **Box 1**.

NEUROCARDIOGENIC SYNCOPE

Neurocardiogenic syncope has been described in association with hair brushing, swallowing, stretching, orthodontic maneuvers, anomalies of the cervical spine, and dental trauma. Many of these episodes may actually be forms of carotid sinus sensitivity. Cough syncope probably is related to prolongation of high intrathoracic pressure that results in decreased venous return and subsequent decreased cardiac output.

BOX 1: Causes of syncope.

- Postural hypertension
- Carotid sinus syncope
- Stokes—Adams attacks in atrioventricular block
- Paroxysmal dysrhythmias
- Cyanotic attacks in congenital heart disease
- Cough syncope
- Micturition syncope
- Breath-holding attack

ORTHOSTATIC SYNCOPE

Conditions that produce hypotension (orthostatic or supine) frequently produce syncope or presyncope. Cardiac function and structure are usually normal before the episode; during the predisposing illness, cardiac filling pressures are often reduced because of reduced venous return from hypovolemia or decreased peripheral vascular resistance (peripheral pooling of blood). Dehydration from diarrhea and vomiting, hyperthermia, hyperpyrexia, heat exhaustion, polyuria (diabetes mellitus) or poor intake from anorexia, together with the systemic effects of the primary illness, may produce orthostatic or true hypotension and syncope. In these conditions, dizziness, hypotension, or syncope occurs rapidly when the patient assumes an upright position (seconds). Prolonged bed rest, combined with poor fluid intake during an illness, may also result in syncope or presyncope when the child arises to leave the bed. In most of these situations, fluid administration is sufficient to restore intravascular volume and venous return to alleviate postural or supine hypotension.

CARDIAC SYNCOPE/SUDDEN CARDIAC DEATH

A variety of cardiac conditions can result in hypotension and syncope. Dysrhythmias are common and are usually silent between episodes. Supraventricular tachycardia, ventricular tachycardia, and heart block are the most common types of dysrhythmia and may be primary or may result from medications or illicit drugs. Any form of acquired heart block carries a high mortality rate. A common cause of acquired heart block is Lyme disease. Heart block may necessitate temporary or permanent electronic pacing to maintain cardiac output.

Cardiac syncopal episodes can be accompanied by brief tonic-clonic seizure activity known as Stokes–Adams syndrome. The seizure activity appears 10–20 seconds after the onset of asystole and is usually of short duration with no subsequent postictal phase. This may explain why many children with cardiac syncope frequently see a neurologist.

Sudden cardiac death is discussed with cardiac causes of syncope because cardiac causes of syncope may also produce sudden death. Sudden cardiac arrest or death is defined as the abrupt and unexpected loss of heart function. Structural causes include valvular aortic stenosis, coronary artery anomalies, cardiomyopathies, and myocarditis. Cardiac arrhythmias associated with sudden death include Wolff–Parkinson–White syndrome and prolonged QT syndrome.

CATAPLEXY

Cataplexy may be confused with syncope and is characterized by partial or complete paralysis of skeletal muscles resulting in a rapid progression of weakness of the face and neck followed by the muscles of the trunk and extremities. The patient loses tone and may fall to the floor but remains awake and immobile for 1–2 minutes. Triggers include intense positive or negative emotions, such as laughing, frustration, fright, or anger.

SUMMARY AND RED FLAGS

Hypotension, both supine and orthostatic, is a major red flag, as are associated palpitations, exertional symptoms, or chest pain; participation in gym class or sports must be restricted until a complete diagnostic work-up is completed. Additional red flags include syncope while supine, a positive family history, prolonged loss of consciousness, prolonged seizures, prolonged post-event neurologic signs, and abrupt onset with no prodrome.

CHAPTER 160

Fasciculation (Muscle Twitching)

This is the contraction of a group of muscle fibers. This comprises the motor unit. It involves one or more motor units but not the whole muscle. These are seen clinically in tongue, deltoid, calf muscle, and quadriceps muscles.

The causes include progressive spinal muscular atrophy, peroneal muscular atrophy, myositis, and collagen vascular disease. It can occur in normal subjects.

161 CHAPTER

Fetal Alcohol Syndrome

The effect of exposure to significant levels of serum alcohol results in pattern of microcephaly, prenatal and postnatal growth deficiency, short palpebral fissures, long smooth philtrum, and a thin upper lip. Other features include short nose and hypoplasia of nails and distal phalanges (particularly fifth toes). On occasion affected infants have eyelid ptosis, epicanthal folds, strabismus, small, raised hemangioma, cervical vertebral abnormalities, and congenital heart disease.

Newborns are small for gestational age and have poor catch up growth postnatally. They have increased or decreased muscle tone and can be irritable and tremulous. Most older children tend to be thin and hyperactive. >80% have delay in development especially in fine motor function. The diagnosis of fetal alcohol syndrome should be reserved for those infants who have history in utero exposure of large amount of alcohol and who have characteristic physical features of the disorder.

CHAPTER 162

Fetal Scalp Blood Sampling

Cervix should be dilated for 2.5 cm. Patient is placed in wide lithotomy position. Vulvar area is cleaned by povidone-iodine solution. Pelvic examination is done to assess the degree of cervical dilation. Membranes are ruptured artificially if cervix is intact. After the correct angling of the amnioscope, its tip is applied over the scalp of the fetus. The scalp is dried with the cotton swab. It is sprayed with ethyl chloride to cause hyperemia. A small amount of silicon gel and liquid paraffin is applied over the scalp to facilitate the formation of the blood drop. This reduces the chance of exposure to air. Common indications are mentioned in **Box 1**.

BOX 1: Indications.

- *Persistent:*
  - Tachycardia >160/min
  - Bradycardia <120/min
- Late deceleration
- Decreased beat-to-beat variability
- Persistent variable deceleration
- Fetal arrhythmias

Scalp should be penetrated to the depth of 2 mm at two points. Care should be taken to avoid the incision over the fontanel or suture line. Some of the contraindications are mentioned in **Box 2**. The blood should be collected in heparinized capillary tube. Hemostasis is ensured by applying pressure with cotton swab. Fetal pH of 7.25 or more is considered as normal.

BOX 2: Contraindications.

- Placenta previa
- Brow and face presentation
- Hydrocephalus
- Umbilical cord prolapse
- Chorioretinitis
- Fetal hemophilia

Fever

Fever is defined as the persistent elevation of body temperature above normal levels in an individual. Fever is the symptom of infection. As a result of infection, the proteinaceous products called pyrogens are released. This will act on thermoregulatory mechanism. This leads to local prostaglandin production, thus generating heat and loss of heat is prevented. Hence body temperature is increased.

PATHOGENETIC MECHANISM OF FEVER

An elevation of body temperature is a sign of illness, particularly of infection. The pyrogens, small proteinaceous products released in response to infections, in neurologic or toxic stimuli, act on thermoregulatory center and information is then transmitted to vasomotor center, possibly by local prostaglandin production. Heat generation is increased, and heat loss is prevented, thus increasing the body temperature. The attempts to achieve the newly "set" point may be by the mechanism of violent muscular exertion-the shaking chill or rigor attempts to dissipate extra body heat, in febrile states may be by diaphoresis and fever "flush."

Temperature is controlled by the thermoregulatory center, located in the preoptic area of the anterior hypothalamus. The thermoregulatory center receives input from peripheral receptors and the temperature of the blood bathing the hypothalamus and acts on autonomic, endocrine, and behavioral mechanisms to maintain the body temperature at a particular set point. The hypothalamic set point normally maintains body temperature around 37°C, but there can be significant variation among individuals. Normal temperatures range from 36 to 37.8°C, depending on the time of day, with the peak in the afternoon (5–7 PM) and the trough in the early morning (2–6 AM). Although the circadian rhythm is not well established in infancy, it becomes more reliable by the 2nd year of life.

METHODS OF MEASUREMENTS OF TEMPERATURE

- *Oral temperature:* Here a mercury glass thermometer is placed under tongue in right or left posterior sublingual pocket. Mouth is closed. Oral temperature ranges are mentioned in **Table 1**.

TABLE 1: Oral temperature ranges.

Temperature	*Degree Fahrenheit*	*Degree centigrade*
Normal	98–99	36.6–37.2
Subnormal	<98	<36.6
Fever	>99	>37.2
Hypothermia	<95	<35
Hyperpyrexia	>107	>41.6

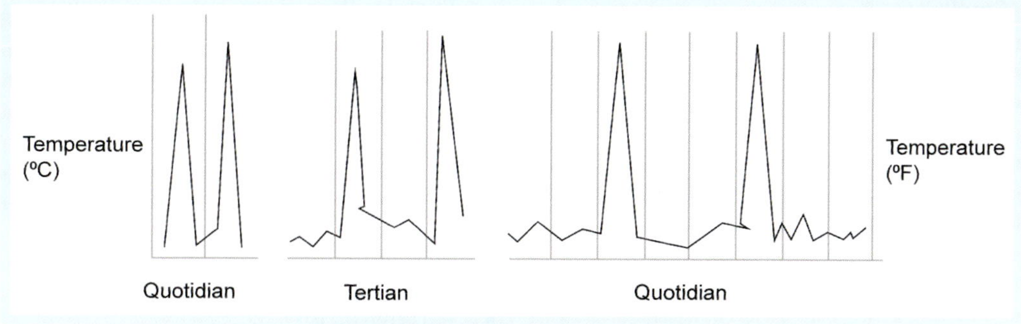

Fig. 1: Types of intermittent fever.

- *Axillary temperature:* Thermometer is placed under the arm with the tip in the center of axilla. It is kept close to the skin. Child's arm is firmly held.
- *Rectal temperature:* Lubricated tip of rectal thermometer is held into the rectum. It should not be inserted >2.5 cm. The child is made to lie on the side in prone position with the knees flexed position. Temperature can also be recorded in groin between and flexed thigh and ear canal (tympanic membrane).

TYPES OF TEMPERATURE

Remittent Fever

Here the diurnal fluctuation of the fever exceeds 1.5°F in 24 hours but does not touch the base line. It is seen in typhoid and infective endocarditis.

Continuous Fever

Here the diurnal fluctuation of the fever is <1.5°F in 24 hours but does not touch the base line. It is seen in lobar pneumonia, typhoid, viral, and infective endocarditis.

Intermittent Fever

Temperature spikes upward during the day, falls back to normal on that same day. Intermittent fever that occurs daily is called "Quotidian", on alternate days "tertian" and on every fourth day "Quartan" **(Fig. 1)**. It is seen in Malaria, Kala azar, and pyemia.

Relapsing Fever

These are several days of fever followed by days in which the patient remains afebrile. This is seen in brucellosis.

Pel-Ebstein Fever

Here the fever takes 3 days to rise, 3 days to remain high, returns to normal in 3 days, and fever for 9 days. It is seen among Hodgkin's disease.

FEVER WITH RIGORS

Thermostatic mechanism, i.e., heat regulation mechanism is disturbed in acute onset of fever, heat is conserved by skin vessels being constricted. Body feels cold and child may shiver, rigors occur.

- Pneumonia
- Viral fever
- Streptococcal throat infection
- Malaria
- UTI
- Infective endocarditis

FEVER WITH RASH

- Chickenpox

- Smallpox
- Measles
- Rubella
- Typhoid

FEVER WITH MEMBRANE ON THROAT

- Diphtheria
- Herpetic angina
- Infectious mononucleosis (IMN)
- Agranulocytosis
- Nonlymphocytic leukemia

CAUSES OF HYPERPYREXIA TEMPERATURE >107°F

- Septicemia
- Encephalitis
- Malaria
- Heat stroke
- Pontine hemorrhage
- Tetanus

Most febrile children have a brief, self-limiting viral infection. Mild localized infection, e.g., otitis media or tonsillitis, may be diagnosed clinically. The clinical problem lies in identifying the relatively few children with a serious infection which needs prompt treatment.

FEVER WITH RASH

Some of the febrile syndromes may be associated with skin rash in which rash is a prominent feature of the presentation. The most life-threatening infections associated with fever and rash include meningococcemia, staphylococcal bacteremia, etc. A list of infectious agents producing fever and rash are given below:

Maculopapular Erythematous

- Enterovirus
- Epstein–Barr virus, cytomegalovirus, and *Toxoplasma gondii*
- Human immunodeficiency virus
- *Salmonella typhi*
- *Leptospira interrogans*
- Measles virus
- Rubella virus
- Hepatitis B virus
- *Treponema pallidum*
- Parvovirus B9
- Human herpesvirus 6

Vesicular

- Varicella-zoster
- Herpes simplex virus
- Coxsackie A virus
- *Vibrio vulnificus*

Cutaneous Petechiae

- *Neisseria gonorrhoeae*
- *Neisseria meningitides*
- *Rickettsia rickettsii*
- *Rickettsia typhi* (murine typhus)
- *Ehrlichia canis*
- Echoviruses
- *Viridans streptococci* (endocarditis)

Diffuse Erythroderma

- Group A streptococci (scarlet fever and toxic shock syndrome)
- *Staphylococcus aureus* (toxic shock syndrome)

Distinctive Rash

- Erythema gangrenosum—*Pseudomonas aeruginosa*
- Erythema chronicum migrans—Lyme disease

FEVER AND LYMPHADENOPATHY

Many diseases are associated with fever and lymphadenopathy. The important causes of fever associated with lymphadenopathy are listed below:

- Viral-Measles, rubella, hepatitis B, Epstein–Barr virus mononucleosis, cytomegalovirus, human immunodeficiency virus
- Bacterial scarlet fever, brucellosis, leptospirosis, tuberculosis, syphilis, Lyme disease, streptococcal, and staphylococcal diseases.
- Parasitic-Acute toxoplasmosis.
- Malignancies—leukemias, lymphomas.

CHAPTER 164

Fibroadenoma of Breast

In adolescents, fibroadenoma accounts for 90% of solid masses. They typically occur after menarche but can precede it by 1–2 years. The average size is 2–3 cm but can be much larger. 10% may have bilateral lesion and 25% will multiply lesions. They are more commonly located in the upper outer quadrant of the breast. They can typically be diagnosed based on physical examination as these masses are smooth, well circumscribed, mobile, and non-tender. There may be some variation with menstrual cycle. Ultrasound may be of useful adjunct and may assist in distinguishing solid from cystic lesion. These lesions can be observed. Surgical excisional biopsy reserved for those with increasing size of mass, tenderness and family history of malignancy.

165 CHAPTER Fits and Convulsions

Convulsions are characterized by chronic recurrent bursts of excessive electrical activity within the brain. Each burst of electrical activity is called seizures. If the seizure arises from motor cortex, that abnormal activity is called convulsion. It is not related to fever.

Clonic movements are rhythmic, non-suppressible, position-independent jerking movements (low frequency and high amplitude) caused by involvement of the motor cortex. They can be unilateral or bilateral and can start with one body part and spread. If bilateral, they are synchronous, and do not alternate from one side to the other in a bicycling fashion. This should be distinguished from clonus, which is rhythmic twitching of a limb, generally the foot, caused by hyperreflexia and lack of descending cortical inhibition due to central nervous system (CNS) injury such as is seen in cerebral palsy or stroke.

The term "tonic" refers to a change in tone as a manifestation of seizure activity, which clinically presents as stiffening or arching. This can occur as the only manifestation of a seizure (tonic seizure), or may be followed by clonic jerking, which is the so-called tonic-clonic seizure (GTC or grand mal).

Atonic seizures refer to seizures where a sudden, brief loss of tone in the neck or entire body causes a head nod or fall to the ground. This type of seizure must be distinguished from falls due to complete loss of consciousness or those due to tonic stiffening of the entire body. With atonic seizures, the loss of tone is sudden but brief, and the patient is quickly responsive afterward.

Automatisms are semi-purposeful movements that usually occur with impairment of consciousness either during or after a seizure and can be very useful for identifying a spell as a seizure. These novel movements are most often a mixture of masticatory, oral, and lingual movements (lip smacking or grimacing) and simple fragmentary limb movements, such as fidgeting with a held object or pulling at clothing. In infants, orofacial automatisms are more likely than complex gestures and must be distinguished from the normal behavior of infants. Automatisms can both be seen in focal seizures, specifically those of temporal lobe onset, as well as in some generalized seizures, specifically absence epilepsy, so they are not specific to a broad category of seizure.

CAUSES OF CONVULSIONS

- Febrile convulsions
- *CNS infections:*
  - Meningitis
  - Encephalitis
  - Abscess
- *Metabolic causes:*
  - Hypoglycemia
  - Hypocalcemia
  - Hypomagnesemia
  - Hyponatremia

- Pyridoxine dependency
- Organic academia
- Storage disorder
- *Inborn error of metabolism:*
  - Maple syrup urine disease
  - Phenyl ketonuria
- *Structural abnormalities:*
  - Sturge weber syndrome
  - Neurofibromatosis
  - Tuberous sclerosis
  - Lissencephaly
- Birth asphyxia
- Trauma
- Hypertensive encephalopathy
- *Drugs:*
  - Theophylline, aminophylline, and barbiturates

CONVULSIONS NOT ASSOCIATED WITH FOCAL NEUROLOGICAL DEFICITS

- Head injury
- Septicemia
- Postictal
- Hypertensive encephalopathy
- Hypoglycemia
- Meningitis
- Subarachnoid hemorrhage
- Hydrocephalus
- Lead poisoning
- Shock
- Renal coma
- Hepatic coma

CONVULSIONS WITH FOCAL NEUROLOGICAL DEFICITS

- Cerebral arterial occlusion
- Todd, paralysis
- Demyelinating disorder
- Cerebral contusion
- Brain abscess
- Subdural emphysema
- Arteriovenous (AV) malformation

166

CHAPTER

Fixed Drug Eruption

These are erythematous and often violaceous plaques, which reappear at the same cutaneous site after exposure to an offending drug. They can affect both the skin and mucous membranes. Post-inflammatory hyperpigmentation can be prominent and may be the only manifestation of the rash during remissions. Morphologically and histologically, the annular and sometimes bullous eruptions of fixed drug reactions may appear similar to erythema multiforme. Common defending drugs include sulfa drugs, nonsteroidal anti-inflammatory drugs (NSAIDs), and pseudoephedrine.

CHAPTER 167

Flaring of Alae Nasi

Any condition that difficulty in breathing can cause nasal flaring, it can be a sign of respiratory distress. Nasi flaring may be caused by asthma flare-up. Blocked airway (any cause) swelling and mucus collection in smallest airway passages in the lungs-bronchiolitis.

Newborns breathe almost exclusively through their nostrils, so when they cannot get sufficient oxygen they tend to flare their nostrils.

Flaring of the alae nasi exists when an enlargement of both nares occurs during inspiration. It is due to contraction of the anterior and posterior dilators nares muscle. The appearance of flaring indicates that accessory muscles are being required for inspiration. It is an excellent sign of dyspnea.

Unilateral flaring is a sign of facial paralysis on the opposite side.

CHAPTER 168

Flat Nasal Bridge

Flat nasal bridge is seen among Carpenter syndrome and Williams syndrome. Depressed nasal bridge is seen among thalassemia, Down syndrome, ectodermal dysplasia, Hurler syndrome, hypothyroidism, and congenital syphilis.

CHAPTER 169

Flow Murmurs

The continuous murmur is a systolic murmur that continues or "spills" into diastolic and indicates continuous flow, such as in the presence of a patent ductus arteriosus or other aortopulmonary communication. This murmur should be differentiated from to-and-fro murmur, where systolic component of the murmur ends at or before S2, and the diastolic murmur begins after semilunar valve closure.

CHAPTER 170

Fluid Thrill

Another maneuver is to test for a fluid wave. This procedure requires three hands, so you will need assistance from the patient or another examiner. With the patient supine, ask him or her or another person to press the edge of the hand and forearm firmly along the vertical midline of the abdomen. This positioning helps to stop the transmission of a wave through adipose tissue. Place your hands on each side of the abdomen and strike one side sharply with your fingertips. Feel for the impulse of a fluid wave with the fingertips of your other hand. An easily detected fluid wave suggests ascites but be cautioned that the findings of this maneuver are not conclusive. A fluid wave can sometimes be felt in people without ascites and, conversely, may not occur in people with early ascites.

It is one more method to test fluid wave. This procedure requires three hands. One hand is placed over the lumbar region on one side. Get the assistant to put side of hand firmly on the midline of the abdomen. Then flick or tap the opposite lumbar region with your other hand. A fluid thrill or wave is felt by a definite unmistakable impulse by the formerly placed hand on the other lumbar region.

The purpose of assistant hand is to dampen any impulse that may be transmitted through the fat of the abdominal wall.

As a rule, fluid thrill is felt only when there is a large amount of fluid present in the abdomen, which is under tension.

Demonstrating shifting dullness is helpful when a small amount of free fluid is present in the abdomen. With massive ascites, a fluid thrill is present but shifting dullness may not be demonstrable, because there is little room in the abdominal cavity for the fluid to shift. In infants and young children, a small amount of ascites can be difficult to confirm by clinical examination, and abdominal ultrasonography may be required.

Folliculitis

It is a superficial infection or irritation of the hair follicles. The scalp, face, extensor surfaces of the extremities, and buttocks are the most common sites of involvement. Patients with dry atopic skin or keratosis pilaris (a condition in which follicles become blocked by keratin plugs) are particularly prone to this problem. Other predisposing factors include seborrhea, excessive sweating, poor hygiene, and topical contact with oils, tars, and adhesives. Obstruction of follicles facilitates inflammation and secondary infection. A superficial erythematous nodule develops around the hair, evolving into a thin-walled central pustule with a narrow, red rim. The lesions may itch or burn and subsequently may drain and crust. Although a lesion may heal in 7–10 days without treatment, multiple crops may occur. Scratching may spread the infection to other areas, and secondary impetiginous lesions may develop. *Staphylococcus aureus* is the typical pathogen, although other skin colonizers may participate. Oral antimicrobial therapy directed at *S. aureus* and avoidance of the predisposing condition are both indicated to resolve the process. Empiric treatment should cover both methicillin-susceptible *Staphylococcus aureus* (MSSA) and methicillin-resistant *Staphylococcus aureus* (MRSA), making knowledge of local staphylococcal epidemiology, and antibiotic susceptibility important.

CHAPTER 172 Fontanels

A diamond-shaped gap between frontal and parietal bones is called the anterior fontanel (AF) and a triangular space between two parietal and occipital bones is called the posterior fontanel.

The fontanels are the gaps between bones in the infant skull where three skull bones meet. Gentle palpation of the fontanels is a routine part of the newborn examination.

There are six fontanels at birth ***(Fig. 1)****:*

- Anterior fontanel
- Posterior fontanel
- Two anterolateral—pair of spheroidal fontanels
- Two posterolateral—pair of mastoid fontanels

The anterior fontanel may vary in size. Persistent delay in closure or unusually large in size indicate increased intracranial pressure or pathological delay in bone growth.

Posterior fontanel is present where the lambdoid and sagittal sutures unite. It is triangular in shape and situated at the junction of occipital and two parietal bone meet. It closes by 2 months. Hypothyroidism should be ruled out when the posterior fontanel persists.

PREMATURE CLOSURE OF ANTERIOR FONTANEL

- Microcephaly
- Craniosynostosis
- Hyperthyroidism

DELAYED CLOSURE OF ANTERIOR FONTANEL

- Rickets
- Hydrocephalus
- Hypothyroidism
- Down syndrome
- Achondroplasia
- Osteogenesis imperfecta
- Hypophosphatasia
- Skeletal dysplasia

Raised intracranial pressure in meningitis is reflected by palpable tension of the fontanel

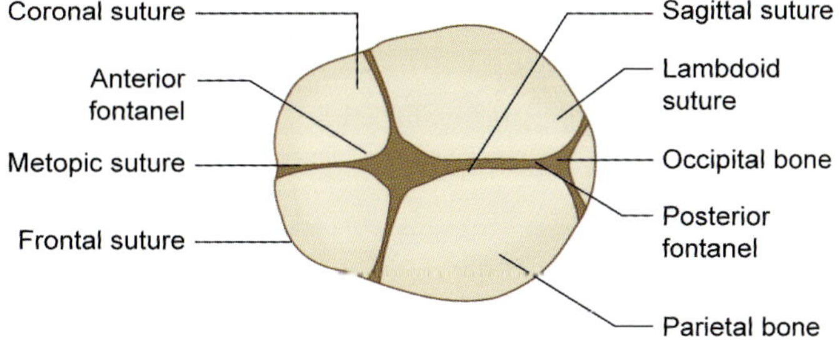

Fig. 1: Newborn skull.

and loss of normal venous pulsation. It is best to assess anterior fontanel when the child is calm and held upright. The sunken fontanel indicates dehydration.

Bulging AF is seen meningitis, congestive cardiac failure (CCF), vitamin A intoxication, lead poisonings, pseudotumor cerebri, and hypophosphatasia. Although a slight depression of the fontanel is common in normal infants, sunken fontanel is a sign of dehydration.

METHOD OF EXAMINATION

- The infant is held in erect position, quiet (not crying).
- The skull is gently palpated in a rotary, gentle movement progressing systematically from front back.
- Right middle finger feels for the "soft-spot" and assesses:
  - Presence (open) or absence (closure)
  - Size of AF (length + width)/2 and plot on normogram. Large if >2 SD.
  - Feel for tenseness, bulging, or depression
  - Feel for other fontanel

Note: Immediately after birth, there is overriding of sutures, and it may conceal the details of AF; hence always examine the child at 24 hours of age when normal separation of sutures has taken place.

Normal

Anterior fontanel closes by 9–18 months.

Posterior fontanel is either closed at birth or closes at 2 months.

173 CHAPTER

Friction Rub

The sound, heard through the stethoscope, made by the rubbing together of the inflamed layers of pericardium in patients with pericarditis or of pleura in patients with pleurisy. A pleural friction rub is an adventitious breath sound heard on auscultation of the lung. The pleural rub sound results from the movements of inflamed and roughened pleural surfaces against one another during movement of the chest wall. The pericardial rub is heard over the left sternal border in end expiration with patient leaning forward. It has a rasping or cracking sound.

It is heard with the diaphragm over the liver and spleen. Friction rub is high pitched sound heard in association with the respiration. This is heard over the enlarged liver or spleen suggestive of perihepatitis and splenitis. It is heard in chronic myeloid leukemia, infectious mononucleosis, malaria, sickle cell anemia, subacute bacterial endocarditis, and liver malignancy.

Frequency of Micturition

It includes urgency, daytime frequency, nocturia, and urge incontinence. It occurs because of the following factors:

- A reduced bladder capacity
- Peripheral edema-particularly dependent edema in old age, or in association with immobility
- Congestive cardiac failure
- Diabetes mellitus and insipidus

These conditions should be treated according to their needs.

CAUSES OF FREQUENCY OF MICTURITION

- Physiological age related
- Stress
- Cold weather
- Emotional attention seeking
- Urinary tract infection
- *Urinary tract abnormalities:*
    - Ureteric reflux
    - Obstruction
        - Neurogenic bladder
        - Posterior urethral reflux
- *Metabolic:*
    - Diabetes mellitus
    - Diabetes insipidus
- Urinary colic
- Pelvic appendicitis

175 CHAPTER

Furuncle

It is a perifollicular dermal abscess that is usually caused by *Staphylococcus aureus*. It may be the result of extension of superficial folliculitis, or of direct inoculation via minor trauma. Hairy areas subject to friction or maceration, as well axillary and inguinal regions with high concentrations of sebaceous glands, are particularly vulnerable. Skin contacts with occlusive agents such as oils, tars, and adhesives are another common predisposing factor. The incidence furuncle is higher in older children and adolescents.

The lesion begins as a small dermal nodule around hair follicle, which initially may produce mild discomfort and itching. As it gradually enlarges, pain worsens and is aggravated by touching and motion of the involved area. With expansion overlying skin becomes reddened, central necrosis begins to occur, and with inflammation and pressure infection begins to increase. Application of warm compresses can hasten this process.

Gag Reflex

The glossopharyngeal nerve conveys motor fibers to the stylopharyngeus muscle; general sensory fibers from the posterior third of the tongue, pharynx, tonsil, internal surface of the tympanic membrane, and skin of external ear. The nerve is gag reflex.

A swab stick touches the posterior pharyngeal wall. It leads to violent contraction of pharyngeal and palatal muscles. There will be symmetric elevation of the palate. The afferent is through the IXth cranial nerve. The reflex center is in the medulla. The efferent impulse is through the vagus nerve IX cranial nerve lesion is commonly associated with Xth and XIIth cranial nerves. The injuries include birth trauma, ischemia, mass lesions, motor neuron disease, retropharyngeal abscess, and Guillain–Barré syndrome.

CHAPTER 177

Gait, Abnormalities

Gait is defined as the propulsive movement of body, characterized by "stance phase" and "swing phase". Gait is formally tested by exposing the lower limbs (by taking off the clothes) and asking the child to walk bare footed, on a flat surface. The child should be asked to walk away from the examiner, to turn round a given point and then to come toward him again. The child is also made to walk on his toes (tests plantar flexion) and heels (tests dorsiflexion) and stand on one leg (tests gluteus medius).

Watching the patient arise, stand and walk forms the most important aspect of neurological examination. A normal gait requires integrity of peripheral nervous system and central nervous system, good proprioception, vision, muscular contraction, reciprocal limb actions, righting reflexes, and coordination of muscular action. Most disorders of muscles, nerves, spinal cord, cerebellum, brainstem, basal ganglia, and cerebrum cause disturbance of gait that are characteristic.

TYPES OF GAIT

Normal Gait

One complete walk cycle consists of a stance phase (when foot is on the ground, supporting as well as propelling the body forward) and a swing phase (when the foot is advanced forward without ground contact). Each leg alternately goes through stance and swing phase rhythmically, carrying the body forward. There is a simultaneous swinging of the arms so as to maintain support. A normal gait requires integrity of peripheral nervous system and central nervous system, proprioceptors, and coordination of muscular action.

Normal gait at different stages

- *1-year-old child:* Wide-based stance, short steps, elbows flexed. No reciprocal arm movement. Foot stroke occurs with initial heel stroke.
- *2-year-old child:*
  - Increased velocity and step length
  - Decreased cadence
- *After 3 years:* Toward adult pattern
- *7 years:* Adult pattern

Abnormal Gait

A child who bears weight for a longer duration on one side than the other, during walking has a painful limp (antalgic gait).

If he walks with the hip markedly flexed, holding his thigh while walking and bears weight on the tip of the toes for as brief a time as possible, he probably has pain in the hip. If he walks on the outer side of the foot, there is probably lifts the whole foot pain in the metatarsophalangeal joint of great toe. If it occurs without a smooth heel-off-toe-off cycle, it indicates a painful foot/stiff knee.

In-toe and out-toe gait: This is determined by asking the child to walk straight. The long axis of the foot is compared with the direction in which the child is walking. If the foot is directed inwardly, it is called in-toe gait (commonly due to internal femoral torsion and internal tibial torsion). If the foot is directed outwardly, it is called out-toe gait (commonly due to external tibial and femoral torsion).

CAUSES OF GAIT

Neuromuscular Causes

- *Hemiplegic gait:* This is also called spastic gait or circumduction gait. There is circumduction movement at the hip joint of the affected side. The patient circumducts a leg dragging the toe, with the ipsilateral arm held in partial flexion. The hip is raised on affected side due to inability to flex the hemiparetic limb. The main causes are congenital cerebral palsy or acute stroke syndrome.
- *Paraplegic gait:* This is also called scissor's gait. This is due to excess adductor tone at hip joint and spasticity. This is seen with cerebral palsy and acquired spastic paraparesis.
- *Ataxic gait (reeling):* It is characterized by unsteady, uncoordinated and cannot walk in a straight line. This is seen in cerebellar ataxia due to cerebellar diseases, periphery sensory loss.
- *Waddling gait, i.e., duck-like-gait:* This is seen in:
  - Duchenne muscular dystrophy
  - Bilateral congenital diaphragmatic hernia (CDH)
  - Polymyositis
  - Myelodysplasia
  - Achondroplasia

Cerebellar Ataxic Gaits (Staggering or Reeling Gait)

Patient walks like a drunken man. Unsteady uncoordinated and cannot walk in straight line or around a chair.

Spastic Gait

Hemiplegic gait (circumduction gait) patient circumducts a leg dragging the toe, placing the ball down without a heel strike, with the ipsilateral arm held in partial flexion.

Paraplegic Gait

- Spastic diplegic gait (scissor gait, due to excess adductor tone at hip joint and crouch gait-with knees flexed while walking)
- Spastic ataxic gait (cerebral palsy and spinocerebellar degeneration)

Parkinsonian Gait

Walks slowly with short steps, lacks arm swing, and turns en-block like a statue.

Festinating Gait

Small short steps as if chasing one's own center of gravity

Choreiform Gait

Choreiform movements increase during walking.

Cerebral Gait (Apraxic Gait)

Dancing bear gait: Stepping on the same spot as if trying to free the feet from thick, sticky mud, e.g., bilateral cerebral lesion such as Alzheimer's disease.

Psychiatric Gaits

Astasia abasia (astasia = not standing; abasia = not walking) in hysteria. Hysterical inability to stand and walk. The patient is ataxic and from the hip rather than ankles. It increases on attention and patient does not hurt himself.

Equinus Gait (Toe-walking)

Toe-walking can be a normal finding in children up to 3 years of age. Persistent toe-walking thereafter or acquired toe-walking at a later age is considered abnormal and necessitates careful evaluation. The differential diagnosis for persistent or acquired toe-walking includes the following:

- Neuromuscular disorders, such as cerebral palsy, Duchenne muscular dystrophy, or spinal cord abnormality resulting from a tethered spinal cord or diastematomyelia
- Congenital Achilles tendon contracture (idiopathic toe-walking)
- Habitual toe-walking
- Lower extremity length discrepancy

Neuromuscular Disorders

The neuromuscular disorder most likely to produce an equinus gait, either unilateral or bilateral, is cerebral palsy. The most common type of cerebral palsy is spastic diplegia, a disorder in which the lower extremities are more involved than the upper extremities. Prematurity is a common risk factor for spastic diplegia. It can be symmetric or asymmetric, with one side being slightly more involved than the other. Spastic diplegia tends to produce a bilateral equinus gait. Spastic hemiplegia, in which only one side is involved, is usually caused by birth trauma (asphyxia), perinatal stroke, or underlying congenital malformation and results in unilateral toe-walking.

Acquired or late-onset toe-walking is usually a result of a developing neuromuscular disorder, such as Duchenne muscular dystrophy. As fat and fibrous tissues replace muscle, equinus and other contractures occur. There is usually a history of progressive clumsiness and frequent episodes of falling. The diagnosis of muscular dystrophy is usually made when the child is between 3 and 5 years of age. The diagnosis is confirmed by markedly elevated creatine phosphokinase levels, by muscle biopsy, or by genetic testing. In a spastic equinus gait without contracture, physical therapy and orthoses (daytime, nighttime, or both) may be beneficial. If a contracture has developed, serial casting may be performed in young children, whereas surgical lengthening of the Achilles is usually necessary in older children.

CHAPTER 178

Gallbladder, Palpable

A grossly distended gallbladder in a thin subject may be visible as a distinct globular swelling in the right upper abdomen. It is felt as an oval, smooth swelling moving downward close behind the anterior abdominal wall. It is attached to the undersurface of a palpable liver in the right nipple line. The tumor generally extends inward as well as downward. It may cross the midline below the level of the umbilicus. It may be large enough to be palpable bimanually in a thin patient. It feels firm and tense rather than hard. An impaired but not quite dull note is obtained on percussion.

The examiner draws a line from the left anterior superior iliac spine through the umbilicus. This line is then extended further so that it meets the right subcostal margin, provided the shape of the abdomen is normal. The gallbladder is better seen than felt when enlarged.

CAUSES OF GALLBLADDER ENLARGEMENT

- Empyema of the gallbladder
- Chronic pancreatitis
- Cholecystitis
- Enteric fever
- Gallstone
- Obstruction of the cystic duct by a gallstone
- Mucocele

CHAPTER 179

Gallop Rhythm

A first sound, second sound, and prominent third sound will cause tripling, as would a fourth sound, first sound, and second sound. The type of tripling commonly called rhythm occurs when the third fourth heart sounds sum in the presence of tachycardia. This may or may not be pathologic. In infants with a physiologically long PR interval and tachycardia, summation tripling can be normal; presence of a pathologic third sound or fourth sound and tachycardia, however, would be abnormal, you must try to identify the sound that causes the tripling. Causes of gallop rhythm include pulses alternans, tachypnea, wheezing, tachycardia, and fatigue.

CHAPTER 180

Gastroesophageal Reflux

Gastroesophageal reflux (GER) is the passage of gastric contents into the esophagus with or without regurgitation and vomiting. GER is a normal physiologic process that occurs several times a day in healthy infants, children, and adults. When this reflex of gastric contents causes troublesome symptoms and/or complications, it is known as gastroesophageal reflux disease (GERD).

Neurologically impaired children like those with cerebral palsy have increased risk of severe GERD due to multiple factors such as low pressure of the lower esophageal sphincter and predominant supine position.

The common symptoms associated with gastroesophageal reflux disease in children are:

- Recurrent regurgitation
- Weight loss or poor weight gain
- Irritability (in infants)
- Heartburn or chest pain (older children)
- Hematemesis, dysphagia, and odynophagia (if complicated by esophagitis or stricture esophagus)
- Wheezing, stridor, cough, and hoarseness
- Sandifer syndrome, an uncommon manifestation, characterized by spasmodic torsional dystonia with arching of the back and opisthotonic posturing

CHAPTER 181 Gastrointestinal Bleeding

Children with gastrointestinal bleeding generally present with hematemesis, hematochezia, or melena. An upper gastrointestinal bleed is bleeding from the esophagus, stomach, or duodenum. Upper sources account for the majority of gastrointestinal bleeds in children. If the site of bleeding is distal to the ligament of Treitz, it is a lower gastrointestinal bleed. Blood passed per rectum can originate from either an upper or lower gastrointestinal source. Occult bleeding may occur from disorders at numerous sites.

HEMATEMESIS AND MELENA—UPPER GASTROINTESTINAL BLEED

Examination

In addition to assessing for pallor, cutaneous lesions may help determine the underlying cause of bleeding. Petechiae can indicate disseminated intravascular coagulation, hypersplenism, or another bleeding abnormality. Hyperpigmented lesions of the oral or anal mucosa may indicate Peutz-Jeghers disease. Cutaneous telangiectasia and hemangiomas may indicate such diseases as Osler-Weber-Rendu syndrome and ataxia-telangiectasia, or they may simply suggest a predisposition for vascular malformations. Palmar erythema, spider angioma, or jaundice suggest underlying liver disease. Scleral icterus may be subtle but can be the first sign of liver disease and may be more easily appreciated than jaundice in darker-skinned individuals.

Differential Diagnosis

In infants, esophagitis, gastritis, and ulcers are the most common causes of upper gastrointestinal bleeding. Esophagitis may be associated with dysphagia, irritability, and arching with feeds. Milk protein sensitivity should be considered as well, although it more often presents with blood in stool. Trauma or infection (such as cytomegalovirus, herpes simplex, or fungal) can cause mucosal irritation presenting as hematemesis. Anatomic abnormalities including duplication cysts or vascular abnormalities may also lead to hematemesis or melena in infants.

In older children, mucosal lesions remain common causes of bleeding. Mallory-Weiss tears are associated with repeated forceful vomiting from a variety of causes (e.g., acute gastroenteritis). The forcefulness of the vomiting causes a tear in the distal esophagus at the level of the lower esophageal sphincter. The history is generally one of frequent non-bloody vomiting that then becomes hematemesis. Prolapse gastropathy, caused by prolapse of gastric mucosa into the distal esophagus, can similarly occur after forceful vomiting and lead to hematemesis. Reactive gastritis secondary to medication [nonsteroidal anti-inflammatory drugs (NSAIDs)] or infection [*Helicobacter pylori* (*H. pylori*)] are also common causes of upper gastrointestinal bleeding. Children with known or unknown liver disease can develop esophageal varices that may lead to large-volume hematemesis and melena (or hematochezia if bleeding is brisk). Ulcers, although rare, can also lead to significant blood loss and may be related to *H. pylori* infection, stress such as surgery or burns, and foreign body ingestion, specifically button batteries, which can lead to significant bleeding.

HEMATOCHEZIA—LOWER GASTROINTESTINAL BLEED

Differential Diagnosis

Anal fissures are probably the most frequent cause of streaks of bright red blood mixed with stool. The bleeding may be associated with hard bowel movements but may occur from straining with normal bowel movements. There is also an association with group A streptococcal perianal cellulitis and bleeding. Anal fissure may be a manifestation of milk protein allergy with resultant perianal inflammation and subsequent constipation to avoid painful defecation. More often, a milk protein allergy will present with specks of blood within the stool. There may be a history of increasing frequency and amount of blood and mucus in the stool. The infant may exhibit cramping with bowel movements and vomiting may be part of the presentation. Often there is a family history of food allergies. Milk protein allergy can be seen in infants fed cow's milk- or soy protein-based formulas, as well as in breastfed infants. Ischemic bowel disease, including necrotizing enterocolitis and volvulus, may lead to rectal bleeding and an acutely ill, sick-appearing neonate, or infant. Risk factors for necrotizing enterocolitis include prematurity, cardiac surgery, polycythemia, chronic diarrhea, and gastrointestinal malformations.

Infectious colitis is common in both infants and children and causes frequent, often watery, bloody bowel movements. There may be cramping pain before and during the bowel movement as a result of the colitis. Common pathogens include *Salmonella* and *Shigella* organisms, especially with dysentery type stools, but *Escherichia coli* (*E. coli*) O157:H7.

For young children, intussusception and Meckel diverticulum are common causes of hematochezia. The hallmark of intussusception is the presence of "currant jelly" stools associated with colicky abdominal pain, lethargy, or irritability. Meckel diverticulum occurs in 1–3% of the population and manifests by the age of 2 years in about 50% of patients.

Juvenile polyps also present with painless rectal bleeding but are uncommon in children <1 year of age with peak incidence between ages 5 and 7 years.

In older children, inflammatory bowel disease becomes a more common cause of hematochezia. The rectal bleeding varies from occult to frank blood in the bowel movements. Blood is present in 100% of cases of ulcerative colitis but in only 30–50% of cases of Crohn disease.

Henoch–Schönlein purpura is a vasculitic syndrome that can cause bloody stools. It is often accompanied by cramping abdominal pain, purpuric rash (palpable purpura), joint swelling, scalp edema (infants and toddlers), and occasionally, nephritis **(Figs. 1A and B)**.

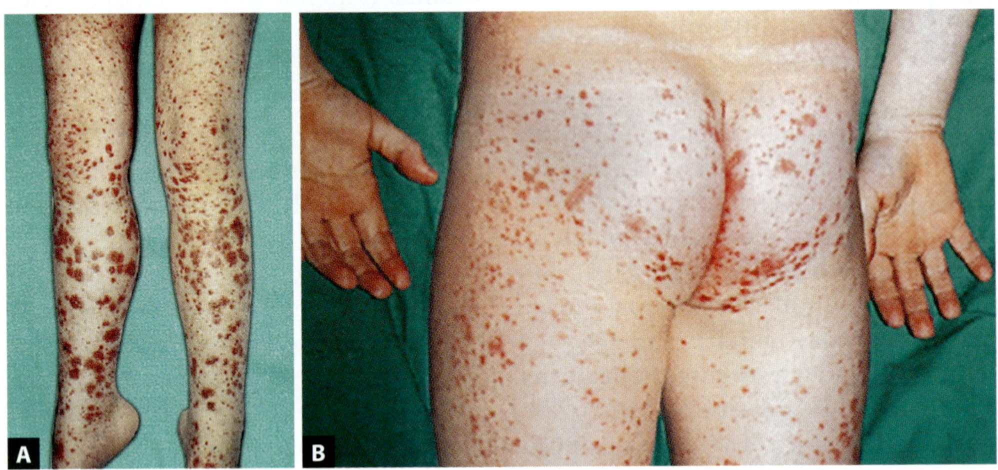

Figs. 1A and B: Henoch–Schönlein purpura.

CHAPTER 182

Genu Valgum

It is seen between 3 and 4 years of age. It occurs when the center of the knee joint is medial to the biomechanical axis to the lower extremity. Clinically, an individual with a distance of >3 cm between the medial malleoli likely has genus valgum **(Fig. 1)**. The maximum valgus of 12° occurs by 3–4 years of age. By 7 years of age, always inspect for varus or valgus misalignment with the knee in a weight-bearing (standing) position (8 degrees in females, 7 degrees in males).

Overall, 95% of cases of developmental physiologic genu varum and genu valgum resolve with growth, even in children with more pronounced physiologic genu varus or genu valgus.

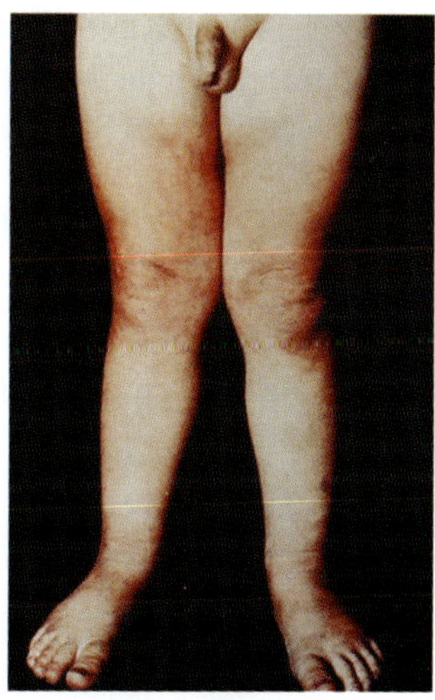

Fig. 1: Genu valgum.

Genu Varus

Genu varus (bowleg) is physiologic in infancy. When the tibiofemoral angle is <15° in varus. The deformity is symmetric **(Figs. 1A and B)**.

GENU VARUM (PHYSIOLOGIC BOWLEG)

Here the center of the knee joint falls lateral to axis connecting the centers of the hip and ankle joints. Space between the medial femoral condyles when standing with feet together is >3–5 cm.

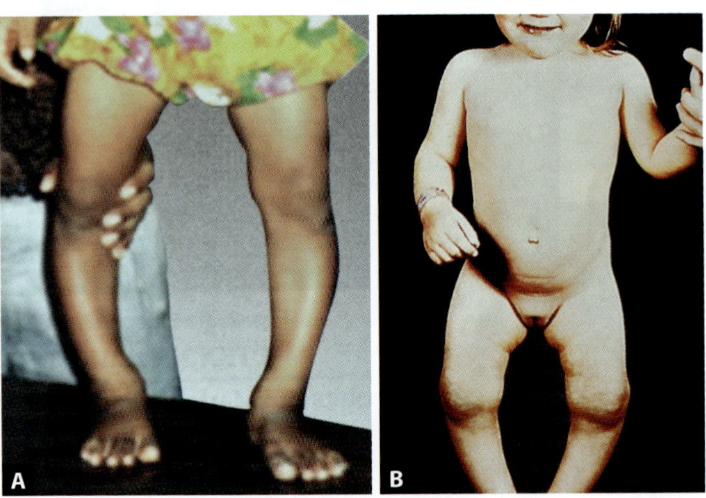

Figs. 1A and B: Genu varus.

184 CHAPTER

Geographic Tongue (Benign Migratory Glossitis)

A patch/patches of the tongue dorsum become depapillated. The patches heal on one side and progress on the another so that they "wander" over the tongue mall, red to purple spots form on the dorsal surface and edges of the tongue, gradually spread out, loose their papillae and form smooth, irregularly shaped, gray to white bordered, black, and inflamed patches **(Fig. 1)**. Although mostly painless, discomfort may be noted when eating spicy or acidic foods.

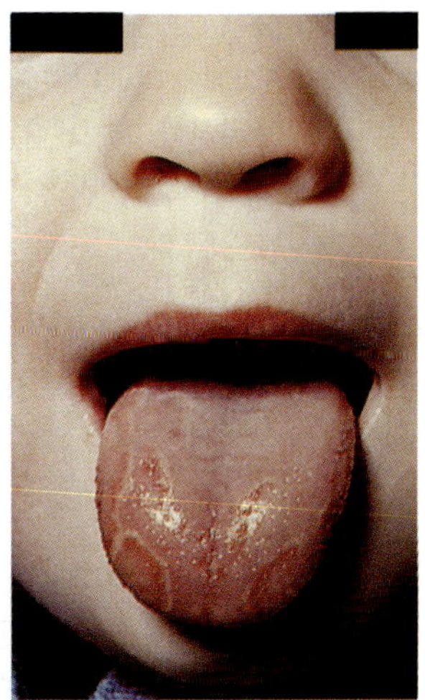

Fig. 1: Geographic tongue.

185 CHAPTER

Glasgow Coma Scale

The Glasgow Coma Scale provides a useful measure to assess the level of consciousness in a person following a traumatic brain injury. Basically, it is used to help gauge the severity of acute brain injury.

It is based on the observation of level of response to graded stimuli in three modes—eye opening, motor function, and verbal utterance. In the first mode, spontaneous eye opening and blinking score the highest grade, eye opening in response to voice the next highest, eye opening in response to painful stimuli the next, and finally no response of eyes opening to stimuli the lowest.

It scored between 3 and 15, with 3 being the worst and 15 being the best. Mild head injuries are generally defined as those associated with a score of 13–15, and moderate are those with 9–12. A score of 8 or less defines severe head injury. A score of 7 or less is considered comatose.

The highest motor response is voluntary movement to command, followed by localizing response to painful stimuli, withdrawal from painful stimuli, a pathological flexor response (sometimes called decorticate), a pathological extensor response (sometimes called decerebrate), and finally no response at all to pain.

CHAPTER 186 Glaucoma

Glaucoma is an increase in the intraocular pressure. It may be either due to an increase in the formation of aqueous humor, or a defect in its exit or due to raised pressure in the episcleral veins. Of these, the first and last are of little importance. It is divided into (1) primary glaucoma which comprises of: (a) simple glaucoma, (b) closed angle glaucoma; (2) secondary glaucoma which is due to a specific anomaly or disease of the eye. The signs and symptoms include epiphora, blepharospasm, hazy cornea, macrocornea, and cupping of the optic disk **(Figs. 1A and B)**.

Pediatric glaucomas result from abnormalities of the aqueous outflow pathways (primary congenital glaucoma) or abnormalities that affect other parts of the eye (secondary glaucoma). Several genes causing primary congenital glaucoma, usually autosomal recessive, have been identified. Primary congenital glaucoma is bilateral in about 65% of patients. It presents as a classic triad consisting of blepharospasm, photophobia, and epiphora. The cornea may be cloudy due to edema resulting from elevated intraocular pressure. The cornea also enlarges, and the axial length of the eye may increase with elevated intraocular pressure. Onset usually occurs in the 1st year of life; only 25% are present at birth. If glaucoma presents after the age of 5 years, it is known as primary juvenile open-angle glaucoma. The natural history of untreated primary congenital glaucoma is blindness resulting from progressive corneal opacification and optic nerve damage.

Secondary glaucoma may present similarly to primary glaucoma but is associated with other factors such as ocular trauma, inflammation, prolonged steroid use, or cataract. Some systemic conditions such as neurofibromatosis are also associated with secondary glaucoma. The differential diagnosis of congenital glaucoma includes

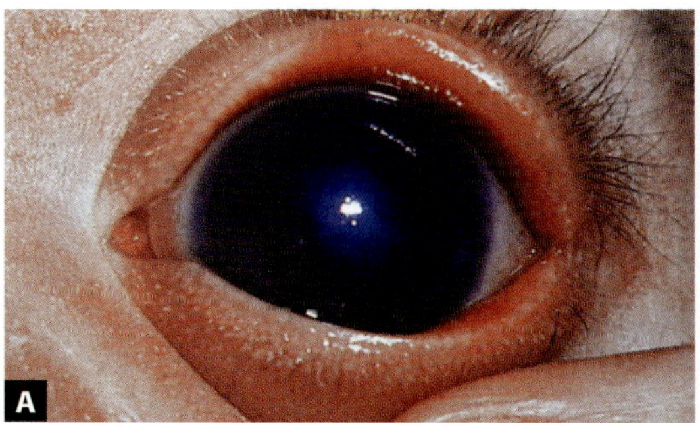
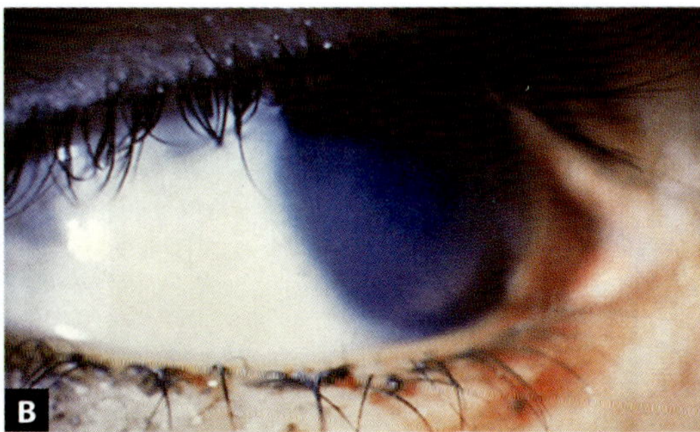

Figs. 1A and B: Glaucoma.

conditions that demonstrate corneal opacities or an enlarged cornea. Epiphora also occurs with conjunctivitis, corneal trauma, and nasolacrimal duct obstruction (NLDO). Photophobia is observed in infants with corneal trauma, corneal deposits, cystinosis, and inflammation (uveitis). Corneal opacification can also be found in infants with corneal dystrophies, metabolic storage diseases such as mucopolysaccharidoses and forceps-related obstetric trauma.

CHAPTER 187

Graves Disease

It is a condition in which a stimulating antibody directed against the TSH receptor (thyroid receptor antibody or thyroid-stimulating immunoglobulin) increases the endogenous production of thyroid hormone. Hashimoto thyroiditis is also the cause of hyperthyroidism. Less common causes include autonomously functioning adenomas, toxic multinodular goiters, activating mutations of the TSH receptor gene, and exogenous intake of thyroid hormones. Exophthalmos is usually less dramatic in children than adults. Proptosis and lid lag are seen in children. The bruit may be heard over the gland. T4 and T3 concentrations are elevated, and TSH concentrations are suppressed.

188 CHAPTER

Gums, Hypertrophy

It is caused predominantly by fibrous tissue and cellular infiltration into the gingival mucosa. This leads to hypertrophy of gums. The important cause is dental infections **(Fig. 1)**.

CAUSES OF GINGIVITIS

- Dental caries
- Overcrowding of teeth
- Scurvy
- Mouth breathing
- Infection
  - Herpes
  - Oral thrush
  - *Staphylococcus aureus*
- Drugs—phenytoin

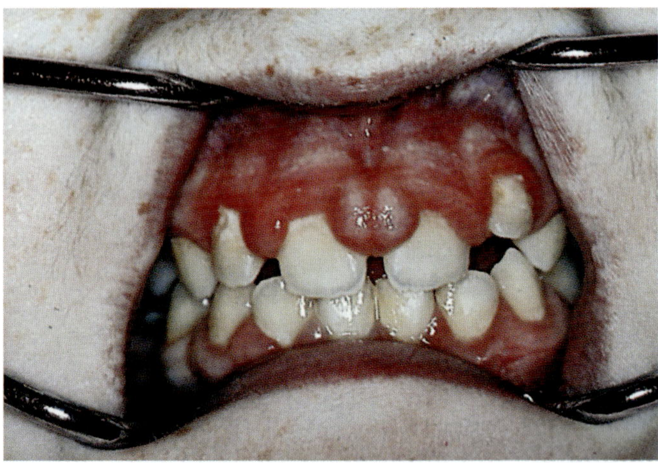

Fig. 1: Hypertrophy of gums.

CHAPTER 189

Gynecomastia

Gynecomastia is common in neonates and at puberty. The cause may be an undue sensitivity of breast tissue to normal circulating hormones; sometimes the enlargement is unilateral.

CAUSES OF GYNECOMASTIA

- Newborn
- Puberty
- Acromegaly
- Thyrotoxicosis
- Hepatic cirrhosis
- Renal failure
- Drugs
  - Digitalis
  - Isoniazid (INH)
  - Gonadotrophins
  - Estrogens
  - Progesterone
  - Spironolactone
- Klinefelter's syndrome
- Adrenal tumor
- Testicular tumor

NEONATAL GYNECOMASTIA

Approximately 70% of male neonates have some breast enlargement. Placental estrogens and human chorionic gonadotropin stimulating the Leydig cells of the baby's testes to produce estrogen will cause neonatal gynecomastia **(Fig. 1)**.

PUBERTAL GYNECOMASTIA

There is a rise in plasm estradiol which anticipates the expected pubertal rise in plasma testosterone. Along with the increased estradiol there is an increase in prolactin, but the levels fall as the gynecomastia develops.

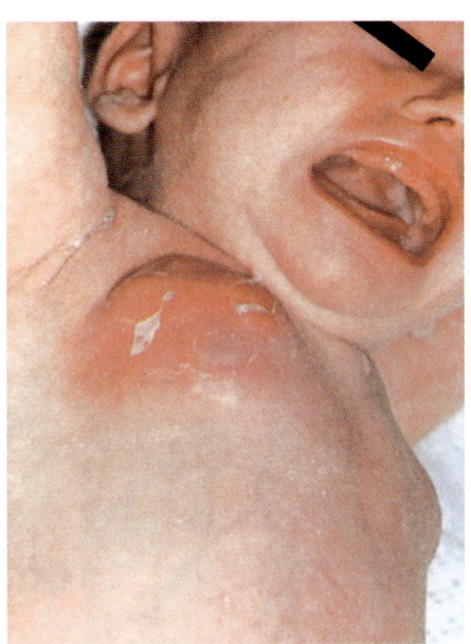

Fig. 1: Neonatal mastitis.

Halitosis

Halitosis (Latin *halitus* means breath) means offensive odor of the breath. Physical examination must in particular aim at excluding orodental conditions which explain halitosis, foreign body in the nose, chronic rhinitis, acute or chronic tonsillitis diphtheria, etc. Lung abscess and bronchiectasis, once suspected from the history, can convincing be excluded or confirmed by chest examination and radiology.

BAD ORODENTAL HYGIENE

The causes of halitosis secondary to bad orodental hygiene include septic tooth, dental canes (which may entrap the food debris), gingivitis, stomatitis, etc.

CHRONIC RHINITIS

Chronic rhinitis, particularly, atrophic, and allergic may be responsible for halitosis. In atrophic rhinitis, fetor is often a remarkable feature. Interestingly, it is taken cognizance by the relatives or the examiner. The patient is virtually of it because of anosmia. The nostrils are widened and the nose broadened. Nasal mucosa appears congested and atrophic.

FOREIGN BODY IN THE NOSE

Halitosis along with unilateral nasal discharge and obstruction make a strong case for a foreign body such as a piece of food, crayon, plastic, bead, etc. in the nose. In addition, there are manifestations such as sneezing, local discomfort, and purulent malodorous or bloody discharge.

INFECTIONS

Halitosis may be encountered in some cases of acute or chronic tonsillitis, diphtheria, Vincent's angina, and infectious mononucleosis.

Vincent's angina, caused by usual oral flora and heavy overgrowth of fusiform bacilli and spirochetes in chronically ill and malnourished children, is characterized by remarkable fetid odor, fever, malaise, and oral lesions consisting of gray necrotic membrane and tiny ulcers over tender, congested gingivae.

BRONCHIECTASIS

Halitosis is a prominent feature of bronchiectasis which is characterized by permanent dilatation of the bronchi and bronchioles as a result of obstruction and/or infection, leading to cavitation of bronchial wall and tissue destruction.

LUNG ABSCESS

Pulmonary abscess not only produces foul-smelling sputum but frequently halitosis as well. The other symptoms of chronic abscess which usually develops insidiously are fever, persistent cough, and at times, dyspnea, and chest pain. Clubbing develops if the child remains without treatment over a prolonged period.

CHAPTER 191

Hamman Sign

It is a mediastinal crunch. It is a crunching rasping sound, synchronous with heartbeat, heard over the precordium in spontaneous mediastinal emphysema. It is felt to heart beating against air filled tissues.

It is found with mediastinal emphysema. There is a great variety of noisy crackles and clicking and gurgling sounds. These are synchronous with the heartbeat and not particularly so with respiration, but sounds can be more pronounced toward the end of expiration. They are easier to hear when the patient leans to the left or lies down on the left side.

CHAPTER 192

Harlequin Color Change

The harlequin color change is a distinctive condition observed in infants lying on their sides. It is characterized by marked erythema on the dependent side of the infant's body with simultaneous blanching of the nondependent side. This phenomenon occurs more often in premature infants but may be observed in full-term newborns.

The change may be caused by autonomic immaturity, which results in an altered peripheral vascular tone. Although it typically occurs within the 1st 3 weeks of life, harlequin color change is most often noted at 2–5 days of age. The changes develop abruptly and usually resolve within 20 minutes. There is generally no need for treatment.

193 CHAPTER

Harrison's Sulcus

It is sequelae to chronic respiratory disease and rickets. A depression may be evident along the lower border of chest at the site of insertion of diaphragm. This appears due to the pull of diaphragm in the weakened chest wall. There is flaring outward of the costal margin **(Figs. 1A to D)**. This is seen in active rickets, is called Harrison's sulcus.

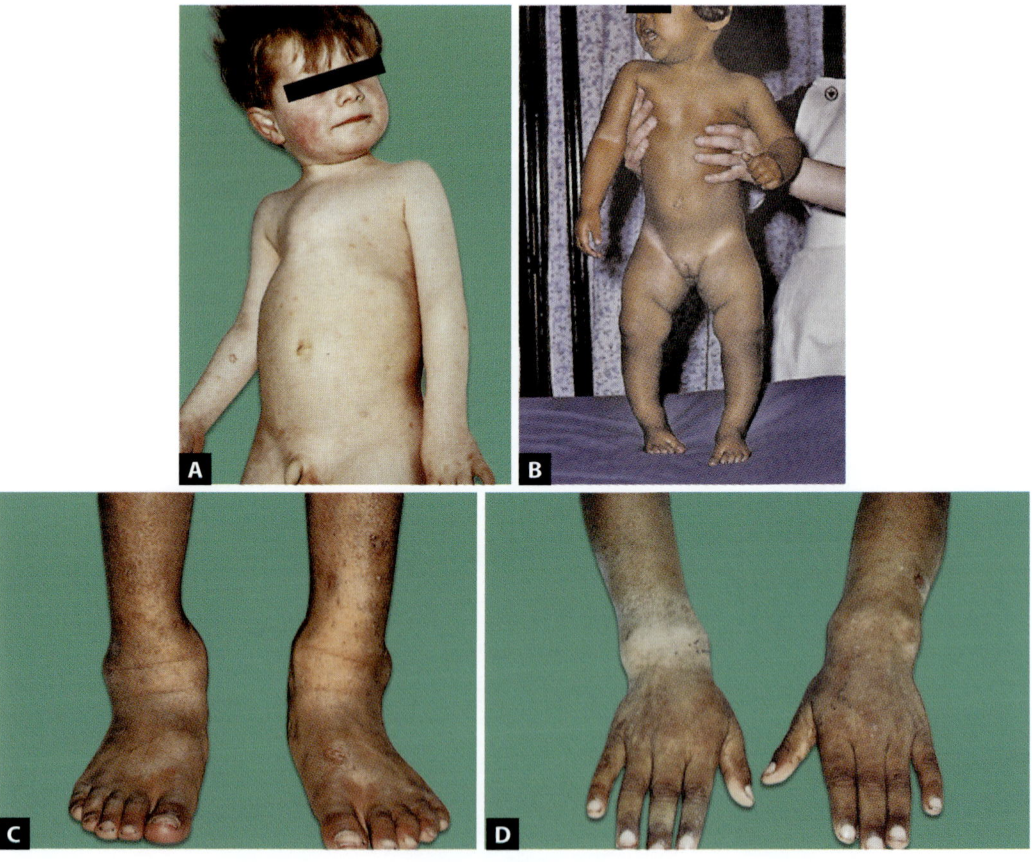

Figs. 1A to D: Rickets.

CHAPTER 194 Head Bobbing

In synchrony with each inspiration, the head is noted to bob forward owing to neck flexion. This phenomenon is probably explained by contraction of scalene and sternocleidomastoid muscle, which are accessory muscles of inspiration.

This is a sign of dyspnea, best observed in an exhausted or sleeping infant lying in its mother's arm. The head must be unsupported except for the suboccipital area.

Head bobbing consists of jerky head movements at a frequency of two to three cycles per second and resembles that of a doll's head atop a spring. In childhood, it may appear as part of spasmus nutans or the bobble-head doll syndrome. Spasmus nutans is a benign disorder of unknown etiology that occurs in early infancy and is characterized by nystagmus (binocular or monocular), head nodding, and head tilt. Neurologic examination is otherwise normal. The syndrome lasts 1–2 years and spontaneously resolves. The bobble-head doll syndrome consists of intermittent head nodding and is seen in association with an underlying central nervous system (CNS) structural abnormality, often a third ventricular cyst or tumor.

Headache

Headache is a frequent complaint of older children (greater than the age of 8 years). It is a much rarer and sometimes ominous complaint in the younger child and must be taken seriously.

Headache, therefore, is a diagnosis that requires attention and good listening skills for the diagnosis of the underlying cause of the headache.

Headache can be either acute or chronic. The various causes of headache are listed in **Box 1**.

- *Vascular-migraine, cluster headaches, and hypertension*
- *Metabolic hypoglycemia*
- *Drugs-alcohol, nitrates, calcium channel blockers, nonsteroidal anti-inflammatory agents (NSAIDs)*
- *Psychogenic-tension headaches, stress, depression, and anxiety*

BOX 1: Acute headache.

- *Infectious:*
  - Any acute infection
  - Meningitis
  - Encephalitis
  - Sinusitis/mastoiditis
  - Brain abscess
- *Post-traumatic:*
  - Concussion
  - Subdural or epidural hematoma
  - Cerebral contusion
- *Vascular:*
  - Subarachnoid hemorrhage
  - Intraparenchymal hemorrhage
  - Vasculitis
  - Migraine
- *Increased intracranial pressure (ICP):*
  - Brain tumor
  - Subdural/epidural hematoma
  - Malignant hypertension
  - Pseudotumor cerebri
  - Trauma (closed head injury)
- *Other:*
  - Acute angle-closure glaucoma
  - Alcohol/drug ingestions
  - Chronic (recurrent) headache

PRIMARY HEADACHES

Tension-type Headaches

Tension-type headache (TTH) occurs in up to 15% of older children. Prevalence increases with age such that TTH is the most frequent headache type in children between 8 and 12 years of age. Younger children also experience both episodic and chronic TTH, usually with mild-to-moderate symptoms.

Tension-type headaches are classified as either episodic or chronic. Both episodic and chronic TTH are further classified as having associated pericranial tenderness or as lacking such tenderness. This tenderness is typically present between headaches and increases during episodes.

Episodic tension-type headache is categorized as either infrequent or frequent. Infrequent episodic TTH is defined as 10 or more episodes total, occurring less than once per month on average. Frequent episodic TTH is defined as 10 or more episodes total, occurring on 1-14 days per month on average for over 3 months.

Individual episodes of either may last from 30 minutes to as long as a week and have at least two of the following features: (1) Bilateral location, (2) pressing or tightening (non-pulsating) quality, (3) mild or moderate intensity, (4) not aggravated by routine physical activity such as walking or climbing stairs. Nausea or vomiting must be absent; if present, migraine should be considered. Either photophobia or phonophobia may be present; if both are present simultaneously, migraine should be considered.

Chronic tension-type headaches are defined as headaches occurring at least 15 days a month for over 3 months, with features otherwise similar to episodic TTH.

MIGRAINE HEADACHES

The diagnosis of migraine headache is typically based on the historical description of episodes. In children, the headaches are less frequent, are shorter in duration, and respond better to treatment. Vomiting and abdominal pain are more common in children than in adults. Pain is more frequently bilateral in children, though tends to become unilateral after the onset of puberty. The pain may be frontal or facial, instead of the more typical temporal location. A family history of migraines is common, with up to 90% of children having a 1st- or 2nd-degree relative with recurrent headaches.

Migraines are categorized based on the presence or absence of an associated aura. Migraine without aura is the most common migraine phenotype in pediatric patients.

Migraine without aura: It has been recognized that children may have shorter-duration headaches, so an allowance has been made to reduce the duration to 2-72 hours or 1-72 hours with diary confirmation **(Box 2)**. The pain typically onsets gradually and is dull and constant. At times, though, the pain of an episode may be sudden and severe, prompting concern for a thunderclap headache. More typically, pain increases in severity over the course of an individual episode and becomes throbbing. As the headache proceeds, the pain may generalize to the entire cranium. Intense nausea often accompanies migraines, with occasional vomiting.

Migraine with aura: In migraine with aura, the headache is preceded by sensory signs or symptoms termed an aura, which is caused by vasoconstriction and diminished blood flow to the affected region of the brain. In migraine with typical aura, the aura is visual and may consist of blurred vision, spreading scintillating scotomas, flashing lights, zigzag lines, and hemianopsia **(Box 3)**. These features typically last <60 minutes. Sensory auras are less common than visual auras and may consist of numbness or tingling. Further types of migraine with aura are classified by the specific aura symptoms.

BOX 2: Migraine without aura.

A. At least five attacks fulfilling criteria B-D
B. Headache attacks lasting 4–72 hours (untreated or unsuccessfully treated)
C. Headache has at least two of the following four characteristics:
   1. Unilateral location
   2. Pulsating quality
   3. Moderate or severe pain intensity
   4. Aggravation by or causing avoidance of routine physical activity (e.g., walking or climbing stairs)
D. During headache at least one of the following:
   1. Nausea and/or vomiting
   2. Photophobia and phonophobia
E. Not better accounted for by another International Classification of Headache Disorders, 3rd edition (ICHD-30) diagnosis

BOX 3: Migraine with typical aura.

A. At least two attacks fulfilling criteria B and C
B. Aura consisting of visual, sensory, and/or speech/language symptoms, each fully reversible, but no motor, brainstem, or retinal symptoms
C. At least two of the following four characteristics:
   1. At least one aura symptom spreads gradually over 5 or more minutes, and/or two or more symptoms occur in succession
   2. Each individual aura symptom lasts 5–60 minutes
   3. At least one aura symptom is unilateral
   4. The aura is accompanied, or followed within 60 minutes, by headache
D. Not better accounted for by another International Classification of Headache Disorders, 3rd edition (ICHD-3) diagnosis, and transient ischemic attack has been excluded

Cluster headache: Cluster headache is categorized as either episodic or chronic. Episodic cluster headaches occur in a series that may last for weeks or months, separated by remission periods of months to years, whereas chronic cluster headaches are defined as occurring for >1 year without such a remission period, or with remission periods that last <1 month. Cluster headaches are more common in individuals who smoke tobacco.

SECONDARY HEADACHES

Headache Associated with Trauma

Acute headache: If a child presents with a headache after trauma and has abnormal neurologic signs or symptoms, non-contrast CT of the head should be obtained emergently to assess for subarachnoid, subdural, or epidural intracranial bleed. Cervical spine radiographs should be obtained if cervical injury is suspected. If the child has focal neurologic deficits indicating possible vascular injury, magnetic resonance imaging (MRI) is indicated, potentially with MR angiography.

Headaches Associated with Vascular Disorders

Acute ischemic stroke: Headache is a feature of up to one-third of acute ischemic strokes. More commonly experienced symptoms are focal neurologic deficits such as weakness of the limbs and face or speech abnormalities; as such, every child presenting with a focal neurologic deficit must undergo evaluation for stroke. The headache in acute ischemic stroke is typically of moderate intensity, and otherwise lacks consistent features, though may occasionally present as a thunderclap headache. Similar headaches may also accompany transient ischemic attacks.

Headaches Associated with Nonvascular Intracranial Disorders

This category includes headaches due to a variety of causes including increased cerebrospinal fluid (CSF) pressure, decreased CSF pressure, noninfectious inflammation, neoplasms, intrathecal injection, seizures, and Chiari type I malformations.

Disorders Associated with Increased Cerebrospinal Fluid Pressure

Pseudotumor cerebri may be either primary or secondary to a variety of medical conditions. In idiopathic intracranial hypertension, a subset of primary pseudotumor cerebri, the typical patient is post-pubertal, obese, and female. Pseudotumor cerebri may also be due to obstructive, toxic, metabolic, or hormonal causes that may often be revealed through a thorough history and physical examination.

Pseudotumor cerebri may be diagnosed in the absence of papilledema if a sixth cranial nerve palsy is present and the patient has a normal neurologic examination, normal neuroimaging (including venography if indicated), an elevated CSF opening pressure, and a normal CSF profile. If the patient does not have a sixth cranial nerve palsy, then the diagnosis may be suggested (but not confirmed) if three of the following imaging requirements are met—empty sella, flattening of the posterior aspect of the globe, distention of the perioptic subarachnoid space with or without a tortuous optic nerve, and transverse venous sinus stenosis.

INTRACRANIAL MASSES

Brain neoplasms are the second most common type of childhood malignancy, though the overall incidence is low. As such, tumor is an infrequent cause of headache in children. The mechanisms by which tumors produce headaches include obstruction of CSF flow leading to hydrocephalus, or direct traction on dural or vascular structures.

Headaches Associated with Epileptic Seizures

Headache may be a preictal phenomenon in patients with focal epilepsy syndromes, or a consequence of an epileptic seizure. Postictal headaches tend to remit within hours of the cessation of seizure activity but may last as long as 72 hours. Headache occurring as an ictal phenomenon in partial seizures remits with or soon after the cessation of seizure activity.

INTRACRANIAL AND SYSTEMIC INFECTIONS

Infectious causes of headache are common and are typically benign, with the most common etiology being a viral upper respiratory tract infection. However, serious and life-threatening infections may present with headache. Meningitis and meningoencephalitis may present with a headache that is acute in onset and generalized. Fever, nuchal rigidity, alteration in sensorium, and abnormal neurologic findings may be present as well.

196 CHAPTER

Head Circumference

When a child's head circumference is two standard deviations or more above the mean, apply a tape measure to each of the parents' heads to see where their measurements fit on the chart before creating anxiety or considering further investigation. Once it has been established that having a large head is a familial characteristic and that the affected parent and child are both otherwise normal, no further investigation is necessary. This normal variant goes by the pretentious name benign familial megalencephaly.

Remember that skull bones grow in a direction perpendicular to the suture lines. The directions in which the skull can and cannot grow after synostosis of a suture are therefore predictable, as is the shape of the resulting cranial distortion. For example, if the sagittal suture fuses prematurely, further lateral growth of the skull is prevented. Anteroposterior growth continues (perpendicular to the coronal sutures), and the skull will become long and narrow (a condition known as dolichocephaly).

HEAD MEASUREMENT

Accurate measurement of the circumference is surprisingly difficult. Measure the largest circumference possible by wrapping the tape around the most prominent parts of the forehead and occiput. You should routinely take three measurements. If these measurements differ, you need to refine your technique. Even a slight variation in the position of the measuring tape changes the result significantly. Many infants and young children actively dislike head circumference measurement.

A single measurement of head circumference may identify significant microcephaly or macrocephaly. Of greater value is the pattern of growth over time. Accurate measurement and charting are critical. An increase in measurement from the 25th to the 75th percentile over a month may lead to early detection of hydrocephalus or to a distressed, angry family if either measurement is inaccurate. More importantly, computed tomography (CT) studies of the infant brain have been implicated in decreased cognitive and intellectual outcomes and increased lifetime risks of cancer. Diagnostic imaging of the young brain should be ordered only when there is reasonable evidence of a significant problem.

At birth, the head circumference is about 34 cm. It is about 2 cm more than the chest circumference. By 6–9 months, the two measurements become equal, after which the chest circumference overtakes the head circumference. In severely malnourished children, this overtaking may be delayed by 3–4 years due to poor development of thoracic cage.

It is measured until the normal child is 3 years of age. It is measured by steel or plastic tape **(Fig. 1)**. The maximum circumference of the head is measured by placing the tape

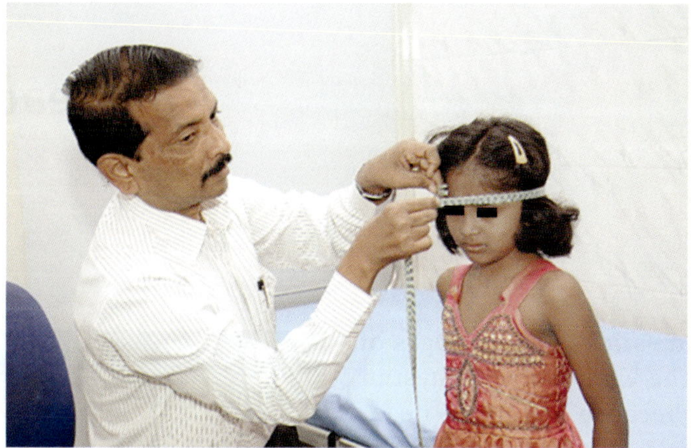

Fig. 1: Head circumference.

anteriorly over the supraorbital ridges and posteriorly over the occipital prominence. If the child has hydrocephalus serial measurements should be made. Tape is positioned so that maximum circumference is obtained.

The neonate's head circumference is 33–35.5 cm. It is larger than chest circumference by 2–3 cm. It grows at the rate of 1–2 cm per month for the first 6 months. Then it grows at the rate of 0.6 cm per month for the next 6 months. Head circumference equals the chest circumference by 1 year. In preterm infants the chest circumference may exceed head circumference by 6–9 months. In malnourished child chest circumference may be significantly smaller than head circumference because brain growth is less affected by malnutrition. The chest circumference is greater than head circumference by about 5–7 cm during childhood.

The formula used to calculate head circumference in the first year of life is:

$$\frac{(\text{Length in cm} + 9.5) \pm 2.59}{2}$$

197 CHAPTER Head Variants

Shape of the head varies in wide ranges of size and shape. The variation is greatest in younger infants because of pliable head, molding of the head occurring during vaginal delivery. Overlapping of some skull bones are common, remolds spontaneously within days.

Premature infants have characteristic head shape. It is flattened along the temporal aspects leading to long, narrow appearance due to increased pliability of the bones **(Fig. 1)**.

The palpation of newborn skull shows two common abnormalities one is *caput succedaneum,* which is a diffuse area of edema over the presenting part of the head. It does not follow any bony landmarks. It resolves by itself. Second is *cephalhematoma,* which is a subperiosteal hemorrhage. It is usually found over the parietal bones posteriorly. These will heal partly through the ossification. This starts around the edges where the periosteum has been lifted away from the skull. They are harmless, never cross the suture line. It may take many months to resolve.

The main determinant of the head size is the growth of the brain. Other important factors include genetic, intracranial pressure, and bony abnormalities.

Hydrocephalus is the abnormal accumulation of cerebrospinal fluid which leads to increased intracranial pressure and rapid expansion of the infant skull.

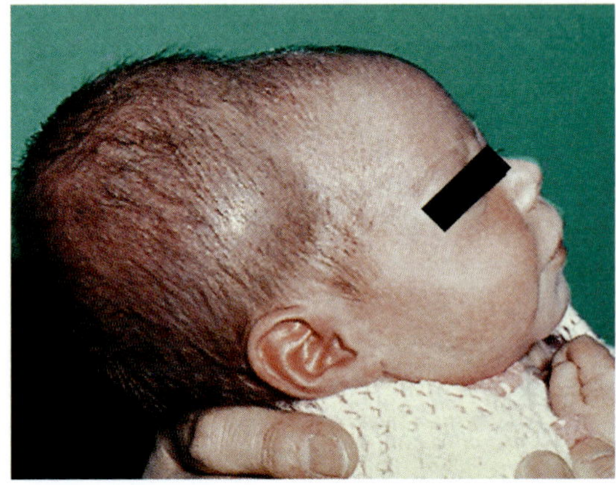

Fig. 1: Cephalhematoma.

Craniosynostosis is the premature fusion of the suture. This will limit skull growth. Abnormal shape of the head occurs. It may be seen secondary to decreased brain growth **(Fig. 2)**.

DOLICHOCEPHALY OR SCAPHOCEPHALY

It is due to premature fusion of sagittal suture. Coronal and lambdoid suture grow. Anteroposterior length is more than width. It is associated with prominent occiput and broad forehead. There is no anterior fontanelle.

BRACHYCEPHALY

It is due to premature fusion of coronal sutures. Brain grows sideways. There is flat

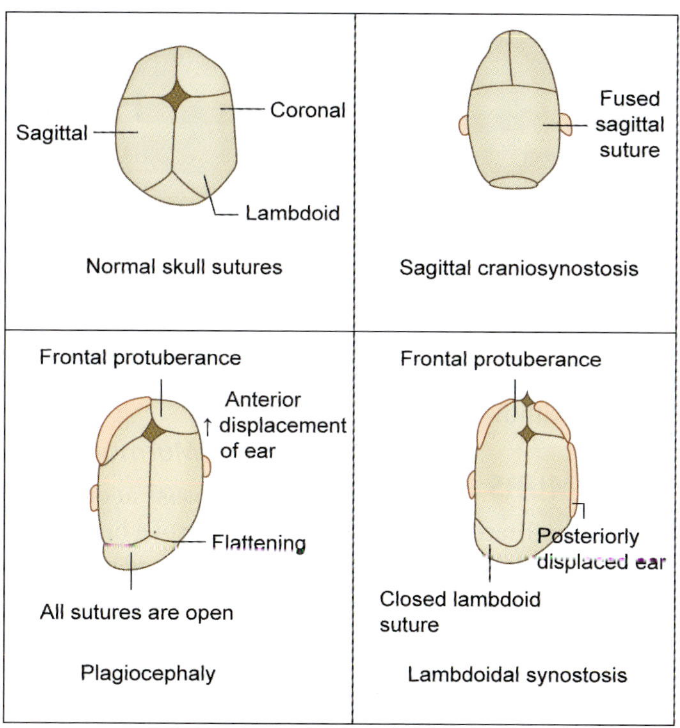

Fig. 2: Craniosynostosis.

forehead, broadening of the skull, decreased anterior posterior diameter.

PLAGIOCEPHALY

Skull is abnormal and asymmetrical in shape. It occurs due to irregular and asymmetric fusion of sutures. It may be of two types, i.e., frontal and occipital plagiocephaly.

OXYCEPHALY

It is due to premature fusion of coronal and lambdoid sutures. Skull is conical in shape and appears like a tower.

TRIGONOCEPHALY

Metopic sutures present between two fontanel bones fuse prematurely. Skull is narrow anteriorly and wide posteriorly.

CHAPTER 198

Heart Murmurs

These are produced by turbulence of the blood flow at or near a valve because of an abnormal communication within the heart.

GRADING OF MURMURS

Murmurs are graded to facilitate communication with colleagues and to make long-term records. An American system of grading is as follows:

- *Grade I:* Audible only with difficulty (on careful examination, i.e., after tuning of ears)
- *Grade II:* Easily heard
- *Grade III:* Between grade II and IV
- *Grade IV:* Murmur with thrill
- *Grade V:* Between IV and VI
- *Grade VI:* Heard with stethoscope off the chest wall

CLASSIFICATION OF MURMURS

Murmurs are broadly divided into:

- Innocent murmurs
- Organic murmurs

Innocent Murmurs

Definition: Murmurs that occur in the absence of either anatomic or physiologic abnormalities of the heart or circulation are called innocent, functional, or physiological murmur.

The innocent murmurs are broadly classified into seven systolic and three continuous murmurs. From this classification, following three innocent murmurs are common in pediatric practice.

Vibratory Murmur Characteristics

- The closest acoustic analogy is like the "buzzing of a bee".
- It is best heard between the apex and lower sternal border with the bell of stethoscope.
- Murmur grade ranges from 1 to 3 and occurs in midsystole.
- Amplitude of murmur increases in the supine position and murmur intensifies during exercise, excitement, or fever.
- Most common murmur under the age of 10 years.

Pulmonary Systolic Murmur

- It is best heard in the second left intercostal space close to the sternum and conducted upward to the infraclavicular region.
- Murmur is crescendo-decrescendo in configuration and occurs in midsystole.
- Murmur is high frequency, blowing ejection systolic murmur with grade ranging from 2 to 3, best heard with diaphragm.
- II heart sound is normally split
- Intensity of murmur increases during exercise, fever, or excitement.

Venous Hum

- Most common type of innocent continuous murmur

- *It is usually present in children and in hyperkinetic conditions such as:* Anemia, thyrotoxicosis, cirrhosis, AV fistula, post-exertion, and anxiety.

Characteristics

- It is best heard in the right supraclavicular fossa but often quite loud below the clavicles.
- Hum is a blowing continuous murmur, typically loud in diastole.
- *Murmur is abolished by the following methods*:
  - Compressing the internal jugular veins
  - Patient turns head from the side to a midline position
  - Supine position
  - By performing Valsalva's maneuver

Organic Murmur

Organic murmurs occur when blood flows through an abnormal valve or an abnormal orifice in the heart or between the great vessels. They are broadly classified into the following:

- Systolic murmur is heard between first and second heart sounds.
- Diastole murmur is heard between second and first sound.
- Continuous murmur heard continuously in both systole and diastole.

Systolic Murmurs

Systolic murmurs are classified as follows:

Ejection systolic murmur: It caused by forward flow of blood through a normal or diseased aortic or pulmonary valve. Murmur is characterized by increasing to a peak or crescendo in midsystole and ending before the second sound. The causes of ejection systolic murmur are given in **Table 1**.

TABLE 1: Causes of ejection systolic murmur.

Aortic area	*Pulmonary area*
Aortic stenosis	Pulmonary stenosis
Coarctation of aorta	TOF
Patent ductus arteriosus (PDA)	Atrial septal defect (ASD)
High output states	• Pulmonary artery dilatation • Pulmonary hypertension • Innocent murmurs • High output states

Pansystolic murmur: It is caused by retrograde flow of blood through an incompetent atrioventricular valve or through a ventricular septal defect. Pansystolic murmurs occupy the whole of systole and continues right up to the second heart sound. In phonocardiogram recordings, murmurs appear as plateau shaped.

Causes of pansystolic murmur:

- Mitral regurgitation
- Tricuspid regurgitation
- Ventricular septal defect
- Patent ductus arteriosus

Diastolic Murmur

Diastolic murmurs occur when the semilunar valves are incompetent, when the atrioventricular valves are narrowed or when they are normal, but there an increased volume of blood flow through them. The three main types of diastolic murmurs are as follows.

Mid-diastolic murmur: These are low pitched, rumbling murmurs associated with the flow of blood through the AV valves during the phase of rapid ventricular filling in diastole. The closest auditory-analogue of mid diastolic rumble is "the thunder of a distant ox cart rumbling over a loose wooden bridge." The characteristic mid-diastolic murmur of mitral stenosis is low-pitched rumbling murmur starting with the opening snap with a clear interval after the second heart sound.

Mid-diastolic murmur is best heard when the patient is in the left lateral position.

Early diastolic murmur: This murmur is caused by regurgitation flow of blood from arterial trunk into ventricle, through an incompetent aortic or pulmonary valve. The murmur starts immediately after a second sound and attains its crescendo, almost at the start of murmur, and then declines to give rise to a decrescendo murmur. Early diastolic murmur is the highest pitched of all cardiac murmurs, best heard with the diaphragm of stethoscope and with the patient sitting up or bending forward and breath held in expiration. The early diastolic murmur of pulmonary regurgitation is known as Graham-Steell murmur.

Causes of early diastolic murmur:

- Aortic regurgitation
- Systemic hypertension
- Pulmonary regurgitation
- Pulmonary hypertension

Atriosystolic or presystolic murmur: These murmurs occur when blood flows from auricle to ventricle during the phase of active atrial systole, which correspond to late diastole or presystole. It is a crescendo decrescendo murmur occurring in late diastole.

Causes of presystolic murmur:

- Mitral stenosis
- Tricuspid stenosis
- Atrial septal defect

Continuous Murmur

A classic continuous murmur rises to peak in late systole, continuous without interruption through the second sound, which it envelops and then declines in intensity during the course of diastole.

Causes of continuous murmur:

- Patent ductus arteriosus
- Aortopulmonary septal defect
- Arteriovenous (AV) fistula or aneurysm
- Venous hum
- Pulmonary atresia with bronchial artery anastomosis

199 CHAPTER Heart Sounds

FIRST HEART SOUND (S1)

S1 marks the onset of systole and is produced mainly by mitral valve closure and to a lesser extent by tricuspid valve closure. It is best heard in the mitral area. The various factors affecting intensity of S are described.

- *Loud S1:*
  - Normally heard in children
  - Sinus tachycardia
  - Mitral and tricuspid stenosis
  - Hyperdynamic state
  - Short PR interval
  - Left atrial myxoma
- *Soft S1:*
  - Long PR interval
  - Second heart sound (S2)
  - Pericardial effusion
  - Emphysema
  - Mitral stenosis with calcified valves
  - Mitral and tricuspid regurgitation
  - Left bundle branch block (LBBB)
  - Myocarditis

SECOND HEART SOUND (S2)

Second heart sound is produced by closure of the aortic and pulmonary valves and it marks the end of systole and beginning of diastole. S2 is best assessed in the pulmonary area. A complete assessment of S2 means, auscultating carefully for aortic and pulmonary components of second heart sound and appreciating splitting of second heart sound.

NORMAL SPLITTING OF SECOND HEART SOUND

A normal splitting of second heart sound means wide splitting during inspiration and narrow split in expiration.

Pathophysiology

As described earlier, second heart sound is produced by the closure of aortic and pulmonary valves. In expiration the closure of both valves is almost synchronous thus producing a single sound. But in inspiration due to increased venous return and more right ventricular filling the pulmonary component is delayed, resulting in splitting of II heart sound.

WIDE INSPIRATORY SPLITTING

- Due to delay in P2
- Causes-pulmonic stenosis

Pathophysiology

In pulmonary stenosis, the right ventricular blood is emptied slowly and thus further delaying the closure of pulmonary valve.

Due to early A2:

- Mitral regurgitation
- Ventricular septal defect

In ventricular septal defect (VSD), the wide inspiratory split is due to the early closure of aortic valves as a result of rapid emptying of blood through the defect into the right ventricle and aorta. Whereas in mitral regurgitation, the blood is rapidly emptied into left atrium and aorta, resulting in early closure of aortic valve.

WIDE AND FIXED SPLIT

This is described as equal split interval between A, and P2 during inspiration and expiration. It is illustrated in the diagram.

Causes of wide fixed splitting:

- Atrial septal defect
- Right bundle branch block (RBBB)
- Total anomalous pulmonary venous return
- Right ventricular failure

Pathophysiology

In atrial septal defect (ASD), there is a wide splitting of second heart sound. This is because the right side of heart receives more blood through the defective atrial septum, which causes delayed emptying of right ventricle and consequently delay in closure of pulmonary valve. The splitting is said to be fixed in otherward there is no inspiratory widening. During inspiration, the small extra return of blood to (right) side of the heart will not have any significant hemodynamic consequence as the right side of the heart has already received large amount of blood through ASD.

REVERSED SPLITTING OF SECOND HEART SOUND

In this P, precedes A, and split is maximum in expiration.

Associated Cardiac Conditions with Reversed Splitting

- LBBB
- Aortic stenosis
- Left ventricular failure
- Patent ductus arteriosus (PDA)

Pathophysiology

Abnormal delay in closure of aortic valves due to mechanical or electrical delay as in cases of PDA and LBBB, respectively.

Single S2

A single S will be heard on inspiration when either A, or P, is inaudible or when the inspiratory separation of A, and P2 is so narrow that the ear cannot distinguish both components. The following are common causes of a single S2.

THIRD HEART SOUND

The third sound occurs in the earlier part of diastole and it coincides with rapid ventricular filling. An audible S may be present in (1) normal heart, (2) diastolic overload states, (3) patients who have LV dysfunction with or without overt congestive heart failure. An exaggerated S is called ventricular gallop.

FOURTH HEART SOUND

The fourth sound (S4) is a low-frequency sound produced by atrial contraction and this sound is heard in late diastole. It follows the P wave by 0.14–0.20 sec and precedes S1. An audible S is usually abnormal and is usually indicative of increased resistance to ventricular filling. The atrial gallop sound may be caused by contraction of left or the right atrium.

Causes of left atrial gallop:

- Systemic hypertension
- Aortic valvular stenosis

Causes of right atrial gallop:

- Pulmonary hypertension
- Isolated pulmonary stenosis

- Atrial septal defect
- Ebstein's disease
- Increased PR interval

OTHER SOUNDS

Opening Snap

The opening snap is a high-pitched loud snapping or clicking diastolic sound, which is best heard, just inside the apex. The diaphragm of stethoscope is more appropriate for detecting opening snap. An opening snap denotes as stenosed, but mobile mitral valve.

Pathophysiology

Opening snap of the mitral valve appears to be due to sudden doming or tensing of stenotic anterior leaflet downward, with a jerk thus producing a click or snapping sound.

Systolic Ejection Click

An ejection click is a high-pitched sound heard best in aortic or pulmonary areas.

Presence of ejection click in aortic or pulmonary area denotes the following cardiac lesions.

Pulmonary Area

- Dilatation of pulmonary artery
- Pulmonary stenosis
- Pulmonary hypertension
- The systolic ejection click is due to sudden doming of stenotic valve, when blood is ejected into the pulmonary artery or aorta, as in cases of PS or AS.

Aortic Area

- Aortic stenosis
- Aortic regurgitation
- Coarctation of aorta
- Hypertension

Midsystolic Ejection Click

It occurs later than S, and it is often localized to the right or left 2nd or 3rd interspaces, where it indicates mitral valve prolapse. It varies with diastolic volume and therefore varies with posture, sustained handgrip, and Valsalva maneuver.

Hematemesis

Gastrointestinal hemorrhage commonly presents as vomiting of blood or blood-stained gastric content; this is defined as hematemesis.

SWALLOWED BLOOD

Bleeding from the nose may be followed by hematemesis when blood has been swallowed and then vomited; this may occur at night when blood has been swallowed during sleep.

CAUSES OF HEMATEMESIS IN NEWBORN

- Regurgitation of swallowed maternal blood
- Hemorrhagic disease of the newborn
- Traumatic bleeding due to stiff catheters
- Disseminated intravascular coagulation (DIC)
- Necrotizing enterocolitis
- Maternal medication
- Congenital anomalies of gastrointestinal (GI) tract
  - Reduplication, Meckel's diverticulum
  - Intestinal obstruction

INFANTS AND YOUNG CHILDREN

Common

- Ingestion of exogenous toxins, e.g., iron, toxins, aspirin, acids, and alkalis
- Coagulation disorders
- Own blood swallowed from nasopharyngeal bleeding
- Nosebleed swallowed
- Oropharyngeal or dental origin
- Localized abnormalities of GI tract
- Cow's milk allergy

OLDER CHILDREN AND ADOLESCENTS

Common

- Exogenous ingestion of drugs and poisons iron, aspirin acids, and alkalies
- Coagulation disorders
- Own blood swallowed from nasopharyngeal bleeding
- Oropharyngeal or dental origin
- Severe vomiting (Mallory-Weiss syndrome)
- Long-standing hepatic disease with portal hypertension
- Esophageal varices
- Localized abnormalities of GIT

CAUSES

- Esophagitis
- Esophageal varices
- Gastric ulcer
- Duodenal ulcer
- Drug-induced gastritis
- Tumors
- Bleeding dyscrasias
- Liver cell failure
- Septicemia

CHAPTER 201 Hematuria

Hematuria is defined as the presence of an abnormal amount of red cells in urine.

Macroscopic hematuria is the reddish or brownish discoloration of urine directly visible to eye. In asymptomatic hematuria, there will be absence of dysuria, oliguria, edema, or any symptom related to the renal system.

Microscopy of the urine is more revealing, but it must be carried out on a fresh specimen. The presence of red cell casts is pathognomonic of glomerular bleeding. A midstream specimen, clean catch is the method of choice. After cleaning external genitalia the midstream portion of the urine is collected in a sterile container. >5 red blood cells (RBC)/high-power field (HPF) are considered for hematuria.

Further investigation of hematuria should usually include a plain supine X-ray of the abdomen (to look for stones or the shadow of a renal mass) and ultrasound scanning of the urinary tract. Intravenous urography (IVU) is less commonly performed nowadays as ultrasonography provides useful information and will pick up urinary tract tumors in the bladder and kidneys.

The main causes of hematuria are summarized in **Table 1**.

TABLE 1: Causes of hematuria.

Renal: • Trauma • Tumors • Calculus • Glomerulonephritis • Polycystic kidneys • Tuberculosis • Pyelonephritis • Infarction • Polyarteritis nodosa *Ureteric:* • Calculus • Tumors	*Vesical:* • Trauma • Tumors • Tuberculosis • Calculus • Cystitis • Foreign body • Disease of adjacent organs *Urethral:* • Urethritis • Calculus • Tumors • Foreign body *General:* • Drugs • Bleeding disorders

CHAPTER 202

Hemiballismus

It is a rare hyperkinetic movement disorder, characterized by violent involuntary limb movements, on one side of the body and can cause significant disability, symptoms can decrease during sleep. It is an abnormal, involuntary, non-repetitive violent flinging movements. It mostly involves the proximal part of the limb. There will be a tendency to rotational movements of the limb and trunk, lesion is in subthalamic nuclei of lays. It is usually caused by a stroke that affects a small area just below the basal ganglia called the subthalamic nucleus helps to control voluntary movements. The causes include tuberculous meningitis and encephalitis.

It is treated with antipsychotics such as haloperidol and clozapine. Thalamic ablation is considered in severe cases if there is no response to medical treatment.

203 CHAPTER

Hemihypertrophy

It is a condition in which one side of the body or apart of one side of the body is larger than the other to an extent considered greater than the normal variation **(Fig. 1)**. It is often associated with overgrowth syndromes such as Beckwith-Wiedmann syndrome, Proteus syndrome, neurofibromatosis type 1, and mosaic trisomy 8.

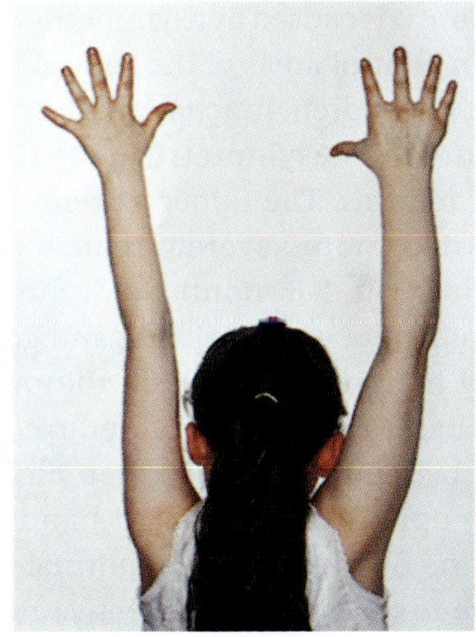

Fig. 1: Hemihypertrophy.

Medullary sponge kidney: This is a congenital abnormality which probably represents a minor form of polycystic kidneys. The condition is not always bilateral and is often associated with the unusual physical sign of body hemihypertrophy. Unless the family history is known, the condition usually presents as renal angle pain, pyuria, supervening upper tract sepsis and ureteric colic. The stones may erode into the pelvic-alycine system and from there make their way along the ureter. The radiological changes are pathognomonic of the condition, showing the typical "bouquet of flowers". Treatment is centered on screening the patient for tumor growth and treating tumors. For abnormal limb size, orthopedic treatment and corrective shoes can be recommended.

CHAPTER 204

Hemiparesis

Hemiparesis is caused by asymmetric damage to motor control areas of the central nervous system. In children, functional discrepancies often predate asymmetrical changes in tone or reflexes. The upper extremities may be affected more severely than the lower extremities. At 4–6 months old, during the development of early reaching and grasping, signs of hemiparesis include the presence of one hand that is fisted, the arm getting caught beneath the body when child tries to prop upon the elbows and hands. Later during the first year of life abnormal include a failure to develop the protective response of lateral propping or the development of an asymmetrical parachute response. In addition, crawling may be uneven, with propulsion coming from one side while the opposite arm and leg are dragged behind.

Walking is typically delayed until 2–3 years old. Usually, the lower limb rotates internally, and the foot may be held in equinus, making it functionally longeron swing through part of the gait. To clear the foot from the floor, the child compensates by swinging the leg farther out in abduction or by circumduction of the affected side. Children may neglect the visual on their affected side. Parents should position their infants so that visual stimulation is provided to the intact visual field.

Hemiplegia

It is a condition caused by brain damage or spinal cord injury that leads to paralysis on one of the bodies. It causes weakness, problems with muscle control, and muscle stiffness. The brain damage disrupts the connection between brain and the muscle on the affected side. The degree of hemiplegia symptoms varies depending on the location and extent of injury. **Table 1** outlines the differences between infantile hemiplegia and adult hemiplegia.

CAUSES OF HEMIPLEGIA

Primary Causes

- Central nervous system (CNS) infection
- Subarachnoid hemorrhage

Secondary Causes

- Congenital heart disease
- Bronchiectasis
- Leukemia
- Thrombocytopenia

TABLE 1: Differences between infantile hemiplegia and adult hemiplegia.

Features	***Infantile hemiplegia***	***Adult hemiplegia***
Site of lesion	Cortical/subcortical area	Internal capsule
Convulsions	Common	Uncommon
Mental retardation	Common	Uncommon
Muscle wasting	Present	Absent
Involuntary movements	Less common	Common
Plantar reflex	Flexor	Extensor
Abdominal reflex	Normal	Lost

206 CHAPTER

Hemoptysis

The coughing up of blood is defined as hemoptysis, a term generally accepted to refer specifically to expectoration of blood resulting from bleeding in the lungs or bronchi.

CAUSES

- *Upper respiratory tract:*
  - Trauma
  - Infection
  - Malignancy
- *Lower respiratory tract:*
  - Respiratory
    - Pneumonia
    - Lung abscess
    - Tuberculosis
    - Bronchiectasis
    - Pulmonary embolism
    - Arteriovenous (AV) malformation
    - Retained foreign body in lungs
  - Cardiac
    - Left ventricular failure
    - Primary pulmonary hypertension
  - Congenital causes
    - Pulmonary sequestration
  - Immunological causes
    - Systemic lupus erythematosus (SLE)
    - Henoch-Schönlein purpura
    - Goodpasture syndrome
  - Bleeding dyscrasias
    - Leukemia
    - Idiopathic thrombocytopenic purpura
    - Anticoagulant drugs
  - Trauma
    - Contusion
    - Fractured trachea of bronchus

CHAPTER 207

Hepatomegaly

The liver may be palpable either because it is enlarged (hepatomegaly) or because it has been displaced downward by thoracic deformities or by flattening of the diaphragm, for example, by a large, right sided pleural effusion or lung hyperinflation (e.g., bronchiolitis).

LIVER SPAN

Begin liver percussion at the right midclavicular line over an area of tympany (always begin with an area of tympany and proceed to an area of dullness, usually heard at the costal margin or slightly below it. Mark the border with a marking pen. A lower liver border that is >2–3 cm below the costal margin indicates organ enlargement or downward displacement of the diaphragm because of emphysema or other pulmonary disease.

To determine the upper border of the liver, begin percussion on the right midclavicular line at an area of lung resonance. Continue downward until the percussion tone changes to one of dullness, which marks the upper border of the liver. Mark the location with the pen. The upper border usually begins at the fifth to seventh intercostal space. An upper border below this may indicate downward displacement or liver atrophy. Dullness extending above the fifth intercostal space suggests upward displacement from abdominal fluid or masses. The upper edge, in the liver should be detected within 1 cm of the fifth intercostal space at the right midclavicular line. It is normally placed in the seventh intercostal space along the right midaxillary line and at the ninth intercostal space along the right posterior axillary line.

HISTORY AND PHYSICAL EXAMINATION

On physical examination, it is important to determine the presence or absence of jaundice, splenomegaly, ascites, change in mental status, tremors, neurologic abnormalities, fever, signs of malnutrition, prominent vascular patterns on the anterior abdominal wall (caput medusae and spider angiomas), arterial hypertension, hypotension, bruising, petechiae, hemangiomas, pallor, obesity, renal enlargement, masses outside of the liver, lymphadenopathy, muscle weakness, cyanosis, heart murmurs, tachypnea, tachycardia, abnormal eye examination (cataracts, Kayser–Fleischer ring), bone and joint abnormalities, and dysmorphic features. A pelvic examination in sexually active females may detect signs of a sexually transmitted infection, which can lead to Fitz-Hugh-Curtis syndrome.

PATHOPHYSIOLOGY

The pathophysiologic mechanisms underlying the enlargement of the liver are complex and heterogeneous. Hepatomegaly may reflect proliferation or enlargement or malfunction of one or more component structures of the liver, including liver parenchyma (hepatocytes), bile ducts (cholangiocytes and cysts), the reticuloendothelial system (Kupffer cells), interstitial tissue (stellate cells and collagen), blood (including hematopoietic cells), and blood vessels (endothelial cells). The liver also increases in size as a result of hepatic tumors, benign cysts, and infiltration of inflammatory or malignant cells.

HEPATOMEGALY IN THE INFANT

Causes of Hepatomegaly in Newborn

- Congestive cardiac failure
- Neonatal hepatitis
- Erythroblastosis fetalis
- Intrauterine infection
- Extrahepatic biliary atresia
- Septicemia
- Galactosemia

HEPATOMEGALY IN INFANCY AND CHILDHOOD

- *Infection:*
    - Bacterial
        - Tuberculosis
        - Enteric fever
        - Brucellosis
    - Viral
        - Hepatitis
        - Infectious mononucleosis
        - Cytomegalovirus
- *Infestation:*
    - Protozoal
        - Amoebiasis
        - Kala azar
        - Malaria
- *Hematological:*
    - Hemolytic anemia
    - Leukemia
    - Thrombocytopenia
- *Vascular:*
    - CCF
    - Constrictive pericarditis
- *Nutritional:*
    - Protein energy malnutrition
    - Hyperalimentation
- *Storage disorder:*
    - Glycogen storage disorder
    - Reye's syndrome
    - Gaucher's disease
    - Hemosiderosis
    - Amyloidoses
    - Wilson's disease
- *Malignancies:*
    - Leukemia
    - Neuroblastoma
    - Wilm's tumor
    - Lymphoma
    - Hepatoblastoma
- *Miscellaneous:*
    - Idiopathic cirrhosis (IC)
    - Congenital cyst of liver
    - Hemangioma of liver

CHAPTER 208

Herpangina

It is a common childhood illness often caused by group A coxsackieviruses. It spreads by airborne droplets, contaminated food, or water, by saliva and skin to skin contact. The other viruses responsible include coxsackie B, coxsackie A16, enterovirus 71, and echovirus.

It is an acute infection of the oral cavity caused by the coxsackie virus. It is mostly seen in children below the age of 5 years. Clinically there is fever, sore throat, and discrete vesicles and ulcers mainly located on the anterior tonsillar pillars. The ulcers are small in size and few in number (1–5). In severe cases, ulcers may involve the soft palate, uvula, tonsils, and posterior pharyngeal wall (**Fig. 1**).

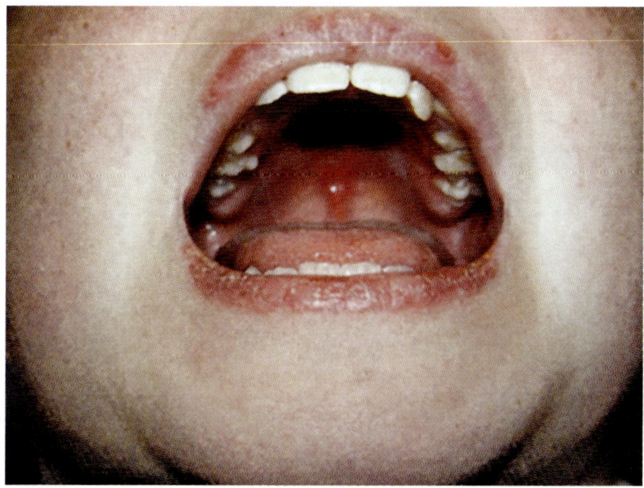

Fig. 1: Herpangina.

Hiccup

Hiccup is very common and is only significant if persistent. It is caused by sudden involuntary contraction of both the diaphragm and external intercostals muscles in association with rapid glottic closure. Hiccups may be induced by stimulating a variety of sensory nerves, particularly the vagus and phrenic. Hiccups usually occur with a frequency of between 4 and 60 per minute.

The most common cause of hiccups is gastric distension after rapid ingestion of food, alcohol, or air. Other common causes include excitement and a sudden change in temperature, either of the environment or of the stomach induced by a hot or very cold meal. However, in persistent cases, the following causes should be considered.

CAUSES

- Newborn—normal after feeds
- Following acute respiratory infection
- Diaphragmatic pleural effusion
- Subphrenic abscess
- Peritonitis
- Uremia
- Encephalitis
- Brain tumor
- Drugs

High-arched Palate

High-arched palate is where the palatal height is >2 cm and narrow. It is usually a congenital developmental defect results from failure of palatal shelves to fuse correctly in development. The same phenomenon leads to cleft palate. When a child has high-arched palate tongue cannot lift to the roof of the mouth. In addition to affecting the shape of palate, it can also feeding and sleep breathing. A child with tongue, i.e., may not be achieve proper latching when feeding.

211 CHAPTER

Hoarseness of Voice

A voice that is rough, harsh, and lower in pitch than normal is usually described as hoarse. The change in the quality of the voice may range from a slight roughness of tone or huskiness to hoarseness or complete aphonia. Hoarseness is usually indicative of some interference with the phonatory function of the larynx. Hoarseness in a newborn baby is likely to be due to trauma or due to a congenital defect. Hoarseness may result from prolonged crying and in the case of an older child, from prolonged shouting, as in games.

CAUSES

In Newborn

- Trauma to the larynx by intubation
- Damage to the recurrent laryngeal nerve or vagus by traction

In Newborn or Later

- Laryngeal web, cyst, tumor, and stenosis
- Weakness of laryngeal muscles (Werdnig-Hoffmann syndrome, Myasthenia gravis).
- Cretinism
- Laryngeal foreign body. Accompanying symptoms include aphonia and drooling.
- Unilateral paralysis of the recurrent laryngeal nerve, at times associated with congestive heart failure (cardiovocal syndrome).

Infection

- Laryngitis or croup (acute epiglottis produces a muffled voice)
- Measles, diphtheria, and laryngobronchial tuberculosis
- Laryngeal fungal infections in patients with chronic mucocutaneous candidiasis or in those who are immunocompromised
- Ectodermal dysplasia
- Lipoid proteinosis
- Thyroid malignancy; chronic lymphocytic thyroiditis
- Ninth and tenth cranial nerve paresis associated with the Arnold-Chiari malformation
- Disseminated lipogranulomatosis (hoarseness may be noted at birth in infants)
- Paralysis of vocal cords-medullary damage (infarction and syringobulbia)
- Spastic dysphonia similar to Writer's cramp

Hoffmann Reflex

It is neurological examination finding elicited by reflex test which can help to verify the presence or absence of issues arising from corticospinal tract.

The terminal phalanx of the patient's middle finger is flicked down briskly. This is done between examiners finger and thumb. The response includes the flexion movements of terminal phalanges and flexion, and adduction of thumb occurs. This reflexive movement is called opposition. The positive Hoffman sign is suggestive corticospinal tract dysfunction localized to the cervical segments of the spinal cord. It is analogous to Babinski sign. This is seen in unilateral pyramidal tract disease, in emotional state. The spinal segments included are C_7, C_8, and T_1. Conditions such as hyperthyroidism anxiety and multiple sclerosis will result in positive sign.

Horner's Syndrome

It is due to paralysis of the cervical sympathetic nerve.

- It consists of slight drooping of upper lid (ptosis).
- Pupillary constriction (miosis)
- Absence of pupillary dilatation on shading the eye or instillation of cocaine
- Absence of ciliospinal reflex
- Absence of sweating on the corresponding half of the face and neck, both in front and behind extending as low as the third rib and the third thoracic spine and over the whole of the upper limb on the same side.

This is a defect in the sympathetic innervation of the eye. The full syndrome consists of ptosis, miosis, and anhidrosis. The upper lid ptosis is mild, and lower lid ptosis creates the false impression of enophthalmos. The anisocoria is of the order of 1 mm, and is less in bright light, greater in darkness **(Fig. 1)**.

The most specific clinical sign of Horner's syndrome is dilation lag of the meiotic pupil compared to the normal pupil when viewed over 15–20 seconds in darkness. The pupillary light reflex and the accommodation reflex are preserved.

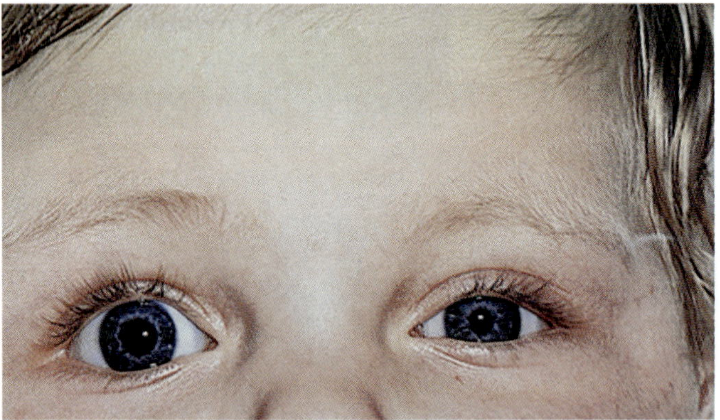

Fig. 1: Horner's syndrome.

CHAPTER 214

Hordeolum

A hordeolum, commonly referred to as a *stye,* is an inflamed gland of Zeis along the eyelid margin. It is a red and painful lump near the edge of the eyelid. They may be painful and produce swelling and erythema of the eyelid. Infection, frequently with *Staphylococcus,* may occur. Some discharge may be seen. Rarely, preseptal cellulitis may occur as a complication. The treatment includes warm compresses and antibiotic eye drops or ointments.

215 CHAPTER

Horseshoe Kidney

It results from the fusion of the lower renal poles during development. Although generally asymptomatic, patients have (1) hematuria after trauma to the pelvic area; (2) midline abdominal mass; or (3) ureteropelvic junction obstruction.

Hydranencephaly

Hydranencephaly is a severe anomaly of the brain characterized by the absence of the cerebral hemispheres despite intact meninges and a normal skull **(Fig. 1)**. Affected children often appear deceptively normal at birth, with little to suggest the presence of a severe brain abnormality. Because newborns function at a subcortical reflex level, even complete absence of the cerebral hemispheres may not interfere with normal reflexes. However, within the first few weeks of life, developmental arrest, decerebration, hypertonia, and hyperreflexia become apparent in the infant with hydranencephaly. Most of these infants do not live beyond 6–12 months old, although survival for several years is occasionally reported. Seizures are common, and progressive enlargement of the head may complicate nursing care.

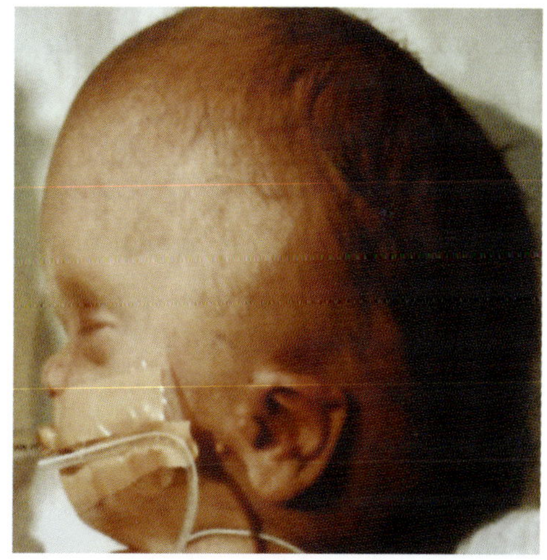

Fig. 1: Hydranencephaly

The diagnosis may be suggested if, on transillumination of the skull, the entire calvarium is lit up. However, severe hydrocephalus and bilateral subdural hygromas may present a similar appearance.

On computed tomography scan or magnetic resonance imaging, cerebrospinal fluid signal intensity replaces the supratentorial brain parenchyma with sparing of the thalami, brainstem, cerebellum, and choroid plexus. The falx is intact, distinguishing this from holoprosencephaly. A thin rim of cerebral parenchyma is lacking, distinguishing this from severe unshunted hydrocephalus. To distinguish this disorder from massive bilateral subdural hygromas, cerebral angiography is required to confirm absence of the cerebrum.

CHAPTER 217

Hydrocephalus

CAUSES

Non-communicating—obstruction in the ventricular system:

- Congenital malformation
- Adequate stenosis
- Atresia of the outflow foramen of the fourth ventricle (Dandy–Walker malformation)

Chiari malformation: *Communicating (failure to reabsorb cerebrospinal fluid):*

- Subarachnoid hemorrhage
- Meningitis

INDICATIONS FOR SHUNT SURGERY IN HYDROCEPHALUS

- Cortical mantle <2 cm on initial imaging in infants <6 months of age at presentation
- Features of raised intracranial pressure
- Evidence of thinning of cortical mantle
- Delayed milestones despite of medical treatment on follow-up.
- Evidence of papilledema or periventricular ooze **(Figs. 1 and 2)**.

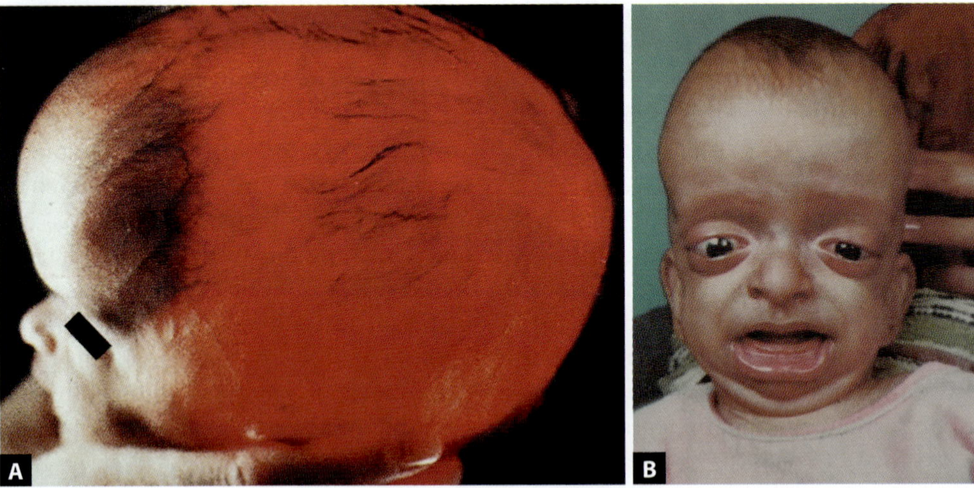

Figs. 1A and B: Hydrocephalus.

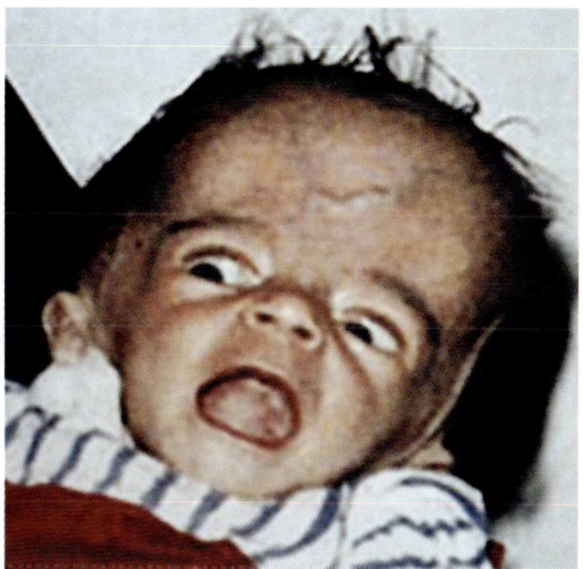

Fig. 2: Congenital hydrocephalus.

CHAPTER 218

Hypertelorism

In hypertelorism (i.e., wide spacing of the eyes), the interpupillary distance is increased. When the inner canthi are laterally displaced but the interpupillary distance is normal, the eyes falsely appear widely spaced; this feature is called tele canthus. In hypotelorism (not shown), the interpupillary distance is decreased.

It is abnormally wide-spaced eyes. There is broadened nasal bridge. This is due to maldevelopment of sphenoid bone. This is seen among cretinism, cerebral gigantism, thalassemia major, and craniofacial dysostosis.

Hypertelorism, i.e., widely spaced orbit is diagnosed by:

$$\frac{\text{Distance between inner canthi}}{\text{Distance between outer canthi}} \times 100$$

Normally it is <40%. In hypertelorism, it is >40%.

Pupillary reflex is present after 28–30 weeks of gestation, while pupillary reflex, i.e., leukocoria is present in congenital cataract, chorioretinitis, and retinopathy of prematurity (ROP).

CHAPTER 219 Hypertrichosis

Hypertrichosis is defined as excessive growth anywhere on the body either in males or females. It is important to distinguish from hirsutism, which is the term reserved for females who grow an excessive amount of terminal hair in androgen-dependent sites.

The causes include:

- Hurler's syndrome
- Cornelia de Lange's syndrome
- Porphyria
- Hyperthyroidism
- Anorexia nervosa

220 CHAPTER

Hydrocele

Hydroceles are fluid accumulations within the tunica vaginalis or processus vaginalis. They may be small or large, are usually painless even if they are large, and they may be tense enough to obscure palpation of the testis. They transilluminate. Simple scrotal hydroceles are common in neonates and usually resolve spontaneously over several months **(Figs. 1A and B)**. When examining an infant with a huge hydrocele, examination of the lower abdomen should be performed to rule out the presence of an abdominoscrotal hydrocele. The presence of an abdominoscrotal hydrocele may be noted if compression of the scrotal hydrocele causes enlargement of a lower quadrant mass. Ultrasound may confirm this finding. Large hydroceles may present in adolescence without an obvious etiology. In adolescent cases, when the testis cannot be palpated, an ultrasound examination should be done to verify that the testis is normal. If the processus vaginalis remains patent, a communicating hydrocele results and may present with periodic increase and decrease in scrotal size. In these cases, thickening of the inguinal spermatic cord may be noted. If a segment of processus vaginalis fails to obliterate, trapping fluid in mid-cord, a hydrocele of the cord may result. These may also communicate with the peritoneum through a patent processus vaginalis and thus may vacillate in size. When the diagnosis of an inguinal mass is uncertain, imaging (ultrasound or CT) or exploration may be warranted because soft tissue sarcomas may originate from spermatic cord and paratesticular tissue.

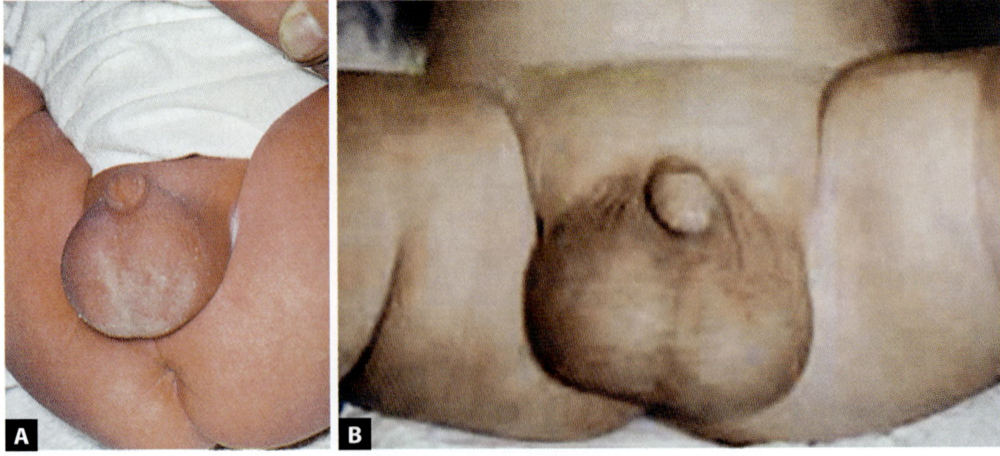

Figs. 1A and B: Hydrocele.

CHAPTER 221

Hypercyanotic Spells

In some forms of congenital heart disease, the degree of cyanosis worsens periodically and can be quite profound, to the point of causing loss of consciousness. These episodes are known as hypercyanotic spells and occur classically in children with cyanotic congenital heart disease that involves narrowing of the infundibulum (the subpulmonary outflow tract) and a ventricular septal defect (VSD), classically tetralogy of Fallot. This clinical phenomenon is caused by either: (1) An increase in pulmonary resistance (resulting from either a subpulmonary infundibular muscle spasm or an increase in peripheral pulmonary vascular resistance) or (2) a fall in systemic vascular resistance. Both mechanisms result in a relative increase in the restriction of blood flow out of the right ventricular outflow and a subsequent increase in right-to-left shunting across the VSD. Spells often are precipitated by crying. After patients with hypercyanotic spells have been stabilized, their condition should always be discussed with a pediatric cardiologist before they are discharged from the hospital or emergency department.

Hypercyanotic spells are a medical emergency and often affect the treatment algorithm. Cases of patients with hypercyanotic spells should be discussed with a cardiologist before the patient is discharged from the hospital or emergency department.

Hyperopia

In patients with hyperopia (farsightedness), parallel rays of light in the non-accommodating eye would, if possible, be focused behind the retina. The process of accommodation (focusing), which alters the shape of the lens, can compensate for some degrees of hyperopia. Because most children have a tremendous range of accommodation, mildly hyperopic children can see clearly without any visual symptoms. Moderate to severely hyperopic children may be unable to fully compensate through accommodation. The greater accommodative effort may lead to symptoms of "eyestrain," which consist of headaches, fatigue, or eye rubbing. These symptoms may lead to a lack of interest in reading or in prolonged close work. Some children may also develop accommodative esotropia. Some children have a decreased ability to accommodate, or accommodative insufficiency, and are symptomatic even with low degrees of hyperopia. If hyperopia produces symptoms or causes esotropia, spherical convex (plus) lenses usually in the form of glasses are prescribed to correct the refractive error.

CHAPTER 223

Hyperthyroidism

Hyperthyroidism refers to excessive thyroid hormone secretion by the thyroid gland. Features of hyperthyroidism include accelerated basal metabolism, tachycardia, weight loss, increased frequency of bowel movements, heat intolerance, nervousness, widened pulse pressure, and tremor. The skin is warm and moist; hair is fine and friable. Separation of the distal margin of the nail bed, Plummer's nails, may be noted. Restlessness, inability to sit still, emotional lability, short attention span, excessive sweating, decreased school performance, and fatigue may be found.

Hyperthyroidism can be due to autoimmune thyroid disease including Graves' disease or the hyperthyroid phase of Hashimoto thyroiditis, commonly called *hashitoxicosis.* Graves' disease is a condition in which a stimulating antibody directed against the TSH receptor [thyroid receptor antibody (TRAb) or thyroid-stimulating immunoglobulin (TSI)] increases the endogenous production of thyroid hormone. The transient hyperthyroidism seen in Hashimoto thyroiditis is related to the release of preformed thyroid hormone from a thyroid gland being disrupted by lymphocytic infiltration. Other, less common causes of hyperthyroidism in children include autonomously functioning adenomas, toxic multinodular goiters, activating mutations of the TSH receptor gene, selective pituitary T3 resistance, and exogenous intake of thyroid hormones. Although rare, thyroid cancer can occur within an autonomously functioning "hot nodule."

Exophthalmos, a characteristic finding of Graves' disease, usually is less dramatic in children than adults, but proptosis and lid lag can be appreciated. The hyperthyroid gland can become quite large, as much as three to four times its normal size and is warm when palpated. A bruit may be heard over the gland. T4 and T3 concentrations are elevated, and TSH concentrations are suppressed.

Hyphema

Any child with blunt trauma to the eye should be evaluated for blood in the anterior chamber of the eye, known as a hyphema. Hyphema appears as a bright or dark red fluid between the cornea and iris, or as a diffuse murkiness of the aqueous humor. Children present with acute loss of vision with or without pain.

The visual acuity of the injured eye should be measured as possible. The anterior segment and pupillary function should be assessed if the hyphema only partially fills the anterior chamber. Fundoscopy should be attempted to look for associated retinal hemorrhage, edema, or detachment.

The treatment involves efforts to minimize the vision threatening sequel, such as rebleeding, glaucoma, and corneal blood staining. Bedrest is necessary, with elevation of the bed to 30°.

CHAPTER 225

Hypospadias

Hypospadias is a common anomaly that occurs in approximately one in 300 male births **(Figs. 1A and B)**. The configuration of the urethra varies from mild glanular hypospadias to severe perineal hypospadias with chordee (ventral penile curvature). In describing the appearance of the hypospadiac penis, it is important to refrain from nonspecific terms such as *first-degree* and *minimal*. Proper definition of the anomaly should give an accurate description of the location of the meatus (glandular, coronal, subcoronal, distal shaft, midshaft, proximal shaft, penoscrotal, scrotal, and perineal) and the presence or absence of chordee. When hypospadias is associated with cryptorchidism, karyotype should be determined. Voiding cystourethrogram (VCUG) is not indicated in hypospadias except in severe lesions or in boys with a history of urinary tract infection. Renal sonography is more likely to be abnormal in boys with proximal hypospadias. Infants with hypospadias should not be circumcised, because the dorsal preputial skin may be necessary for urethral and penile reconstruction. Repair is usually undertaken at approximately 6 months old.

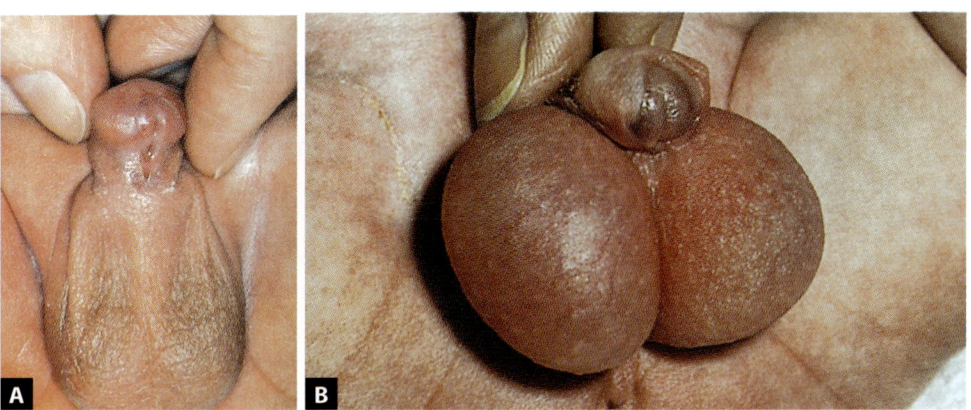

Figs. 1A and B: Hypospadias.

CHAPTER 226

Hypotonia

Hypotonia, or abnormally diminished muscle tone, is defined as decreased resistance to passive movement of a limb through its range of motion. Hypotonia affects children of all ages and may be acute or chronic, progressive, or static, isolated, or part of a complex clinical situation, and may or may not be associated with weakness.

Loss of resistance through movement. Heel does not lift off the bed when knee is lifted quickly. Decreased tone is noted in all lower motor neuron (LMN) disorders, shock period of upper motor neuron (UMN) lesion (few minutes to weeks), in certain brain lesions, and systemic disorders [protein-energy malnutrition (PEM), rickets, etc.].

Marked loss of tone is called flaccidity.

CAUSES

Combined central and peripheral nervous system disease:

- Adrenoleukodystrophy
- Cerebello-thalamo-spinal degeneration
- Infantile neuroaxonal dystrophy
- Metachromatic leukodystrophy
- Krabbe's disease
- Prader-Willi syndrome
- Zellweger syndrome

UPPER MOTOR UNIT DISEASE

- *Any acute cerebral insult:* Cerebrovascular accident (CVA), hypoxic-ischemic encephalopathy (HIE)
- Infections like (viral, bacterial, fungal, and parasitic)
- *Chromosomal anomalies:* Down's syndrome and Prader-Willi syndrome
- *Congenital motor disease:* Atonic or ataxic cerebral palsy
- Incontinentia pigmenti
- *Metabolic diseases:* Carnitine deficiency, gangliosidosis, hypercalcemia, hyperglycinemia, hypocalcemia, Niemann-Pick disease, organic acidemias, and renal tubular acidosis
- *Toxicity:* Bilirubin, magnesium, phenobarbital phenytoin, and sedative drugs
- *Trauma:* Brain and spinal cord injury

LOWER MOTOR UNIT SYSTEM DISEASE

- Arthrogryposis multiplex congenita
- Carnitine deficiency
- Connective tissue disease—Ehler-Danlos syndrome
- *Anterior horn cel:*
    - Spinal muscular atrophy
    - Poliomyelitis
- *Peripheral nerve:*
    - Familial dysautonomia
    - Guillain-Barré syndrome
    - Polyneuropathies
- *Neuromuscular junction:*
    - Botulism
    - Myasthenia gravis syndrome

- *Muscle:*
  - Congenital myopathies
  - Glycogen storage disease
  - Hypothyroidism
  - Polymyositis

The extent to which the joints may be extensible provides an indirect clue to the presence of hypotonia. Examination of mobility at the elbows, wrists, hips, and knees is helpful. The hypotonic infant may assume unusual postures in the presence of joint hyperextensibility. The "scarf sign" is a useful sign of hyperextensibility in the young infant. With the infant in a semi-reclining position, the hand is pulled across the chest toward the opposite shoulder and the position of the elbow is noted. If the elbow passes the midline, then there is hypotonia.

POSTURAL REFLEXES

Traction response (pull-to-sit): The traction response is the most useful and most sensitive of the postural reflexes in infants. With the infant lying supine, the infant's hands are grasped, and the infant is pulled up to a sitting position. Once the sitting posture is attained, the head is held erect in the midline.

COMMON DISORDERS

Hypoxic-ischemic encephalopathy: Brain injury resulting from asphyxia, hypoxia, or ischemia is an important cause of neonatal neurologic morbidity. Tissue oxygen deficiency is presumed to underlie the neurologic injury caused by hypoxic-ischemic insults. An oxygen deficit may be incurred by either hypoxemia or ischemia. Hypoxemia is defined as diminished oxygen content of blood. Ischemia is characterized by reduced blood perfusion in a particular tissue bed. Hypoxemia and ischemia often occur simultaneously or in sequence. Ischemia is likely to be the more important of these two insults.

Asphyxia denotes an impairment in gas exchange, which results not only in a deficit of oxygen in blood but also in an excess of carbon dioxide and thereby acidosis. Furthermore, sustained asphyxia usually results in hypotension and ischemia, which is consistent with the likely predominant importance of ischemia as the final common pathway to brain injury. Asphyxia is the most common clinical insult resulting in brain injury during the perinatal period.

CEREBRAL CAUSES

Several clues suggest that hypotonia is caused by an abnormality of cerebral function. The presence of associated symptoms attributable to dysfunction of the cerebral cortex is the most useful:

- Acute impairment of consciousness
- Acute or chronic impairment of cognitive abilities (mental status examination or poor school grades, respectively)
- Seizures

Delayed language and social development are typical chronic problems. The presence of microcephaly or macrocephaly is also an important clue. The presence of brisk reflexes, clonus, an asymmetric tonic neck response, and the Babinski sign suggests possible cerebral cortical dysfunction. The presence of dysmorphism or of congenital malformations suggests the possibility of a cerebral malformation. Congenital ocular malformations (e.g., microphthalmia or optic hypoplasia) are frequently associated with congenital brain malformation.

The presence of hypertonia mixed with signs of hypotonia strongly suggests a cerebral origin. This may seem paradoxical, but it is often overlooked that many children

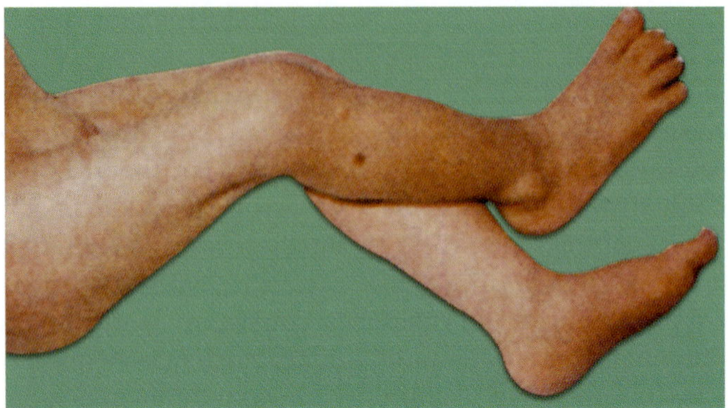

Fig. 1: Cerebral palsy.

with cerebral causes of hypotonia have signs of hypertonia as well. This may occur as an evolutionary phenomenon in the development of spasticity; cerebral palsy is often characterized by hypotonia in infancy with later development of spasticity **(Fig. 1)**. In some children with cerebral dysfunction, the coexistence of hypotonia and hypertonia is persistent. Thus, an infant with hypotonia of the neck and trunk musculature who also exhibits scissoring of the lower extremities or persistent fisting of the hands (typical signs of hypertonia) can be presumed to have cerebral dysfunction.

Signs of cerebellar dysfunction (ataxia, nystagmus, titubation, dysmetria, and impairment of coordination) are often useful diagnostic clues. The cerebellum helps maintain normal muscle tone, and diseases of the cerebellum typically are associated with some degree of hypotonia.

SPINAL CORD DYSFUNCTION

Classically, spinal cord dysfunction produces spastic weakness of all four extremities or paraparesis of the lower extremities. However, particularly after acute injury to the spinal cord and in some chronic disorders of the spinal cord, hypotonia may be the prominent motor sign. The typical associated findings of hyperreflexia, clonus, Babinski signs, and sensory loss (with a sensory level) are important clues, as is the disparity between the weakness and sensory impairment of the extremities in contrast to the normal strength and function of the head and neck.

Spinal cord injury resulting from birth trauma is frequently overlooked as a cause of hypotonia in the newborn. A history of a lengthy or difficult (breech or vertex) delivery should suggest spinal cord injury, and care should be taken not to falsely attribute motor dysfunction in these infants to anoxic brain injury. The bones of the cervical spine are *normal*, but MRI demonstrates the cord lesion. This diagnosis should never be missed because neurosurgical intervention is often required. To make matters more confusing, many neonates with spinal cord injuries also have anoxic encephalopathy because of the traumatic nature of the delivery.

ANTERIOR HORN CELL CAUSES

The functional unit of the anterior horn cell, peripheral nerve, neuromuscular junction (NMJ), and muscle fiber makes up the motor unit. Disorders that affect the motor unit produce a common clinical picture characterized by preservation of cognitive function and alertness, absence of seizures, characteristically diminished or absent muscle stretch reflexes, and hypotonia. *Muscle atrophy* is frequently associated with motor unit disorders, but it can also occur in cerebral causes of hypotonia.

It is not always easy to determine which component of the motor unit is abnormal (anterior horn cell, peripheral nerve, NMJ, or muscle), but the following guidelines are useful.

Anterior horn cell disease is suggested by hypotonia, weakness, absence of reflexes, and fasciculations. The presence of fasciculations of muscle usually cannot be appreciated in infants because of the presence of subcutaneous fat. Fasciculations might be seen on the tongue, but they must be distinguished from normal quivering movements. Muscle enzymes are usually normal but can sometimes be mildly to moderately elevated, and nerve conduction studies are usually normal. The electromyogram (EMG) may demonstrate fibrillations and large motor unit potentials that are reduced in number.

Immotile Cilia Syndrome

It is a defect in the component of mucosal barrier and mucociliary transport. Kartagener syndrome consists of situs inversus, chronic sinusitis, and bronchiectasis. These patients are infertile because of poorly motile spermatozoa. The resultant ciliary dysfunction impedes mucous clearance and produces a combination of signs and symptoms.

Clinical features include early onset of chronic rhinorrhea, chronic otitis media, and chronic sinusitis. Chronic productive cough, bronchiectasis, digital clubbing, and nasal polyps are present. This disorder should be suspected in any child with chronic or recurrent upper or lower respiratory tract infection.

CHAPTER 228

Imperforate Anus

Because of common embryologic origins and the anatomic proximity of the genitourinary and lower gastrointestinal tracts, children with imperforate anus have a high incidence of genitourinary and lower spinal abnormalities. A high imperforate anus (at or above the levator ani) is associated with a 50% incidence of genitourinary anomalies, mainly unilateral renal agenesis, neurogenic bladder, or vesicoureteral reflux (VUR). In boys, one usually finds a fistulous communication between the blind end of the rectal pouch and the prostatic urethra. In girls, the rectum often communicates with the vagina or posterior fourchette. All children with imperforate anus should undergo renal ultrasonography and must be monitored for urinary tract infection (UTI) **(Fig. 1)**.

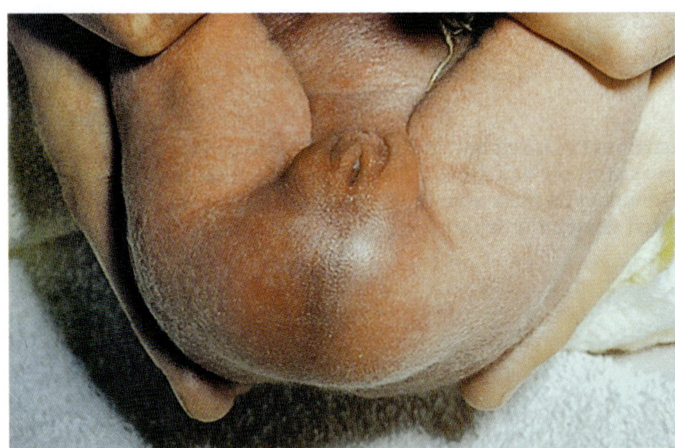

Fig. 1: Imperforate anus.

229 CHAPTER

Impetigo

Impetigo is a superficial infection of the epidermis caused by streptococci, staphylococci, or both. Exposed portions of the body including the face, extremities, hands, and neck are the most common sites of involvement **(Figs. 1 to 4)**. Lesions teem with organisms and serve as a potential source of transmission to others. The disorder has a peak incidence in summer and early fall in temperate climates because of increased exposure to insect bites, injury, and colonization by pathogenic organisms. In tropical climates, impetigo is prevalent year-round. Impetigo was traditionally considered a streptococcal disease. However, in more recent decades, *Staphylococcus aureus (S. aureus)* has eclipsed *Streptococcus pyogenes (S. pyogenes)* as the predominant cause of impetigo. Accordingly, microbiologic culture is helpful for treatment choices, particularly if severe enough to warrant systemic antibiotics. In patients without preexisting dermatitis, lesions tend to be localized, but if the child has an antecedent condition (such as, eczema), the infection can spread rapidly to involve extensive areas.

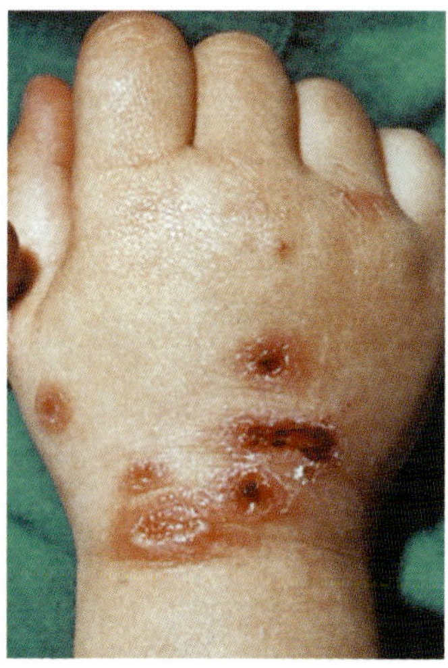

Fig. 1: Bullous impetigo.

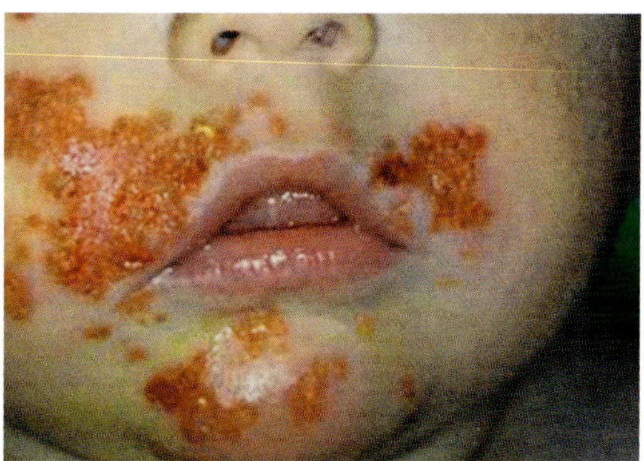

Fig. 2: Bullous impetigo.

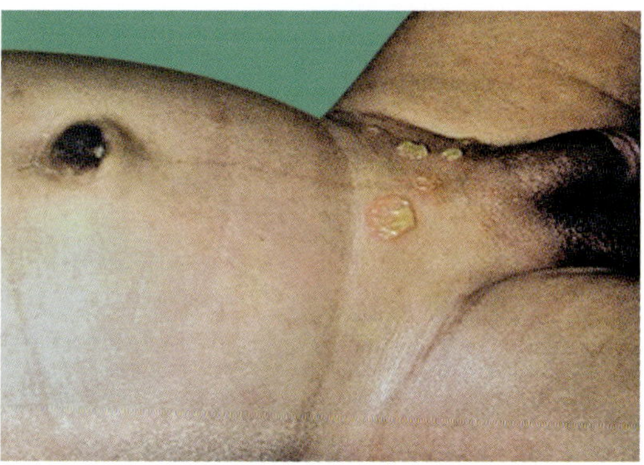

Fig. 3: Bullous impetigo.

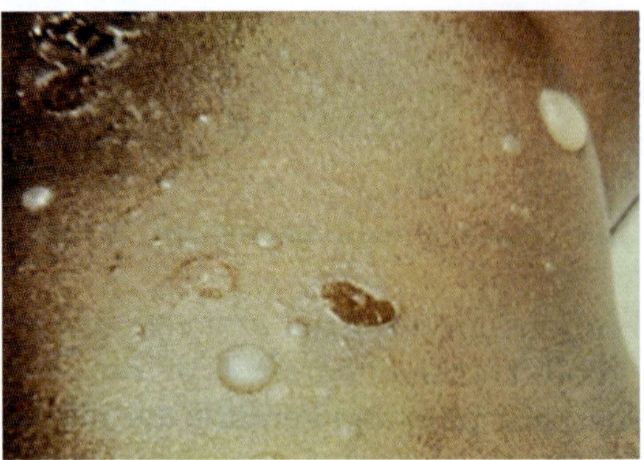

Fig. 4: Bullous impetigo.

Contagious superficial infection caused by streptococci, staphylococci, or both occurring frequently on the exposed parts of the body, begins with 1–2 mm erythematous macules and develops into thin-roofed vesicles/bullae surrounded by erythema. These rupture to form honey-colored crusts.

- *Bullous impetigo:* Staphylococci, streptococci.
- *Vesiculopustular impetigo:* Beta hemolytic streptococci.

Infantile Hemangioma

The infantile hemangioma is the second most common vascular anomaly with an incidence of 4.5% in the general population with a female predominance. The classic understanding of infantile hemangioma is a benign endothelial tumor that is usually absent at birth or present as a premonitory mark with rapid postnatal growth followed by slow involution. To expand upon this understanding, the clinician starts with understanding that infantile hemangioma has varied presentations in quality, location, size, and progression. These four areas also provide the key in clinically describing an infantile hemangioma.

These are proliferative benign vascular tumors of vascular endothelium may become apparent in the 1st or 2nd week of life.

They should be classified as superficial, deep, or mixed.

Innocent Murmurs

It originates from a normal heart. The characteristics of innocent murmur are as follows:

- Asymptomatic child
- Grade I and II
- Alters with postures
- Cardiovascular system is normal
- X-ray chest and ECG are normal.

CHARACTERISTICS OF INNOCENT MURMUR

- Asymptomatic
- Short systolic
- Varies with posture
- Soft blowing murmur
- Left sternal edge
- Normal heart sounds
- No parasternal thrill
- No radiation.

TYPES OF INNOCENT MURMUR

- Still's murmur: It is a mid-diastolic murmur. It is musical in character. It is heard over the lower left sternal edge or apex.
- Pulmonary flow murmur: It is an ejection murmur. It is heard over the pulmonary area. It is found commonly in infancy (0–6 months).
- Innocent systolic murmurs: An ejection systolic murmur is commonly heard in fit children or young adults, particularly after exercise or vasodilatation. Characteristically, the murmur is soft, best heard in the second left intercostal space, and becomes louder on inspiration; the second sound is normally split, and there are no other abnormal signs.

Insect Bite

Insect bites, most commonly caused by mosquitoes, fleas, mites, and fleas, tend to produce mild acute local reactions including erythema, edema, and urticarial papules that are typically pruritic. A tiny central crust or hemorrhagic punctum may be apparent on close inspection. On occasion, patients develop more intense hemorrhagic reactions.

Although mosquito and mite bites occur only during the warm months of spring, summer, and fall, flea bites can occur year-round, typically in households with pets or in apartments or homes recently vacated by previous tenants or owners whose pets had fleas. Young children who only visit on occasion with friends or relatives who have pets are also susceptible. Bites are usually found on the lower legs above the sock line but can be more diffusely distributed on crawling infants and toddlers. Like those of bedbugs, flea bites often appear in clusters of three (a clinical finding termed "breakfast, lunch, and dinner"). This stems from the fact that although fleas can jump, they cannot fly. Hence, they tend to produce a localized series of bites in the same vicinity before jumping on to a new area. Excoriation caused by scratching makes them prone to secondary impetiginization. It should also be noted that not all members of a household may be sensitive to flea bites, and therefore some may "appear" to be spared. This can be a source of confusion for people who assume that if fleas are the source, everyone should be affected.

On occasion, the bites of grass or sand mites can produce frank blistering because the venom they inject contains a blistering agent that affects sensitive individuals.

Biting flies include sandflies, blackflies, horseflies, and gnats. The bite itself causes immediate pain and is usually followed by the development of a painful papule that sometimes vesiculates centrally.

Intraosseous Transfusion

Intraosseous needles (for intramedullary venous plexus access) are special rigid large bore needles. If venous access is not available within approximately 1 minute in a child with cardiopulmonary arrest, an intraosseous (IO) needle should be placed in the anterior proximal tibia. This should penetrate the anterior layer of the compact bone; its tip is advanced into spongy interior of bone. All medications, blood products, including medications required for emergency resuscitation.

Infusion site is identified. Fractured bones should be avoided. Skin is cleaned over the chosen site. Needle is inserted at 90° to the skin. Needle is advanced until the "give" away sensation is felt as cortex is penetrated. A 5-mL syringe is attached. Aspirate or flush confirms the positioning. A 20-mL syringe is attached, and fluid is infused.

Intrauterine Transfusion

This is used for prophylactic administration of anti-D immunoglobulin to Rh-negative mother. It is a life-saving procedure. It helps to correct anemia to prevent hydrops. The indication is the critical titer of the indirect Coombs test and amniotic fluid optical density difference (ODD) at 450 mm at 20–22 weeks. It is the intrauterine transfusion of packed RBCs to correct anemia.

CHAPTER 235 Involuntary Movements

These are the muscular contractions involving a part of the body. These movements cannot be stopped. These are due to structural or biochemical lesion usually in the basal ganglion, reticular formation, and cerebellum.

Involuntary movements involve the part of the body as well as muscle fibers.

TREMORS

Rhythmic and regular oscillations of a body part are discussed here.

Types

- Resting tremors [3–5 cycles per second (CPS)] often seen in Parkinsonism, has low amplitude and regular frequency of five CPS, disappear during intentional movement and increases during emotional stress.

There are two descriptive types:

1. *Pill-rolling*
2. *Drum beating*
   - Parkinsonism tremors are often associated with lead-pipe or cogwheel rigidity, overall bradykinesia, akathisia (an irresistible need to move).
   - Intentional (ataxic tremor) regular tremor of low or moderate amplitude that appears during intentional movement (Finger-Nose test).
   - *Positional or postural tremor:* It occurs in maintaining a certain posture, e.g., holding head up or out stretching of hand. These are seen in cerebellar lesions or in their pathways. A combination of resting tremor, intention tremor, postural tremor constitutes "rubral tremor" due to a lesion in dentatorubral or dentatothalamic tract.
   - Tremors of anxiety, hypoglycemia, and hyperthyroidism are fine and fast (10 CPS)

It may be defined as a regular rhythmic oscillation of one part of the body from a fixed point usually in one plane.

It results from alternating or synchronous contractions of reciprocally innervated antagonistic muscles. The most affected parts of the body include limbs, neck, tongue, chin, or vocal cords.

There are three basic types of tremors:

1. *Resting tremor:* This is present when the relevant body point is rested completely.
2. *Postural tremor:* This is elicited by extending a limb against gravity.
3. *Intention tremor:* This is elicited by moving a limb to and from a target.

Athetosis

These are abnormal, non-repetitive, involuntary slow writhing movements of the periphery. These involve mostly fingers and wrists. These involve distal parts of the limb leading to rotation of limb and spreading toward the proximal part of the limb and trunk. The site of lesion is basal ganglia especially putamen. The causes are Wilson disease, tuberculosis, kernicterus, birth asphyxia, encephalitis, measles, and diphtheria.

Dystonia

These are prolonged slow alternating contraction and relaxation of agonists and antagonists. This frequently occurs in proximal joints. This causes abnormal posturing of limbs. This includes twisting for a prolonged period of time. The causes include benign dystonia of infancy, cerebral palsy, ataxia telangiectasia, and encephalitis.

Hemiballismus

It is an abnormal, involuntary, and non-repetitive violent flinging movement. It involves one side of the body. It mostly involves the proximal part of the limb. There will be a tendency to rotational movements of the limb and trunk, lesion is in subthalamic nuclei of lays. The causes include tuberculous meningitis and encephalitis.

TICS

It is spontaneous stereotyped muscle contraction. It involves the face. These can be stopped momentarily by volition. They are often associated with obsessive compulsion disorder. Causes include encephalitis, head injury, Sydenham chorea, and carbon monoxide poisoning.

Convulsions

This is the most common involuntary movements in childhood. It is an abnormal involuntary, repetitive, jerky vigorous movement (clonic) or sustained clonic (tonic) of a part or whole of the body. This may be with or without loss of consciousness.

Fasciculation

This is the contraction of a group of muscle fibers. This comprises the motor unit. It involves one or more motor units but not whole muscle. These are seen clinically in tongue, deltoid, calf muscle, and quadriceps muscles.

The causes include progressive spinal muscular atrophy, peroneal muscular atrophy, myositis, and collagen vascular disease. It can occur in normal subjects.

Fibrillation

It is the contraction of individual muscle fibers. It cannot be diagnosed by electromyography (EMG) and not clinically.

SECTION 10

Jaundice

Jaundice may be caused by a raised conjugated or unconjugated bilirubin. Unconjugated hyperbilirubinemia may be due to excessive production of bilirubin (hemolysis), reduced uptake of bilirubin, or a failure of conjugation by the liver. Conjugated hyperbilirubinemia results from hepatocellular damage or obstruction of the bile ducts, either within the liver (intrahepatic cholestasis) or of a major bile duct (extrahepatic obstruction jaundice). Jaundice is also often classified into pre-hepatic (hemolysis), hepatic, and extrahepatic types.

HISTORY

Chronic fatigue, though nonspecific, is a common symptom of liver disease and should trigger at least a basic evaluation including aminotransferases even in the absence of overt jaundice **(Flowchart 1)**. Myalgias, nausea, vomiting, and fever are often seen in patients with viral hepatitis or autoimmune hepatitis.

Acute biliary obstruction is signaled by right upper quadrant pain, vomiting, fever, and acholic stools in addition to jaundice.

Flowchart 1: Evaluation of cholestatic jaundice.

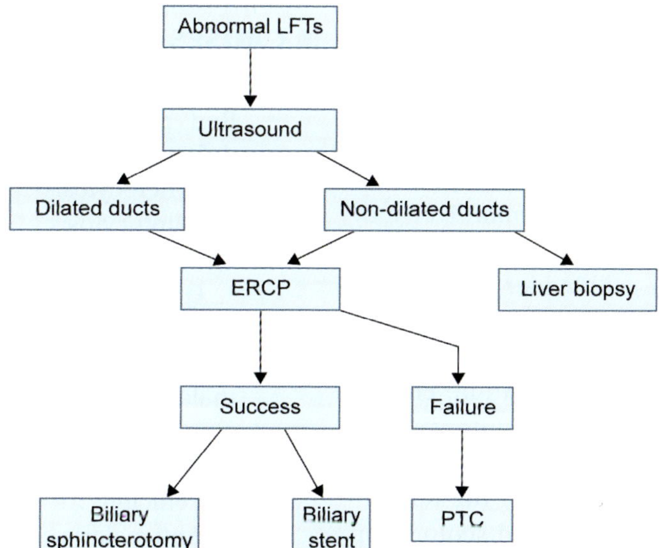

(ERCP: endoscopic retrograde cholangiopancreatography; LFTs: liver function tests; PTC: percutaneous transhepatic cholangiography)

Neurologic and psychiatric symptoms may be among the manifestations of Wilson disease. Autoimmune hepatitis may be accompanied by manifestations of other autoimmune disorders.

The child's age at the onset of symptoms may be helpful. Wilson disease commonly manifests in school-aged children and adolescents. Similarly, autoimmune hepatitis is most prevalent in school-aged children and adolescents with female predominance. A thorough history should include past and present use of prescription, over-the-counter (e.g., acetaminophen), and street drugs.

Symptoms of cholestasis such as jaundice, dark urine, steatorrhea, symptoms of fat-soluble vitamin deficiency, failure to thrive, and pruritus should be explored in detail.

CLINICAL FEATURES

The clinician should focus on signs of portal hypertension—spider angiomas, palmar erythema, dilated abdominal veins, ascites, and splenomegaly with a small liver **(Figs. 1A and B)**. Cutaneous excoriation as evidence of pruritus, xanthomas, and jaundice support cholestasis. Clubbing of digits may suggest hepatopulmonary syndrome. A large, tender liver is suggestive of acute viral hepatitis or congestive heart failure. A small liver may be found in patients with severe hepatitis or cirrhosis. A tender gallbladder is indicative of choledocholithiasis or cholecystitis. Abnormal neurologic findings, including tremor, fine motor incoordination, clumsy gait, and choreiform movements, suggest Wilson disease. A slit-lamp examination should be included to look for the Kayser–Fleischer rings (a brownish discoloration at the periphery of the cornea) of Wilson disease.

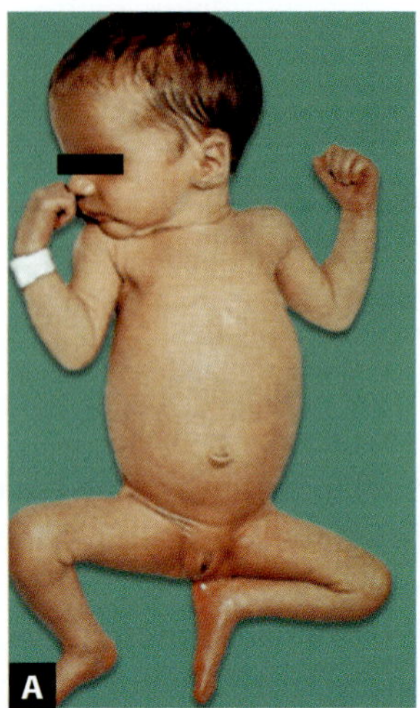

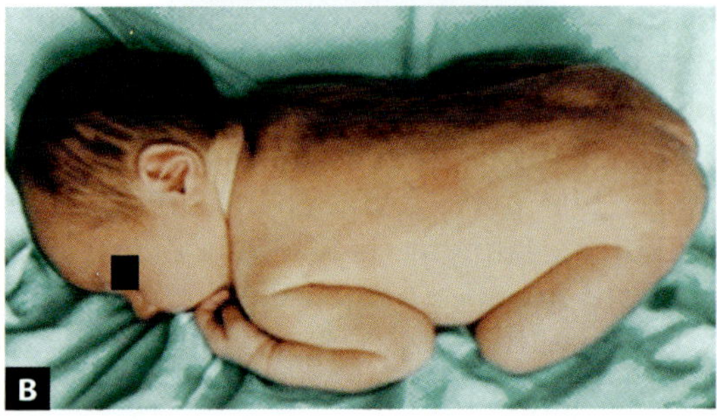

Figs. 1A and B: Jaundice.

CAUSES

- *Hemolytic (pre-hepatic):*
  - Red blood cell (RBC) membrane defects
    - Spherocytosis
    - Elliptocytosis
  - RBC enzyme defects
    - Glucose-6-phosphate dehydrogenase (G6PD) deficiency
  - Globin chain synthesis defect—thalassemic
  - Acquired hemolysis
    - Drug—surfs
    - Penicillin
    - Anti malaria
- *Liver cell disease:*
  - Neonatal jaundice

- Viral hepatitis
- Crigler–Najjar syndrome
- Gilbert's disease
- Galactosemia
- Hypothyroidism
- Intrauterine infection

▪ *Obstructive (posthepatic):*
- Biliary atresia
- Choledochal cyst
- Instigated bile
- Stricture and calculus in biliary tree
- Alpha-1 antitrypsin deficiency
- Dubin–Johnson syndrome
- Rotor syndrome

UNCONJUGATED HYPERBILIRUBINEMIA

A complete blood count with evaluation of the smear, reticulocyte count, and Coombs test can differentiate hemolytic from non-hemolytic disorders.

Erythrocyte membrane defects (spherocytosis) and enzyme defects (pyruvate kinase deficiency, G6PD) may not be apparent until childhood or adolescence. Acquired autoimmune hemolytic anemia is characterized by pallor, abdominal pain, fever, and dark urine in addition to jaundice. Laboratory studies document anemia and reticulocytosis. The direct Coombs test result is positive. Hemolytic anemia can be associated with infection, immunodeficiency, malignancy, hemolytic uremic syndrome, or other autoimmune disorders, such as systemic lupus erythematosus, rheumatoid arthritis, thyroid disorders, and autoimmune hepatitis.

Unconjugated hyperbilirubinemia can be caused by congestive heart failure and infection should in such circumstances extra-hepatic symptoms, cardiac failure, or sepsis dominate the picture. If no other explanation is found, Gilbert syndrome or Crigler–Najjar syndrome type II should be considered.

This condition is due to:

▪ *An increased production of bilirubin:*
- Inefficient marrow production
- Increased breakdown (hemolysis)
  - Hemoglobinopathies
  - Antibody-mediated
  - Drug-induced

▪ Decreased uptake of bilirubin into the liver; Gilbert's disease

▪ *Decreased conjugation of bilirubin in the liver:*
- Crigler–Najjar syndrome
- Neonatal jaundice
- Drugs
- Lucey–Driscoll syndrome

Viral Hepatitis

Infection

Infections are a common cause of jaundice in the child and adolescent. The most important step is to evaluate patients for synthetic liver failure and for signs of chronicity (portal hypertension, growth failure, risk factors for blood-borne, or sexually transmitted disorders). Patients with synthetic liver failure should be referred for urgent evaluation by the liver transplant center.

Hepatitis A virus (HAV) infection is usually anicteric or asymptomatic in children <5 years of age. About 2–7 days before the onset of jaundice, there is a flulike illness with symptoms that can include malaise, headache, myalgias, anorexia, vomiting, diarrhea, right upper quadrant pain, and fever. Some children present with cough and coryza. The urine becomes dark, and jaundice and pale or acholic stools develop. Aminotransferase levels are 10–100 times normal. The diagnosis is confirmed by an HAV IgM study. Children generally recover within 2 weeks.

Acute hepatitis C virus (HCV) infection is often mild and usually subclinical. Jaundice is unusual. Screening for hepatitis uses anti-HCV antibodies, and infection is confirmed via polymerase chain reaction (PCR) for HCV RNA. Transmission may be parenteral due to IV drug use or exposure to blood, or sexual or vertical transmission is also possible.

Wilson's Disease

Wilson disease is an autosomal recessive disorder of copper metabolism. As a result of ATP7B mutation, copper cannot be excreted and it accumulates in the liver, which causes hepatic steatosis and necrosis. Copper is then released into the circulation and is ultimately deposited in the central nervous system, kidneys, and cornea. The hepatic manifestation predominates in childhood; a neuropsychiatric manifestation becomes more common later, in adolescence and adulthood. The liver involvement may manifest as acute hepatitis, fulminant hepatic failure, chronic hepatitis, cirrhosis, or asymptomatic elevation of serum aminotransferases. Neurologic symptoms such as dysarthria, clumsiness, tremor, and mood disorders may or may not be present. In the kidney, the result is tubular dysfunction; in the cornea, the result is Kayser–Fleischer rings. Hemolysis can be present as a result of copper toxicity. The diagnosis is supported by documenting a low serum ceruloplasmin level, high urinary copper excretion, and increased hepatic copper concentrations on liver biopsy.

Autoimmune Hepatitis

Autoimmune hepatitis (AIH) is a common cause of chronic liver injury. The most frequent course is insidious with fatigue as a dominant symptom. Autoimmune hepatitis can present acutely with malaise, anorexia, nausea, vomiting, and jaundice. Autoimmune disorders such as arthritis, thyroiditis, vasculitis, nephritis, hemolytic anemia, or diabetes mellitus are often associated with AIH.

Biliary Disease

Primary Sclerosing Cholangitis

Primary sclerosing cholangitis (PSC) is characterized by focal dilatation and stenosis of the intrahepatic or extrahepatic bile ducts with surrounding fibrosis resulting from an inflammatory process. It can manifest from early childhood through adulthood.

Extrahepatic Biliary Obstruction

Gallstones

Gallstones are particularly common in children with hemolytic disorders, such as sickle cell disease, thalassemia, erythrocyte membrane defects, erythrocyte enzyme defects, and autoimmune hemolytic anemia. The mean age at presentation is 12 years. Gallstones are also associated with anatomic abnormalities of the biliary tract, cystic fibrosis, ileal dysfunction, obesity, parenteral nutrition, sepsis, prematurity, and pregnancy.

JAUNDICE IN THE NEONATE AND INFANT

Physiologic and Breast Milk Jaundice

In neonates, increased bilirubin production is caused by the normally increased neonatal red blood cell mass and the decreased life span of the red blood cells (80 vs. 120 days). Albumin binding is decreased because of lower albumin concentrations and diminished binding capacity, which results in decreased transport of unconjugated bilirubin (UCB) to the liver with increased deposition in tissues. Uptake of bilirubin by the hepatocytes during the 1st weeks of life is defective. Low levels of glutathione S-transferase B decrease intracellular binding, which may impede the transport of UCB to the endoplasmic reticulum. Conjugation is impaired by decreased activity of uridine diphosphate glucuronosyltransferase (UDPGT). Secretion into the canaliculi is impaired. There is increased enterohepatic circulation of unconjugated bilirubin as a result of increased concentrations of β-glucuronidase in the intestinal lumen and as a result of decreased intestinal bacterial flora, leading to diminished urobilinogen formation.

These features contribute in varying degrees to physiologic jaundice, characterized by a peak bilirubin level of <13 mg/dL on postnatal days 3–5, a decrease to normal by 2 weeks of age, and a conjugated fraction of <20%. In premature, breastfed infants of diabetic mother, the peak is higher and lasts longer. Conjugated bilirubin should be checked if there is any question of the nature of jaundice.

Breastfeeding has been associated with an increased incidence of unconjugated hyperbilirubinemia outside the expected range (>13 mg/dL). Jaundice of this level may occur in 10–25% of breastfed infants, in contrast to 4–7% of formula-fed infants. It can occur within the 1st 5 days of life and is referred to as "early" or "breastfeeding" jaundice. Breastfeeding jaundice is seen in infants who are not feeding adequately and may be dehydrated or malnourished. In a second group of breastfed infants, the jaundice develops slowly, occurring after the first week of life, and peaks between the 2nd and 3rd weeks of life at 10–20 mg/dL. This is referred to as "late" or "breast milk" jaundice. The precise cause of increased bilirubin levels in this latter setting has not been established; alternative theories include inhibition of glucuronosyltransferase activity and increased enterohepatic circulation of UCB. Kernicterus appears to be very rare but has been reported in association with breastfeeding. No treatment is necessary for physiologic jaundice **(Fig. 2)**.

Polycythemia: Neonatal polycythemia, defined as a hematocrit >65% by venipuncture, can be caused by maternal diabetes, maternal-fetal, or twin-twin transfusion, intrauterine hypoxemia, endocrine disorders, and delayed cord clamping. Polycythemia results in increased bilirubin production because of the increased red blood cell mass.

Hemolytic disorders: Reticulocytosis, unconjugated hyperbilirubinemia, and an increased nucleated red blood cell count, with either a low or normal hematocrit, suggest hemolysis. This can result from isoimmunization; erythrocyte membrane, hemoglobin, or enzyme defects; or sepsis with disseminated intravascular coagulation.

Isoimmune hemolytic disease: In this group of disorders, maternal antibodies

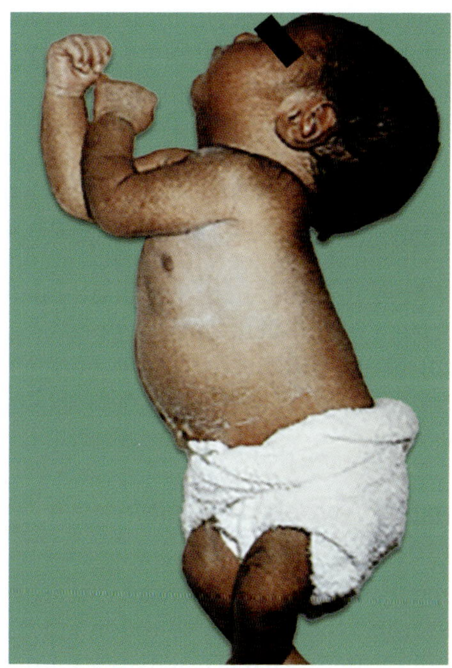

Fig. 2: Kernicterus.

(immunoglobulin G) to the infant's erythrocytes cross the placenta, resulting in red blood cell destruction. The administration of anti-D gamma globulin [RhO(D) immune globulin (RhoGAM)] after delivery to women who are Rh-negative has reduced the incidence of Rh sensitization and erythroblastosis fetalis.

The diagnosis is confirmed by demonstrating that the infant is Rh-positive, that the direct Coombs test result is positive, and that maternal antibody is coating the infant's red blood cells.

ABO blood type incompatibility causes a less severe form of isoimmune hemolytic disease with a less rapid development of jaundice. It is more common in infants with blood type A or B who are born to mothers with blood type O.

Erythrocyte enzyme defects: G6PD deficiency is common. Jaundice is seen more frequently in persons with a Mediterranean or Far Eastern ancestry who have a complete absence of the enzyme. In these individuals, hemolysis can occur without a precipitant. In African-American patients, the disease is generally less severe, and hemolysis is rare without exposure to a drug, toxin, or infection that causes an oxidant stress. G6PD deficiency can manifest as neonatal jaundice on day 2 or 3 after birth; alternatively, it may not manifest until later in childhood, when jaundice is associated with an acute hemolytic crisis. The diagnosis of G6PD deficiency is confirmed by documenting deficiency of the enzyme in red blood cells.

Familial Disorders of Bilirubin Metabolism

Gilbert syndrome is a heterogeneous group of disorders that have in common at least a 50% decrease in UDPGT activity as a result of a defect in the gene responsible for this enzyme. In 20–30% of individuals with Gilbert syndrome, there is also a decrease in hepatocyte bilirubin uptake. Affected individuals are generally asymptomatic and may not present with jaundice until the 2nd or 3rd decade of life. Gilbert syndrome may be responsible for some cases of neonatal jaundice. Mild jaundice with a bilirubin level up to 7 mg/dL can occur transiently with fatigue, exercise, fasting, febrile illness, and alcohol ingestion in older patients.

Crigler–Najjar syndrome: Crigler–Najjar syndrome types I and II (also known as Arias syndrome) are rare autosomal recessive conditions caused by mutations (different alleles from those of Gilbert syndrome) in the gene coding for UDPGT.

The onset of Crigler–Najjar syndrome type II is usually at birth, although it can be in late childhood. There is <5% of the normal UDPGT activity. Bile contains bilirubin monoglucuronides. Bilirubin levels, generally 8–25 mg/dL, respond to phenobarbital administration with a significant decrease. Neurologic disease is rare.

Lucey-Driscoll syndrome: Lucey-Driscoll syndrome is a transient familial neonatal hyperbilirubinemia that appears in the 1st few days of life and resolves by 2–3 weeks of age. This results from the inhibition of UDPGT by a substance that has been found in both maternal and infant serum.

Neonatal Conjugated Hyperbilirubinemia

Common to all of these conditions is the potential for hypoprothrombinemia. If the PT is prolonged, the infant should be treated with intravenous vitamin K to avoid spontaneous hemorrhage, particularly intracranial. Depending on the degree of hepatocellular damage, vitamin K may not correct the PT.

Hypoglycemia is another danger that is associated with diseases that cause severe hepatic dysfunction, metabolic disorders as well as with hypopituitarism. The infant may be relatively asymptomatic despite significant hypoglycemia. The serum glucose level can be measured before a feeding. If hypoglycemia is present, the infant should receive frequent feedings, continuous feedings, or intravenous dextrose infusions. Glucose level should always be the part of the evaluation of conjugated hyperbilirubinemia.

Obstructive/Anatomic Abnormalities, Idiopathic Cholestasis, and Idiopathic Neonatal Hepatitis

Biliary atresia: Untreated biliary atresia is lethal, and only prompt diagnosis and surgical treatment can prevent mortality. Biliary atresia accounts for approximately 30% of cases of neonatal cholestasis seen at major referral centers. It occurs in one in 8,000–15,000 live births. It is the result of a progressive inflammatory process leading to obliteration of the lumen of the extrahepatic duct. It is the leading indication for liver transplantation in the pediatric population. Infants are less often icteric from birth and more often develop jaundice at 2–6 weeks of age. Infants are usually full term and initially appear healthy except for jaundice, dark urine, and acholic stools. The family history usually is negative for liver disease. There appear to be two forms of biliary atresia:

BOX 1: Conditions not to miss in infants with conjugated hyperbilirubinemia.

- *Priorities:*
  - Hypoprothrombinemia
  - Hypoglycemia
  - Extrahepatic biliary atresia
- *Infections:*
  - Sepsis
  - Urinary tract infection
  - Syphilis
  - Toxoplasmosis
  - Herpes simplex virus
- *Endocrine disorders:*
  - Hypopituitarism
  - Hypothyroidism
- *Metabolic disorders:*
  - Galactosemia
  - Hereditary fructose intolerance (fructosemia)
  - Tyrosinemia
- *Other:*
  - Neonatal hemochromatosis
  - Bile acid abnormalities
  - Choledochal cyst
  - Intestinal obstruction
  - Familial hemophagocytic syndromes
  - Heart disease
  - Toxins

1. In the "embryonic" or "fetal form," which occurs in 15–30% of cases, there is no jaundice-free period. There are often associated defects, including cardiac defects, polysplenia, malrotation, and situs inversus.
2. In the "perinatal form," there may be a jaundice-free interval after resolution of the normal physiologic jaundice, and there are no associated anomalies.

There are a few conditions "Not to Miss in Infants with Conjugated Hyperbilirubinemia" given in **Box 1**.

237 CHAPTER

Jugular Venous Pressure

The pressure is noted in the internal jugular vein. Its pulsations are observed. It is underneath the sternomastoid muscle. It clinically assesses the right atrial pressure which is directly transmitted into internal jugular vein.

Clinical recording of the jugular venous pressure is done when the child is at 45° inclined position. The neck muscles should be relaxed. The upper border of jugular venous pulsation should be looked for.

The horizontal plane at the upper border of pulsation, by placing the measuring scale is made to contact and cut the vertical plane at sternal angle, i.e., by placing another measuring scale. The distance between the sternal angle and the meeting point between the two planes is the measurement of jugular venous pressure.

When the jugular venous pressure is raised.

- Pulsation is visible in sitting position at the lower part of the neck.
- The vertical measurement of the upper border of venous pulsation made at sternal angle is >4 cm at 45°.

CAUSES OF RAISED JUGULAR VENOUS PRESSURE

- *Common causes:*
  - Congestive cardiac failure
  - Over-transfusion
  - Cor pulmonale/right heart failure
  - Tricuspid regurgitation
- *Less common causes:*
  - Pericardial effusion
  - Massive pulmonary embolism
  - Constrictive pericarditis
  - Tricuspid regurgitation
- *Rare causes:*
  - Restrictive cardiomyopathy
  - Carcinoid syndrome
  - Right atrial tumors

238 CHAPTER

Jugular Venous Pulsations

For practical purposes, the jugular venous pressure may be regarded as raised if jugular pulsation is visible, or the internal jugular vein is seen to be distended, with the patient sitting erect. This is more reproducible than the older criterion of 4 cm above the sternal angle with the patient lying at 45°, and a grossly elevated venous pressure is less likely to be missed.

The first major distinction is between non-pulsatile and pulsatile elevation of the venous pressure.

ABNORMALITIES OF THE JUGULAR VENOUS PULSE

- Congestive failure
- Tricuspid regurgitation
- Right atrial hypertrophy
- Complete heart block
- Ventricular tachycardia
- Pacemaker, etc.
- Constrictive pericarditis
- Tricuspid stenosis

The differences between jugular venous pulsation (JVP) and carotid artery pulsation are elaborated in **Table 1**.

WAVES

The pulse has three positive waves "a", "c", and "v" and two negative waves or "x" and "y" wave is due to atrial contraction. The "c" waves are due to bulging of valve apparatus into the atrium during the onset of valve apparatus into the atrium during the onset of ventricular asystole.

The "v" wave is due to venous inflow and rise in pressure in the atria during ventricular systole. The "x" descent is due to atrial relaxation and also due to ventricular contraction pulling down the floor of atrium toward the ventricular aspects. The "y" descent is due to rapid atrial emptying in the early part of ventricular diastole **(Fig. 1)**.

Three Positive Waves and Two Descents

Three positive waves are:

a: Corresponds to atrial contraction

c: Corresponds to AV valve closure

v: Corresponds to atrial filling when AV valve is closed.

Large v: Waves are seen tricuspid regurgitation.

TABLE 1: Difference between jugular venous pulsation (JVP) and carotid artery pulsation.

	JVP	*Carotid artery pulsation*
Position	Lateral	Medial
Visible and palpable	Better seen	Better felt
Wave form	Multiple wave form	Single brief pulsation
Respiration	Decreased in inspiration Increased in expiration	No change

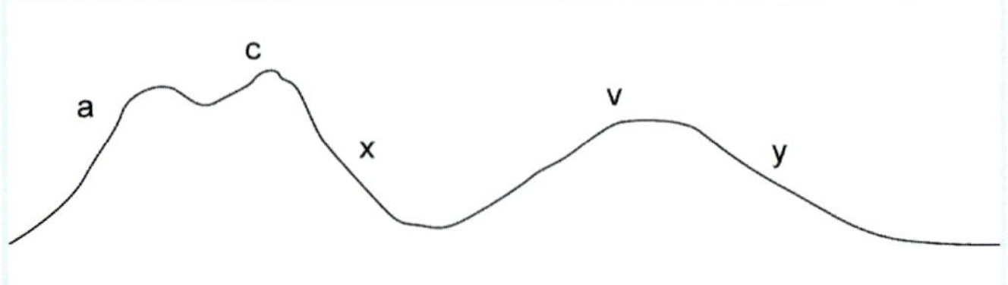

Fig. 1: Jugular venous pulse wave form.

Two descents are:

x: Corresponds to atrial relaxation

y: Corresponds to the opening of AV valve and to passive filling of right ventricle at the start of diastole. Decreased Y descent is due to obstruction to right ventricular filling.

Giant a waves: This occurs when the right atrium contracts against higher ventricular and diastolic pressure.

- Pulmonary hypertension
- Pulmonary stenosis
- Pulmonary atresia

CANNON WAVES

Cannon *a* wave is a giant *a* wave and occurs in cases with atrioventricular dissociation, where the area contracts against a closed tricuspid valve. Independent of the ventricular contraction. It is seen in complete heart block and ventricular tachycardia with atrioventricular dissociation.

KUSSMAUL SIGN

Normally during inspiration there is negative intrathoracic pressure leads to increased venous return; this leads to fall in jugular venous pressure. If there is a reverse, i.e., during inspiration the jugular venous enlargement increases. The phenomenon is called Kussmaul sign. This occurs in pericardial effusion and constrictive pericarditis. As this is hindrance to drainage of superior vena cava into the right atrium, the increased venous return in response to negative intrathoracic pressure during inspiration is to be accommodated within the vein itself.

Kussmaul's sign can occur in right heart failure and restrictive cardiomyopathy.

HEPATOJUGULAR REFLEX

Right hypochondrial is pressed for 30 seconds so that the liver is pressed. Normally there will be a rise in JVP by 3 cm. This is followed by gradual fall, which occurs even if the pressure is sustained. Hepatojugular reflex is said to be elevated if it is >3 cm and, does not fall even, instead there is sustained rise in JVP, for >15 seconds. Hepatojugular reflex is elevated in right heart failure, tricuspid regurgitation.

Keloid

Keloids are firm, rubbery nodules or plaques that result from the proliferation of fibroblasts and deposition of collagen after injury to the skin. They can be pruritic or tender, especially during the active growing phase, and they may extend well beyond the margins of the original wound. This latter trait distinguishes keloids from hypertrophic scars, which remain confined to the wound margins and flatten partially within 6 months of the injury. In predisposed individuals, keloids often occur after minimal injury, such as abrasions, minor lacerations, acne papules, insect bites, and ear piercing. Fortunately, they are not commonly seen on the midface. Keloids may soften or regress with topical or intralesional steroid injections alone or in combination with surgical excision. However, recurrences, especially following surgery, are common.

CHAPTER 240

Kidney: Palpable

Kidneys are rarely palpable in healthy children. A kidney may be enlarge because of an obstruction (hydronephrosis), an infection, a cyst, or a tumor. Bilateral renal enlargement suggests either polycystic kidney or bilateral obstructive uropathy due to posterior urethral valves.

Kidneys are palpated bimanually. To palpate the right kidney, keep the right hand over the right lumbar region and the left hand behind the right loin at the renal angle. The renal angle is formed in the back by the lower border of the twelfth rib and outer border of erector spinae muscle. Press the right hand deep into the abdomen to push the kidney posteriorly during expiration when the abdominal muscles are relaxed. The left hand is used to push the kidney anteriorly. Try to feel for the lower pole of kidney as the child takes deep breaths.

Kidneys are usually ballot able, i.e., can be pushed between the two hands. To elicit ballot ability, push the kidney down with the right hand, and feel by your left hand kept in the loin when it strikes posterior surface of the abdomen. A renal lump will also move with respiration. The lower pole of the right kidney may be palpable in thin patients.

Palpate the left kidney in a similar way by keeping the right hand in the left lumber region and the left hand posteriorly in the left loin. You can stand either on the right or the left side of the patient.

A renal lump is palpable in following situations—Wilms tumor, perinephric abscess, hydronephrosis, renal cysts, congenital anomalies, and ectopic kidney.

The differences between an enlarged spleen and an enlarged kidney are highlighted in **Table 1**.

Based on the above physical characters, a renal tumor should present little difficulty in diagnosis; however, a tumor possessing several of these characters may often create considerable doubt as to the nature of the organ from which it has arisen. The following points will assist in the differentiation of renal swellings from other tumors with which they may be confused.

TABLE 1: Differences between enlarged spleen and kidney.

	Spleen	***Kidney***
Direction of enlargement	Toward the right iliac fossa	Loin
Splenic notch	Present	Absent
Hand insinuation	Not possible	Possible
Percussion	Dull	Resonance

241 CHAPTER

Knock Knees

The knees are closed to each other and the intermalleolar distance is increased. It is seen in congenital condition, a normal variant and in rickets.

Knock knee in child younger than age 7 should be ignored **(Fig. 1)**. There is asymmetric angular deformity or evidence of knee instability, with a lateral thrust (bow leg) or medial thrust (knock knee) that occurs immediately on weight bearing.

Joint is palpated for the evidence of effusion. *Bulge sign* is elicited to detect a small-to-moderate effusion by milking fluid out of medial recess in suprapatellar pouch and then stroking the lateral recess in downward direction to move the fluid back into the medial recess. The later maneuver creates a fluid bulge in the knees medial aspect between the patella and femur.

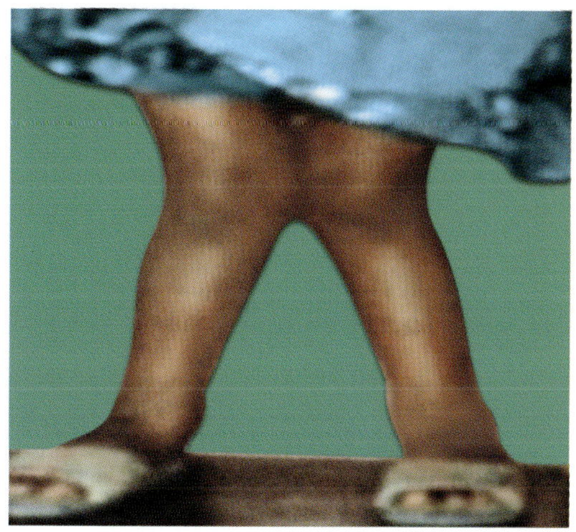

Fig. 1: Knock knee.

Laryngomalacia

Laryngomalacia, a congenital condition, accounts for >70% of cases of persistent inspiratory stridor in infants. The problem is the result of unusual flaccidity of the laryngeal structures, especially the epiglottis and the arytenoid cartilages. The supraglottic structures hang over the airway entrance. Stridor is inspiratory, hence does not represent true wheezing.

CHAPTER 243

Length and Height

RECUMBENT LENGTH VERSUS HEIGHT

Babies younger than 10–12 months cannot stand alone and most toddlers refuse to stand. Hence, any child younger than 2 years should be measured for length in the recumbent position. Standard growth charts for young children are based on the measurement of recumbent length.

There are two types of length **(Figs. 1A and B)**:

1. *Crown-heel length*: It is the measurement from the crown of the head to the feet of the infant. Here, the child's body is fully extended by flattening the knees and maintaining the head in midline position. The head piece is fixed to the measuring table at zero mark. The foot piece is made to slide along the measuring board till it touches against the sole of the feet.
2. *Crown rump length*: It is the measurement from the crown of the head to the rump in the infant. It is equivalent to sitting height in the older child.

HEIGHT MEASUREMENT

Standing height can be measured when the child can stand straight and can hold the head so that the line of vision should be parallel to floor surface. The child stands in bare foot against the wall on which there is a ruler. The child's occiput, upper back, buttocks, and heels touch the wall. A flat object is placed on the head and against the ruler to obtain the accurate measurement **(Fig. 2)**. Older child may stand on the scale.

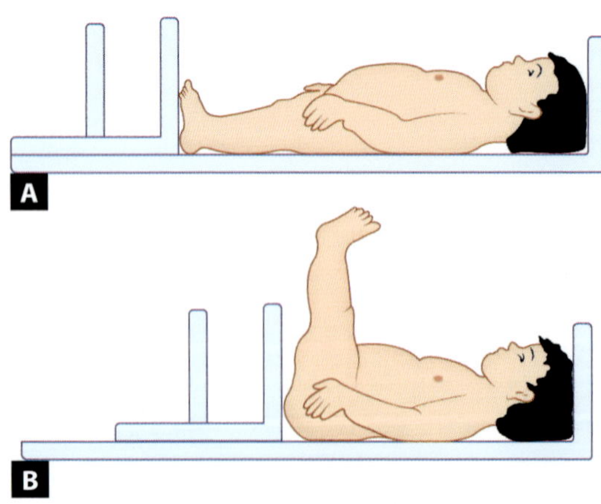

Figs. 1A and B: Types of length. (A) Body length measurement; (B) Crown–rump measurement.

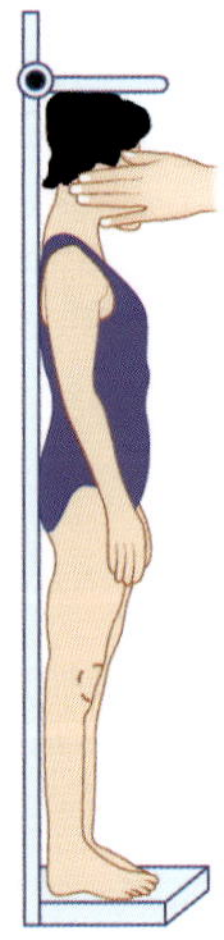

Fig. 2: Measurement of height.

The difference in the height and length can be up to 2 cm, as ligaments are compressed in standing posture.

Nutritional deficiency for long term will affect the linear growth. Acute malnutrition will result in wasting of subcutaneous tissue and muscle mass.

Formula to calculate the expected height:

2–12 year : Age (year) × 6 + 77 cm

Height (Length)-for-age

Height should be taken in a standing position without footwear. If the height machine is not available, the measuring scale fixed to the wall can be employed. This arrangement is suitable for children 2 years and above. The measuring scale should be capable of measuring to an accuracy of 0.1 cm. A very great effort should be made to measure children accurately. Errors in the measurement of a young child may lead to significant errors in the classification of the nutritional status. The WHO standards for height-for-age are given in **Table 1**.

The length of a baby at birth is about 50 cm. It increases by about 25 cm during first year, and by another 12 cm during the second year. During growth spurt, boys add something like 20 cm in their height, and girls gain 16 cm. The spurt is followed by a rapid slowing of growth. Indian girls reach 98% of their final height on an average by the age of 16.5 years, and boys reach the same stage by the age of 17.75 years.

Height is a stable measurement of growth as opposed to body weight. Whereas weight reflects only the present health status of the child, height indicates the events in the past also.

Low Height for Age

This is also known as nutritional stunting or dwarfing. It reflects past or chronic malnutrition. The cut-off point commonly taken for the diagnosis of stunting is 90% of the height-for-age values. Waterlow recorded the use of 2SD below the median reference as the cut-off point.

TABLE 1: WHO standards for length/height for age of boys and girls up to the age of 5 years (cm).

		Boys			Girls	
Age (months)	–2SD	Median	+2SD	–2SD	Median	+2SD
0	46.1	49.9	53.7	45.4	49.1	52.9
4	59.7	63.9	68.0	57.8	62.1	66.4
8	66.2	70.6	75.0	64.0	68.7	73.5
12	71.0	75.7	80.5	68.9	74.0	79.2
16	75.0	80.2	85.4	73.0	78.6	84.2
20	77.7	83.2	88.8	76.7	82.7	88.7
24	81.7	87.8	93.9	80.0	86.4	92.9
28	83.8	90.4	97.0	82.2	89.1	96.0
32	86.4	93.4	100.4	84.9	92.2	99.4
36	88.7	96.1	103.5	87.4	95.1	102.7
40	90.9	98.6	106.4	89.8	97.7	105.7
44	93.0	101.0	109.1	92.0	100.3	108.6
48	94.9	103.3	111.7	94.1	102.7	111.3
52	96.9	105.6	114.2	96.1	105.0	114.0
56	98.8	107.8	116.7	98.1	107.3	116.5
60	100.7	110.0	119.2	99.9	109.4	118.9

Leukemoid Reaction

A leukemoid reaction, which is characterized by a high WBC count (usually >50,000/mm^3) also must be distinguished from leukemia carefully. Although this is definitively accomplished by a bone marrow aspirate, peripheral blood studies can assist a diagnosis. Patients with Down syndrome may experience a transient leukemoid reaction (called *transient myeloproliferative disorder*) in the newborn period. Some red flags of malignancy are mentioned in **Box 1**.

BOX 1: Red flags of malignancy.

- Pallor, fatigue
- Petechiae
- Fever without source
- Bone pain, limp
- Weight loss
- Anorexia
- Headache, vomiting, and lethargy
- Lymphadenopathy
- Hepatomegaly
- Splenomegaly
- Abdominal mass
- Testiculomegaly

245 CHAPTER

Leukocoria (White Pupillary Reflex)

Leukocoria is the term used to describe an abnormal white papillary reflex **(Fig. 1)**. Leukocoria or "white pupil" is a sign, not a specific disease. True leukocoria mandates prompt referral to an ophthalmologist as the causes may threaten either vision and/or life. Retinoblastoma is the most feared cause of leukocoria because of its potential to metastasize and cause death. It is the most common malignant ocular tumor of childhood, with an incidence of about 1/15,000. Leukocoria, the most common presenting sign, is caused by light reflection from the tumor's white surface as opposed to the usual red reflex from the retina. Approximately, 25% present with strabismus. Less common presentations include periocular inflammation, glaucoma, and proptosis.

Normally, the ophthalmoscope will elicit a red pupillary reflex due to the reflection of a vascular retina and choroid through a clear lens, anterior and posterior chambers. When it is not possible to clearly visualize the fundus, the least that should be done is to observe this red reflex. Obtaining a white pupillary reflex signifies that a lenticular opacity (cataract) is present or that some other intraocular pathogenesis is present.

Disorders associated with white pupillary reflex include cataracts, colobomas, retrolental fibroplasia, chorioretinitis, retinoblastoma, organized vitreous hemorrhage, congenital retinal fold, intraocular foreign body, retinal detachment, metastatic retinitis and endophthalmitis, external exudative retinitis of Coats, larval granulomatosis (*Toxocara canis or cati*), and persistent primary vitreous. Differential diagnosis of leukocoria is mentioned in **Box 1**.

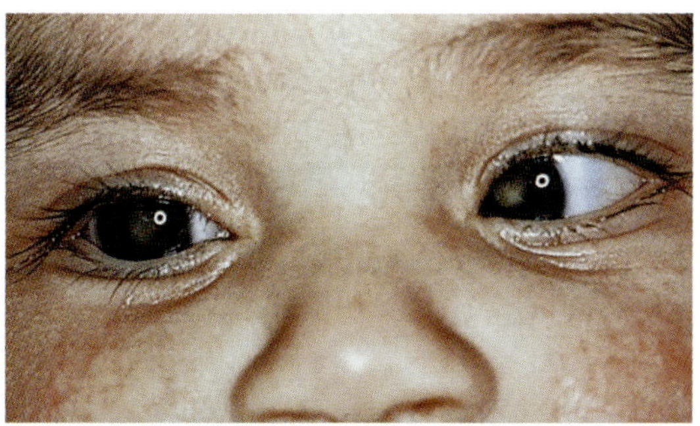

Fig. 1: White pupillary reflex.

BOX 1: Differential diagnosis of leukocoria.

- Angiomatosis retinae
- Cataracts
- Coats disease
- Colobomas
- Congenital retinal fold
- High myopia
- Incontinentia pigmenti
- Medulloepithelioma
- Myelinated nerve fibers
- Persistent hyperplastic primary vitreous (PHPV)
- Retinal detachment
- Retinal dysplasia
- Retinoblastoma
- Retinopathy of prematurity (ROP)
- Toxocariasis
- Uveitis
- Vitreous hemorrhage

246 CHAPTER

Lips: Affections

Lips should be examined for cleft lip **(Fig. 1)**, unilateral/bilateral, micro- or macrocheilia, congenital pits, or fissures.

Examine the lips for texture, color (cyanosis, anemia), abnormal pigmentation (Peutz–Jeghers syndrome; **Fig. 2)**, swellings, ulcers, blisters, and cracks.

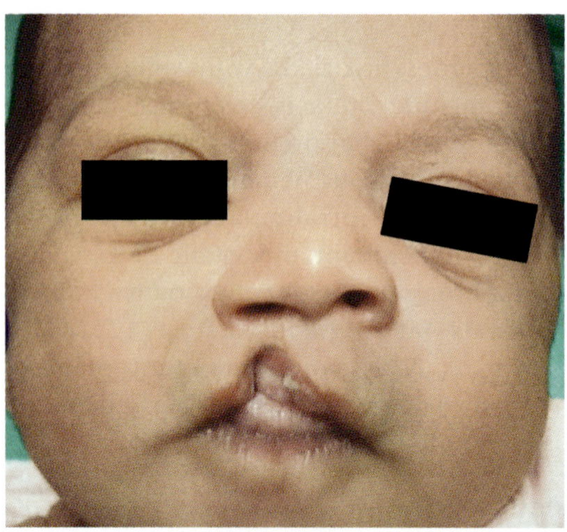

Fig. 1: Cleft lip.

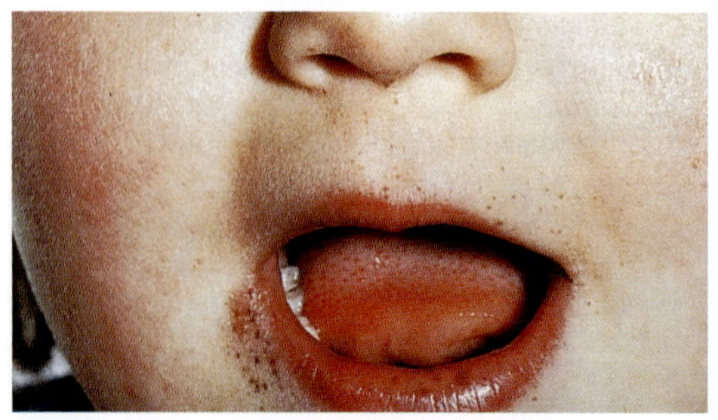

Fig. 2: Peutz–Jeghers syndrome.

Alteration in color may indicate anemia and cyanosis. Circumoral pallor should be noted and seen in scarlet fever. Chapping, flaking, and cracking may denote a recent fever, Herpes labialis, constant mouth breathing, or something as simple as outdoor activity with too much exposure to wind or sun. Lips may be large in case of Hurler's syndrome, angioneurotic edema, or as simple as racial macrocheilia.

The most commonly troublesome lesion affecting the lips is angular cheilitis, deep folds at angles of mouth become traumatized as a result of continual wetting of saliva and get secondarily infected.

CAUSES AND ANGULAR CHEILITIS

Generalized swellings of the lips may occur from trauma, bites, stings, lymphangitis, lip abscess, intraoral abscess, or angioneurotic edema.

Localized swellings may arise from the same cause and additionally from herpes simplex, mucous cysts, pyogenic granuloma, hemangiomas, lymphangiomas, or other tumors.

The frenulum should be examined for any extensions palatally or lingually between the teeth.

CHAPTER 247

Light Reflex

The light reflexes must be tested in a dimly lit room. Patient is instructed to look straight ahead and focus at a point in the distance (to avoid constriction of the pupil that accompanies convergence). The examiner may place the edge of one hand against the nose and forehead to prevent light from reaching the other eye. The other eye should remain open during the test. The examiner brings the bright light of a pen torch from the side of the patients head into one eye. Pupillary reactions in both eyes should be examined and duly recorded.

Afferent pathway is through the optic nerve-pretectal nucleus—Edinger-Westphal nucleus. Efferent fibers are carried by the oculomotor nerve through the ciliary ganglion.

Iridoplegia describes a condition in which the pupil does not react to light. Amaurotic pupil is one that does not constrict in response to light (complete destruction of retina or optic nerve).

248 CHAPTER

Lisch Nodules

These are the pigmented hamartomas of iris, are seen in more than 90% of patients with neurofibromatosis 1 who are older than 6 years, and can be found in nearly one-third of younger individuals. Although these hamartomas are asymptomatic and do not correlate with extent and other manifestations, they are helpful in establishing diagnosis.

CHAPTER 249

Lordosis

There is a smooth extension curve. Normal cervical or lumbar lordosis describes the standing posture of these two areas of the spine. Compensatory lordosis indicates an increased curve secondary to a structural kyphosis of the thoracic spine.

Lordosis causes an unusually large, inward arch on lower back, just above the buttocks. The condition may cause lower back pain. When the lordosis at your lower back or your neck becomes too much pronounced low back pain, numbness and weakness may occur.

Gradual kyphosis (round kyphosis) is due to partial or complete collapse of more than two vertebrae, e.g., ankylosing spondylitis.

An abnormally prominent spinal convexity anteriorly is known as lordosis. Some amount of lordosis is normally present in the lumbar and cervical regions (in tetanus there is posterior curving of whole back opisthotonus).

In lumbar lordosis, due to disease, the abdomen becomes prominent. If the central furrow is deeper, it indicates that the lordosis is exaggerated and if there is no central furrow, there is complete obliteration of the lordosis and flattening of the back. Look for any swelling, sinuses, depression, scar, nevus, tuft of hair (e.g., spina bifida occulta), note any globular swelling, with or without skin cover (spina bifida manifesta, meningomyelocele), compensatory lordosis may be due to bilateral CDH.

250 CHAPTER

Low-set Ears

Because the ear has a complex origin, it is subject to a wide variation in position, size, and structure and is almost as individual as fingerprints. Assessing ear position and rotation often is extremely subjective and imprecise. A scrupulous examination technique is required to conclude that a child has "low-set" ears. The ears must be examined at an appropriate angle. If examined from the front with the child's neck extended, the ears will appear low. If the ears are examined from the side, assessment of their set is subjectively influenced by its relation to the vertex above and the chin and shoulder below **(Fig. 1)**. In infants, in whom the mandible and neck are small in relation to head, this circumferance often results in an incorrect judgement of low-set ears.

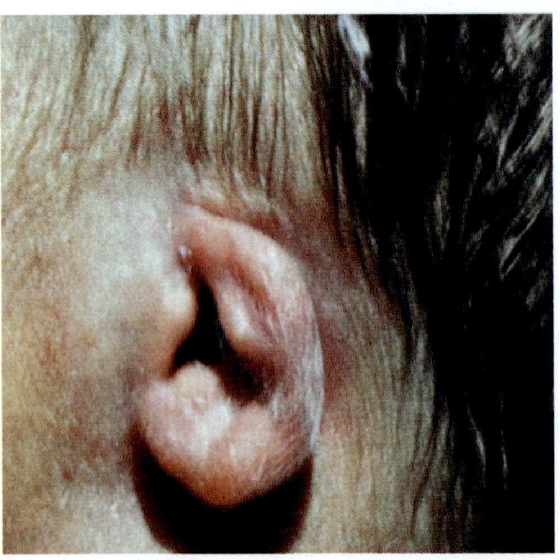

Fig. 1: Low-set ears.

The ears also appear low set if—(1) the head shape and size are unusual; (2) the helix is poorly developed; (3) the mandible is particularly small; or (4) frequently, no matter the angle from which the ears are examined, they are rotated posteriorly.

The best way to assess the set of the ears is to examine the child from the front, with the child's head held erect and the eyes facing forward. Then draw an imaginary line between the inner canthi of the eyes and extend it around the head. The superior attachment of the pinna of the ear should be at or above the line.

Next, note the size and shape of the ears. Interestingly, the right ear often is slightly larger than the left ear. Examine the preauricular region carefully for tags, pits, and fistulas. These finding can be important clues to other abnormalities, especially those involving the branchial arches and, often, hearing deficits.

CAUSES

- Apert syndrome
- Cri-du-chat syndrome
- Carpenter's syndrome
- Mucopolysaccharidoses
- Noonan's syndrome

CHAPTER 251

Lumbar Puncture

This is the method of choice for the collection of cerebrospinal fluid (CSF). This is easier to perform in older children. The key to success is to get the baby in correct position. Local deformities such as spina bifida make the procedure difficult. Spinal cord ends at relatively lower level in relation to the lumbar vertebrae during early fetal life. It extends to the level of third lumbar vertebrae in a term infant at birth. This difference in anatomy when compared to the older children must be kept in mind. This can be done in an infant lying down or sitting up. Most of the infants are generally ill and procedure should be carried out gently.

The baby has to be placed on firm surface. It should be held by a nurse at the edge of the table. Spine should be flexed as far as possible **(Fig. 1)**. Child must be curled into a flexed fetal position. The infant should be in a lateral position. The position is to have the plane of his back at 90° to the bed to avoid rotation on spine. In general, babies tolerate the lumbar puncture in upright position. The landmark is the right iliac crest. Tubercle of the crest is felt as it is the highest landmark. A vertical line is drawn from this point. It crosses the spine through the fourth lumbar vertebrae or in the space between the fourth and fifth lumbar vertebrae. Intervertebral spaces are relatively large in the newborn, vertebral canal is narrow, and accurate localization is necessary. The space used for the procedure is L_{3-4} or L_{4-5}. The skin is sterilized.

New disposable needle is used. The needle is held so that the beveled edge is seen. Thin ligaments are made to split rather than torn. The needle must go in parallel to the bed at 90° to the plane of the body's back. The needle passes through the skin, subcutaneous tissue, spinal ligaments, epidural space, and finally through the dura into subarachnoid, where CSF is situated. It requires only 1 cm to reach the subarachnoid space in newborn

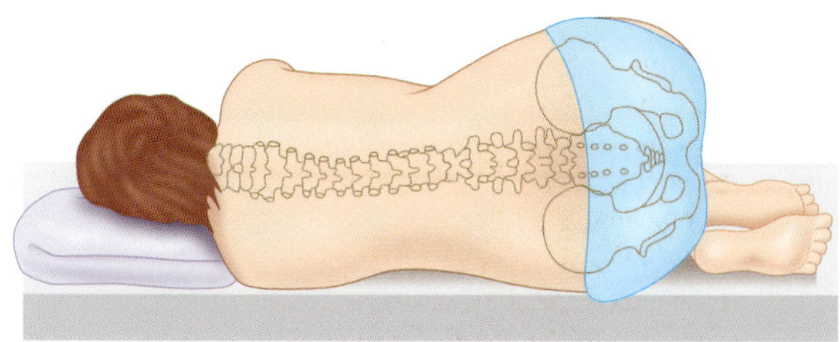

Fig. 1: Lumbar puncture site.

and 5–7 mm in a preterm baby. A feeling of giveaway sensation is felt once the dura mater is entered. Further proceeding with the needle will hit the vertebral venous plexus and blood flows back. CSF should be allowed to drop slowly into the appropriate container. 1 mL of CSF is adequate for all the procedures. Puncture site is covered with adhesive dressing. Contraindications are mentioned in **Box 1.**

BOX 1: Contraindications for lumbar puncture.

- Prolonged or focal seizure
- Focal neurological sign
- Glasgow coma score <13
- Pupillary dilatation
- Impaired oculocephalic reflexes
- Abnormal posture
- Papilledema
- Hypertension
- Coagulation disorder

Lymphadenopathy

Generalized lymphadenopathy, defined as the presence of enlarged or abnormal lymph nodes in two or more noncontiguous lymph node groups (with or without hepatosplenomegaly), is often indicative of a systemic response to an infectious or otherwise inflammatory process but may also indicate malignant proliferation of lymphocytes **(Fig. 1)**.

Infectious diseases produce inflammatory lymphadenopathy which will develop rapidly over several days. Progressive enlargement of multiple noncontiguous nodal groups over the course of weeks suggests a systemic illness such as lymphoma or tuberculosis.

CAUSES OF GENERALIZED LYMPHADENOPATHY

- *Infection*:
  - *Bacterial*:
    - Tuberculosis
    - Typhoid
    - Brucellosis
    - Pyogenic
  - *Viral*:
    - Rubella
    - Measles
    - Cytomegalovirus
- *Collagen*: Still's disease
- *Malignancies*:
  - Leukemia
  - Lymphoma
  - Histiocytosis
- Chronic granulomatous disease
- Storage disorder
  - Gaucher's disease
  - Niemann-pick disease
- *Drugs*: Phenytoin

CAUSES OF LOCALIZED LYMPHADENOPATHY

- Infection
- Malignancies
- Lymphoma
- Kawasaki

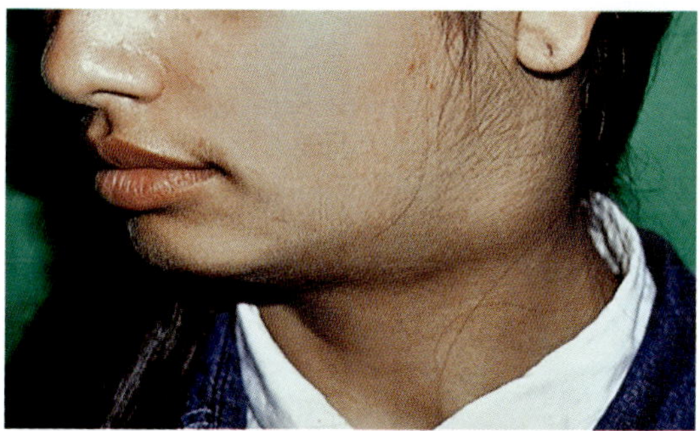

Fig. 1: Cervical lymphadenopathy.

Macewen's Sign

It is the sign used to help to diagnose hydrocephalus and brain abscess. Tapping the skull near junction of the frontal, temporal, and parietal bones produces cracked pot sound. *Macewen's sign*, i.e., resonant note on percussions of the skull is noted. The eyes appear to be pushed down; the sclera becomes visible above the cornea—sun-setting sign. Later, papilledema occurs once the size stops increasing and sutures cannot be widened. An increase in head circumference in the first 3 months of life by >1 cm every fortnight may arouse suspicion of hydrocephalus. Accurate serial recording of head circumference is required for early diagnosis of neonatal hydrocephalus. Widening of squamoparietal suture is not physiological and should be considered as a suspicion of hydrocephalus.

CHAPTER 254

Macrocephaly

Head is measured at a largest circumference by wrapping the tape around the most prominent part of the forehead and occiput. Head size tends to follow the familial pattern.

Head circumference is ideally measured every month for first 6 months, then every 2 months for the next 2 months. Large head or big head, i.e., macrocephaly is defined as an occipitofrontal circumference more than 2SD of the normal for the age, sex, and gestational age. The causes include Beckwith-Wiedemann syndrome, familial, subgaleal hemorrhage, hydrocephalus, achondroplasia, and cerebral gigantism.

An increase in the head circumference of >2 cm per month in the first 6 months shows raise suspicion of macrocephaly. The head circumference of preterm infants may appear large. But it should be confirmed by anthropometry.

Macrocephaly is defined as a head circumference more than two standard deviations above the mean for age, gender, and gestation. This abnormality can be caused by a myriad of conditions, including hydrocephalus [excessive accumulation of cerebrospinal fluid (CSF)], intracranial mass lesions (i.e., tumors, subdural effusions), thickening or enlargement of the skull (primary skeletal dysplasias), and a true increase in brain substance (megalencephaly). The latter is seen in soto syndrome, achondroplasia, neurocutaneous syndromes, and certain lipidoses, leukodystrophies, and mucopolysaccharidoses. Primary megalencephaly may occur as a benign familial trait.

Evaluation of the child with a head that is abnormally large or appears to be growing at an excessive rate should include the following:

- *Serial measurements of head circumference:* Measurement of the parents' head circumferences and exploration of family history for evidence of macrocephaly or neurologic and cutaneous abnormalities
- Developmental history
- Careful examination for evidence of increased intracranial pressure, developmental delay, skeletal dysplasia, abnormal transillumination, cranial bruits, ocular abnormalities, or organomegaly

Plain skull radiographs may provide evidence of increased intracranial pressure, identify intracranial calcification, or detect primary skeletal dysplasias. CT or MRI scans allow assessment of ventricular size and permit detection of intracranial mass lesions and chronic subdural effusions. CT is the method of choice for demonstrating intracranial calcification as seen with congenital cytomegalovirus infection and detecting fresh blood.

CAUSES OF A LARGE HEAD

Must be evaluated in proportion to length, birth weight, chest circumference, fontanelles and sutures:

- *Large for gestational age infant*: Has a proportionally large head with normal sutures and fontanelles
- *Beckwith–Wiedemann syndrome*: Macrocephaly with macroglossia, large kidneys, pancreatic hyperplasia, adrenocortical cytomegaly, and hypoglycemia
- *Familial macrocephaly*: Head is disproportionately large, apparently no neurological deficit, and autosomal dominant. An autosomal recessive variant is associated with mental retardation.
- *Subgaleal hemorrhage:* Misshapen head, ill-defined suture lines and fontanelles, and fluctuant soft tissue on palpation. History of traumatic vertex delivery, rapidly increasing head size, falling hematocrit (Hct), pallor, and hypotension
- *Hydrocephalus:* Widely separated sutures with sun-setting sign, large head with full bulging fontanelle. May be:
  - Isolated congenital malformation
  - Associated with spina bifida
  - Chromosomal aberration
  - Intrauterine infection
  - Postnatal intraventricular hemorrhage
  - Meningitic sequalae
  - Cerebral edema

CHAPTER 255

Macroglossia

It is a disorder in which tongue is larger than normal. Symptoms may include noisy, high-pitched breathing (snoring), and/or feeding difficulties. In some cases, the tongue protrudes from the mouth.

CAUSES

- Acromegaly
- Mongolism
- Cretinism
- Hemangioma
- Cystic hygroma
- Angioedema

Marasmus

Marasmus, defined as predominantly caloric/energy deficiency, is characterized by marked emaciation; loss of subcutaneous fat and muscle; brittle, sparse hair; and poor nail growth. Diarrhea is common as intestinal cell turnover slows, resulting in blunted intestinal villi and a secondary malabsorptive state. Secondary effects of marasmus, such as hypothermia and bradycardia, occur late in the clinical course. Marasmus is usually seen within the 1st year of life at the time of weaning, during famine, or at any time when there is a consistent and extreme deprivation of calories. It is the consequence of poor caloric, protein, vitamin, and mineral intake. Kwashiorkor, on the other hand, results from a diet rich in calories but lacking protein. The initial "moon face" of kwashiorkor is often mistaken for proper nutrition. The child is often edematous, which becomes strikingly apparent after nutritional repletion. Hepatomegaly and mental status changes are common. Skin changes in patients with kwashiorkor include hyperpigmentation or hypopigmentation with a scaly, weeping dermatitis that may ulcerate and desquamate.

CHAPTER 257

Marcus Gunn Pupil

This is relative afferent pupillary defect (Marcus Gunn pupil) and indicates an asymmetric, prechiasmatic, and afferent conduction defect. It is best demonstrated by the swinging flash light test, which allows comparison of the direct and consensual pupillary response in both eyes. With patients fixing on distant target (to control accommodation), a bright focal light is directed alternatively into each eye in turn. In presence of afferent lesion, both the direct response to the light in the affected eye and the consensual response in the other eye are subnormal. Swinging the light to the better or normal eye causes both the pupils to react (constrict) normally. Swinging the light back to the affected eye causes both the pupils redilate to some degree, reflecting defective conduction. This is a very sensitive and useful test for detecting and confirming optic nerve and retinal disease. This test is only abnormal if there is a "relative" difference in the conduction properties of the optic nerves. Therefore, patients with bilateral and symmetric optic nerve disease will not demonstrate an afferent pupillary defect. A subtle relative afferent defect may be found in some children with amblyopia.

Chapter 258 Mastitis

Mastitis is a bacterial infection of the breast. It can result from blocked ducts or from ascending infection due to cracked nipples. Mastitis presents as acute onset of fever, chills, and extreme breast tenderness over an area of induration and firmness, usually on one breast **(Fig. 1)**. This is not a reason to cease breastfeeding. In fact, the treatment includes frequent emptying of the breast, oral antibiotics to cover penicillin-resistant staphylococcal and streptococcal species (e.g., first-generation cephalosporin or dicloxacillin), analgesics, rest, and adequate fluid intake. However, mastitis can progress to breast abscess, which requires incision and drainage and antibiotics. In the case of an abscess, milk should be expressed and discarded from the affected side until no longer draining, and the baby fed only from the unaffected side. Many women report a temporary decrease in milk supply on the side impacted by mastitis or abscess; milk supply increases again if women continue to empty milk from the affected side.

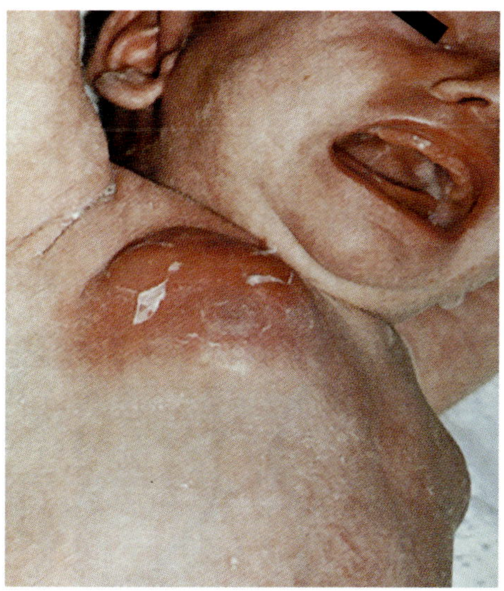

Fig. 1: Mastitis.

Melena

Melena is the term applied to the black bowel motion resulting from hemorrhage. Melena is most commonly due to bleeding from the stomach or duodenum, or more rarely from the esophagus.

CAUSES OF MELENA IN NEWBORN

- Swallowed maternal blood
- Infection
- Necrotizing enterocolitis
- Trauma due to hard stools
- Cow's milk allergy
- Hemorrhagic disease of newborn
- Meckel's diverticulum

MELENA IN INFANCY AND CHILDHOOD

- Constipation
- Anal fissure
- Dysentery
- Salmonellosis
- Meckel's diverticulum
- Intussusception
- Cow's milk allergy
- Rectal polyp
- Ulcerative colitis
- Anaphylactoid purpura
- Bleeding disorder

CHAPTER 260 Menorrhagia

Menorrhagia refers to excessive menstrual flow, or undue prolongation of the time during which it takes place. Excess of menstrual loss in women without abnormal physical is believed to be endocrine in origin, and is called "dysfunctional menorrhagia". Acute endometritis of gonococcal or pyogenic origin tends to cure itself owing to the shedding of the endometrium during menstruation.

Menorrhagia in relation to the menopause and in the years preceding is the result of increasing failure of the ovarian functions and consequent upset in balance between the secretion of estrogen and progesterone.

Polymenorrhea is the name given to a form of irregular and excessive menstruation in which the cycle is shortened from the usual 28 to 21 days, or even less. This is due to a disturbed balance of internal secretions, causing ovulation to occur too early in the cycle; in some cases, two corpora lutea have been found at the same stage of development, and fibroids are present in many cases.

PELVIC PATHOLOGY

Menorrhagia can be associated with fibroids (benign leiomyomas), adenomyosis, infection, endometrial polyps, endometriosis, and the presence of an intrauterine contraceptive device (IUCD). Of all the causes of pure menorrhagia, leiomyoma (fibroids) of the uterus stands out as the only important growth associated with this symptom, and is simple bimanual examination (as a rule) suffices to show that such a tumor exists. The size and shape of the uterus is dependent on the number and size of the fibroids, as there may be more than one tumor in the uterus; its shape may be exceedingly irregular. The uterus feels firm and, in most cases, is mobile. The only difficulty in diagnosis, as a rule, lies in distinguishing a leiomyoma of the uterus from an ovarian cyst. Sometimes, this is difficult, for it is not always possible to say that a given tumor is actually the enlarged uterus. Ultrasound scanning is helpful in the diagnosis of fibroids because it is possible by using this method to determine if a pelvic swelling is both uterine and solid. Fibroids may be submucous, intramural, subserosal, or pedunculated. Distortion of the uterine cavity with an increase in the surface area from which menstruation occurs will lead to menorrhagia.

Chronic salpingo-oophoritis (in the form of a pyosalpinx, a hydrosalpinx, a tubo-ovarian abscess, or chronic interstitial salpingitis) and ovarian endometriosis both give rise to menorrhagia due to pelvic congestion, but dysmenorrhea, pelvic pain, dyspareunia, and backache are usually more prominent symptoms. In either case, a firm tender swelling in the pouch of Douglas is felt on bimanual palpation. It is unusual to encounter menorrhagia under these conditions without bleeding at other times of the cycle.

Adenomyosis is a condition which can present with menorrhagia and pain at the time of menstruation, and no examination the uterus may be tender. The diagnosis can only be confirmed histologically as endometrial tissue is found in the myometrium. The condition is more common in parous women, and in essence there has been bleeding in the myometrium which gives rise to the pain and tenderness.

CLOTTING DEFECTS

There are certain hemorrhagic disorders that can cause excessive menstrual loss; these include thrombocytopenic purpura, von Willebrand's disease, and Christmas disease. These women may suffer excessive menstrual loss and may require surgical intervention. In thrombocytopenia, the blood loss relates to the platelet level, and in some cases, splenectomy for the underlying pathology has improved the menstrual symptoms.

Anticoagulation in women who are receiving long-term anticoagulants after prosthetic heart valve implantation, previous pulmonary embolism or, in some cases, with antiphospholipid syndrome, may develop significant period problems depending on the INR level.

Severe menorrhagia may complicate thrombocytopenia, but as soon as it is cured, the period blood loss becomes normal.

MEDICAL DISORDERS

The function of the thyroid and adrenal glands can influence menstrual loss, though the mechanism is unknown. Menorrhagia tends to be more common in hypothyroidism than thyrotoxicosis, and is not uncommon with Cushing's disease.

Memory

Memory is the retention of learned experience. The following are four different types of memory:

1. *Short memory:* This is tested by giving a set of numbers and child is asked to respect them forward and backward.
2. *Immediate memory:* This is tested by telling the story and asking the child to repeat it.
3. *Intermediate memory:* Here, a name of the fruit or flower is told before the examination. Child is asked to repeat the name of the flowers and fruits being told after the examination.
4. *Long-term memory:* This is examined by asking the child regarding the home, school, and siblings.

CHAPTER 262

Meningococcal Exanthem

Neisseria meningitidis is capable of producing several clinical syndromes. Two major syndromes—acute meningococcemia and chronic meningococcemia (or meningococcosis)—are characterized in part by a generalized exanthem. Meningococcus colonizes the upper respiratory tract of asymptomatic humans who may transmit the organism via respiratory droplets to close contacts. Most people become colonized without clinical disease. Clinical illness is most common in children younger than 5 years old, with a peak incidence between 6 and 12 months old.

A secondary peak of lesser magnitude but significant mortality is seen during adolescence and young adulthood, leading to adolescent vaccination recommendations. Susceptibility to disease appears to be related to a lack of bactericidal antibody or to a failure to produce antibody in response to infection. Antecedent viral respiratory tract infection can be a predisposing factor.

Although meningococcal infection occurs year-round, the peak season is late winter and early spring. Invasive disease occurs both endemically and epidemically. Persons who have intimate contact with infected patients (such as other members of the same household) or persons in "closed communities" (such as military barracks, dormitories, or daycare centers) are at highest risk of becoming secondarily infected and should receive antimicrobial prophylaxis if exposed to a case.

The incubation period after exposure ranges from 1 to 10 days, with most cases developing in <4 days. Secondary attack rates are highest during epidemic outbreaks. Any mucosal surface is subject to colonization, which may remain localized or may serve as the source of invasive disease **(Figs. 1 to 3)**.

- Hutchinson teeth—the upper central incisors are smaller than normal, barrel shaped, and notched in the center of the incisal surface
- Mulberry molars—abnormal cusp development results in the formation of multiple peripheral cusps and a central cusp

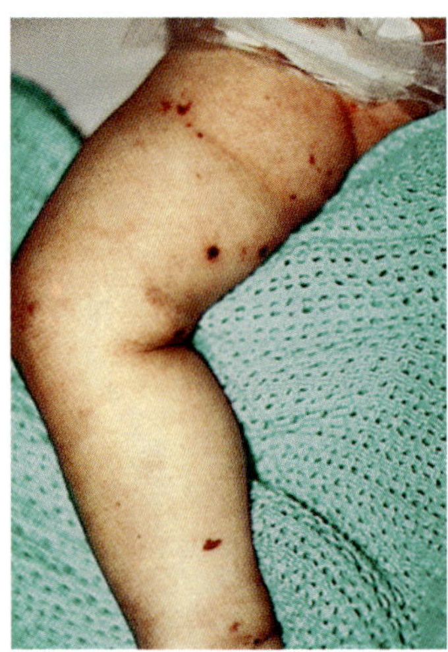

Fig. 1: Meningococcemia.

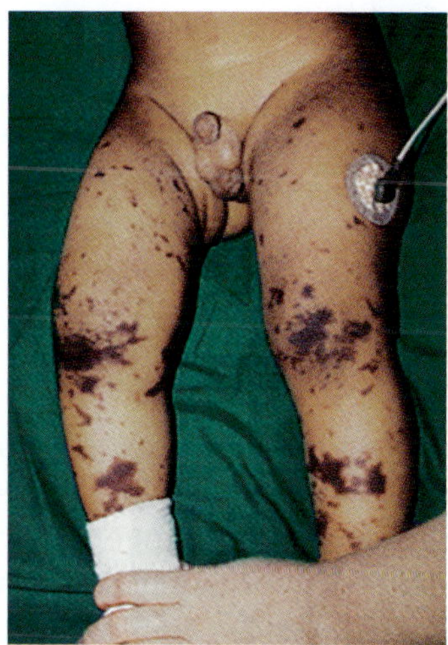

Fig. 2: Meningococcal exanthem.

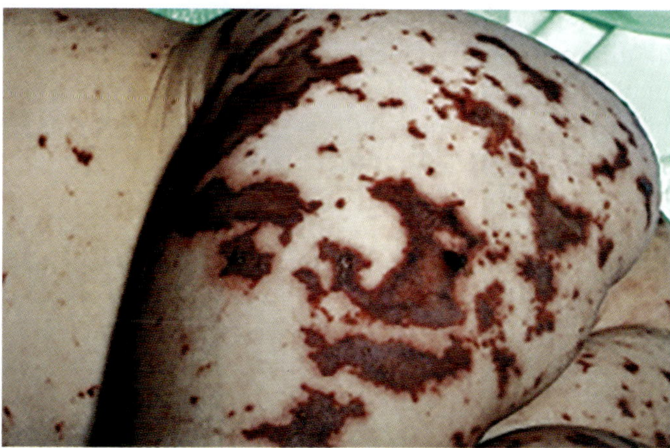

Fig. 3: Meningococcal lesions.

CHAPTER 263 Microcephaly

Microcephaly is defined as a head circumference more than two standard deviations below the mean for age, gender, and conceptual age. Premature fusion of sutures, fontanelle closed, orbits flat, and protruding eyes are present **(Figs. 1A and B)**.

Apart from cases resulting from premature closure of the sutures (generalized craniosynostosis), microcephaly reflects an abnormally small brain and can be a symptom of any disorder that impairs brain growth. The neurologic manifestations range from minor (e.g., poor fine motor skills, mild intellectual impairment) to profound (e.g., decerebration, chronic vegetative state). Diagnostic evaluation should include a family history, prenatal history, a search for associated congenital anomalies, karyotyping, as well as oligo array, amino acid screening, and serologic studies for intrauterine infection, such as congenital cytomegalovirus and Zika virus infection. Plain skull radiographs can detect craniosynostosis, whereas CT scan is useful in identifying intracranial calcifications. MRI is preferred for delineation of recognizable patterns of central nervous system (CNS) dysmorphogenesis.

CONDITIONS CAUSING MICROCEPHALY

Primary Microcephaly

- Microcephaly vera (genetic)
- Chromosomal disorders
- Defective neurulation:
  - Anencephaly
  - Encephalocele

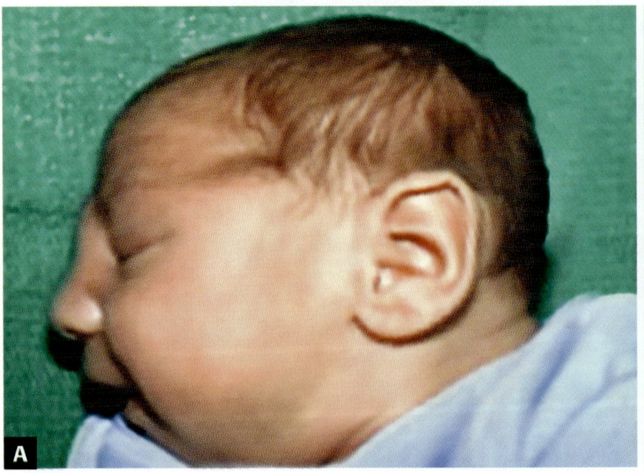

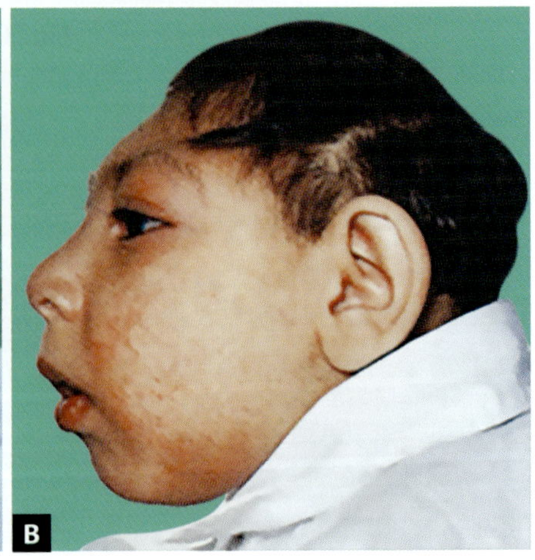

Figs. 1A and B: Microcephaly.

- Defective prosencephalization:
  - Holoprosencephaly (arhinencephaly)
  - Agenesis of the corpus callosum
- Defective cellular migration

Secondary Microcephaly

- Intrauterine disorders:
  - Infection
  - Toxins
  - Vascular
- Perinatal brain injuries:
  - Hypoxic–ischemic encephalopathy
  - Intracranial hemorrhage
  - Meningitis and encephalitis
  - Stroke
- Postnatal systemic diseases:
  - Chronic cardiopulmonary disease
  - Chronic renal disease
  - Malnutrition

The difference between primary and secondary microcephaly and their causes have elucidated in **Tables 1 and 2**.

TABLE 1: Difference between primary and secondary microcephaly.

Features	*Primary microcephaly*	*Secondary microcephaly*
Appearance	Low crown, receding forehead, occipital flattening and wrinkling of the skin	Small head
Onset	Present since birth	May be present at birth or evident later on by 1st year
Predisposing factor	No predisposing factor	Malnutrition, TORCH, alcohol, antiepileptic drugs, hypothyroidism

TABLE 2: Causes of primary and secondary microcephaly.

Causes of primary microcephaly	*Causes of secondary microcephaly*
• Down syndrome • Craniosynostosis • Smith–Lemli–Opitz syndrome • Rubinstein–Taybi syndrome • Batten diseases	• Cerebral dysgenesis • Cerebral hypoplasia • TORCH infection • Hypoxia • Hypothyroidism • Malnutrition • Phenylketonuria • Trauma—birth injuries

CHAPTER 264

Microcornea

It is present when the horizontal corneal diameter is 9 mm or less. Microcornea can be isolated or associated with glaucoma, cataracts, iris abnormalities, or anterior segment dysgenesis. The abnormalities necessitate further tests to exclude glaucoma. If the anterior segment of the eye is severely disorganized, the cornea is opaque, or glaucoma exists surgical reconstruction and repair is indicated.

CHAPTER 265 Microphallus

Microphallus (micropenis) is a small, normally formed penis more than 2.5 standard deviations below the mean (<1.9-cm stretch length in neonates) **(Fig. 1)**. It is important to obtain an accurate penile stretch length and corporal shaft diameter by using a rigid ruler placed on the pubic symphysis and stretching the penis to extend the glans as far as possible along the ruler, while not stretching the prepuce. Microphallus is thought to result from failure of normal penile growth after 14 weeks' gestation. Two primary causes of the failure of penile growth may be hypogonadotropic hypogonadism [failure of the hypothalamus to produce gonadotropin-releasing hormone (GnRH)] and primary testicular failure (deficient testosterone production) (hypergonadotropic hypergonadism). Karyotype should be determined. Follicle-stimulating hormone (FSH), luteinizing hormone (LH), and testosterone levels should be measured in addition to a diagnostic human chorionic gonadotropin (hCG) stimulation test to assess testicular function. Evaluation of pituitary/hypothalamic function should be carried out by review of newborn screening; measurements of serum glucose, sodium, potassium, cortisol, and thyroid hormone levels; and brain MRI scan to assess the anatomy of the hypothalamus and midbrain. Although controversy exists regarding penile growth at puberty and the appropriateness of female gender reassignment in infancy, most authors suggest a diagnostic trial of testosterone for 3 months before making a final decision about gender assignment. An increasing trend is toward the male sex of rearing.

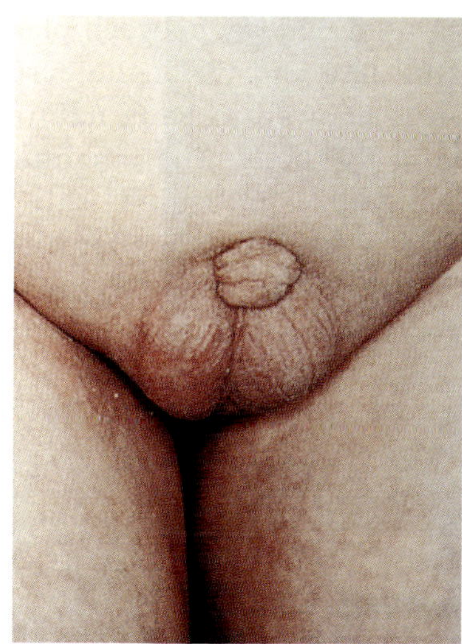

Fig. 1: Microphallus.

CHAPTER 266

Midarm Circumference

It is measured midway between olecranon process of ulna and tip of the acromion. Left arm is allowed to hang naturally by the side of the body. The circumference of the midpoint is measured. This is also considered as age-independent criteria. It has significance between the age of 1–5 years. It gives information about the nutritional status of the young children. It is a good indicator of muscle mass. The normal midarm circumference is 13.5–17 cm. Less than 12.5 cm indicates malnutrition. It is a very useful indicator to follow-up the child with malnutrition on treatment. It does not apply to the child above 5 years.

Milia

Milia are tiny (1–2-mm), whitish-yellow papules that develop spontaneously on the face in neonates. They are firm and, unlike pustules, are not easily denuded by pressure. Milia consist of tiny epithelial-lined cysts arising from hair follicles **(Fig. 1)**. They can be persistent, although they may resolve spontaneously after months to years. In newborns, they usually arise without any apparent cause, although in older infants and children, they are often seen after skin injury, such as that caused by blistering eruptions or abrasions.

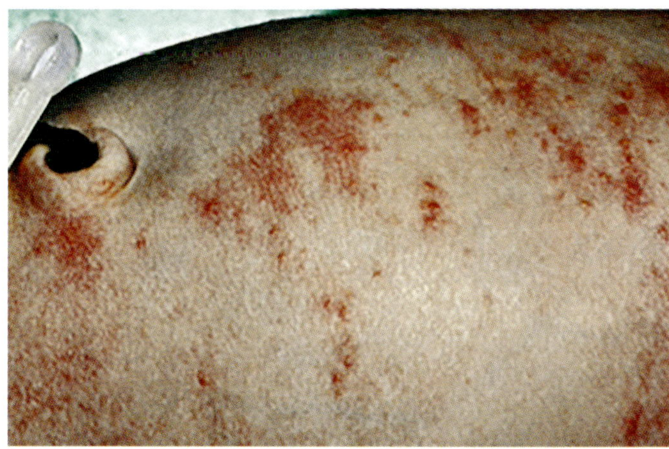

Fig. 1: Milia.

CHAPTER 268

Mongoloid Slant

Mongoloid slant is slanting downward from the lateral to medial canthus. The outer canthi lie above the line joining the inner canthi. There is upward slanting of the eyes. It is seen among Down syndrome, Mongolian race, ectodermal dysplasia, and Prader-Willi syndrome.

269 CHAPTER

Mongoloid Spots

Mongolian spots are flat, slate-gray to bluish-black, and poorly circumscribed macules. They are located most commonly over the lumbosacral area and buttocks, although they can appear anywhere on the body **(Figs. 1A and B)**. The spots range in size from 1 to 10 cm and may be single or multiple. No risk of malignancy is known, and Mongolian spots usually fade without therapy by 7 years old. Special variants of Mongolian spots, including nevus of Ota (involving the face, particularly the periocular area) and nevus of Ito (involving the shoulder), may persist indefinitely. Rarely, when present along with vascular malformations, they can be part of a syndrome called *phakomatosis pigmentovascularis,* which can have associated internal abnormalities.

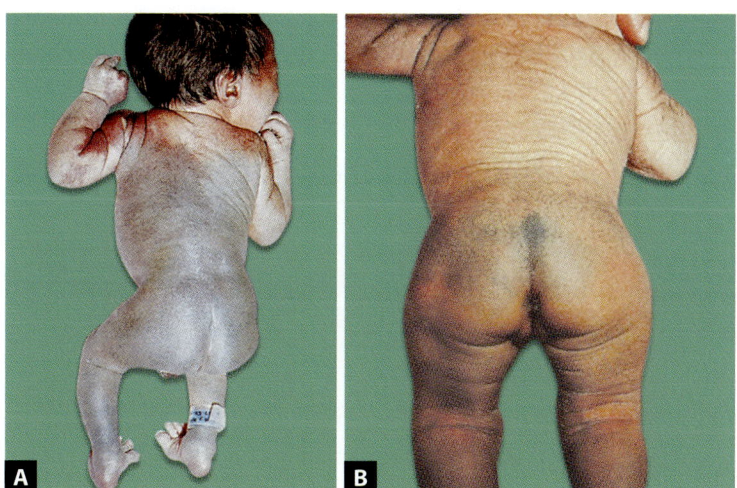

Figs. 1A and B: Mongolian spots.

CHAPTER 270

Motor Reflexes

Certain motor reflexes of the face are affected in facial nerve lesions. These usually indicate a premature nervous system, regression to an infantile status or frontal lobe lesions.

GLABELLAR REFLEX

- Elicited by gentle repeated percussion with a finger over the root of the nose.
- Normal response is brisk closure of the eyes during the first two or three taps. Persistent response without extinction on repeated taps is abnormal.

SNOUT REFLEX

- Consists of puckering of the lips in response to a tap over the upper lip. This reflex is not elicited normally

CHVOSTEK'S SIGN

- Elicited by tapping the facial nerve in front of the ear
- Marked contraction and spasm following such tapping indicate hypocalcemia.
- It is a response due to increased irritability of the nerve fibers to mechanical stimulation.

271 CHAPTER Mouth Pigmentation

It is best to approach the examination positively. Show the child the flashlight or otoscope light without a tongue depressor in sight. Allowing some children to assist by placing a hand on the light or even on the tongue depressor gives them a sense of control. Infants are best examined supine with the arms restrained. Beyond early infancy, it is best to examine infants and children in the sitting position. Encourage the child to open his or her mouth widely and vocalize "aaahhh." In many children, the soft palate rises and the tongue descends spontaneously when the mouth is fully opened, allowing a clear view, which may include the epiglottis.

In other children, even with their full cooperation, it will be necessary to depress the base of the tongue with the tongue depressor to view the full oral cavity. Any pressure at the base of the tongue results in a brief gagging response, which causes the soft palate to rise and allows brief inspection of the posterior pharyngeal wall.

If the child refuses to open his or her mouth, it is still possible to complete the inspection. You will need willing assistants to ensure appropriate restraint of the child (with similar positioning as in the ear examination) and ongoing calming conversation to distract from the examination. Insert the tongue depressor behind the posterior teeth and quickly slip it medially to depress the base of the tongue. The procedure will allow a few seconds of full vision and may result in a gag response and/or vomiting. A typical gurgle preceded an episode of vomiting, which may be aborted by rapid withdrawal of the tongue depressor, closure of the mouth, and tilting the chin upward. Always reassure the child that he or she was very good and brave. Future cooperation with any part of the physical examination depends on your ability to relate to the child after a painful or resisted examination has been completed.

Mucocele and Ranula

A mucocele is a painless, translucent, or bluish lesion of traumatic origin, most often involving minor salivary glands of the lower lip. The lesion may alternately enlarge and shrink. The treatment of choice is surgical excision of the lesion and the associated minor salivary gland.

A simple ranula is a retention cyst in the floor of the mouth that is confined to sublingual tissues superior to the mylohyoid muscle. It appears clinically as a bluish, transparent, thin-walled, fluctuant swelling. Herniation of the ranula through the mylohyoid muscle results in a cervical or plunging ranula that becomes more apparent in the oral cavity with the muscle contraction associated with jaw opening. Simple incision and drainage of the ranula is not an acceptable treatment because healing is followed by recurrence. The ranula must be removed in total along with the associated salivary gland to avoid recurrence.

273 CHAPTER

Murphy's Sign

Severe pain will be present in acute inflammation of gallbladder, i.e., acute cholecystitis. Here, acutely inflamed gallbladder is walled off by greater omentum. This can be felt as tender indefinite mass.

If the gallbladder is tender, the examining finger over the gallbladder point coming in contact with tender gallbladder on deep inspiration will cause pain. This will be maintained as a gasp in breathe with tensing of the abdominal wall muscle. This sign is not found in chronic cholecystitis or uncomplicated cases of gallstones.

CHAPTER 274

Muscular Hypertrophy

INCREASED TONE

Resistance increases suddenly (the catch), heel leaves easily when knee is lifted (spasticity).

- Increased through whole range of movement, as if bending a lead pipe (lead pipe rigidity), i.e., increased tone both in flexors and extensors throughout the movement.
- Regular intermittent break in tone throughout the whole range of movement (cogwheel rigidity). In pyramidal lesion, flexor muscle in upper limbs and extensor muscles in lower limbs will show increased tone. Spasticity is exaggeration of stretch reflexes and expresses itself as: (1) diminished voluntary movements, (2) Increased resistance to passive movement, and (3) Increased reflexes and clonus. Development of spasticity is selective and involves the extensors of the legs and flexors in the arms. Loss of movement is proportional to the degree of spasticity.

The following types of hypertonicity are seen:

- *Clasp knife (spasticity)*: Sign of upper motor neuron type of lesion.
- *Cogwheel rigidity*: Intermittent action of agonists and antagonists—valuable sign of extrapyramidal involvement.
- *Lead pipe rigidity*: Characteristic of extrapyramidal but may also be seen in extreme spasticity of upper motor neuron (UMN) type.
- *Decerebrate rigidity*: All limbs extended, arms pronated, fists closed, and feet plantar flexed. Lesions of brainstem
- *Decorticate positioning*: Upper limbs are flexed, lower limbs extended, seen in extensive lesions at the level of basal nuclei or between basal nuclei and cortex

275 CHAPTER

Muscle Power

This is to find out whether the muscle power is normal or any part of the body is weak or paralyzed.

Weakness or paralysis of any part of the body is assessed by observation of the child's activities. Any asymmetry in the movements of the limbs is to be noted. Walking or gait discloses any hemiparesis. There will not be any spontaneous movements of the part of the body in case of paralysis and paresis. Asymmetry in primitive reflexes in case of small infants will suggest weakness and paralysis.

The following ranges of movements are asked to perform at each joint:

- *Shoulder joint:* Abduction, adduction, flexion, and extension
- *Elbow:* Flexion and extension
- *Forearm:* Pronation and supination
- *Metacarpophalangeal and interphalangeal joint:* Flexion and extension
- *Thumb and finger*: Abduction and adduction
- *Hip joint*: Flexion, extension, abduction, and adduction
- *Knee*: Flexion and extension
- *Ankle*: Dorsi flexion and plantar flexion
- *Foot*: Inversion and eversion
- *Toe*: Dorsiflexion and plantar flexion
- *In the neck*: Flexion, extension, lateral bending, and rotation

GRADING OF MUSCLE POWER

- *Grade 0:* No movements, fully paralyzed
- *Grade 1:* Flicker of contraction
- *Grade 2:* Movement with the gravity eliminated
- *Grade 3:* Movement against gravity, but not against resistance
- *Grade 4:* Movements against gravity and some resistance
- *Grade 5:* Normal power

CHAPTER 276

Myalgia

In the child with extremity pain, muscle pain needs to be distinguished from joint pain, bone pain, and the less common neuropathic pain. If the complaint is localized to the muscles, the differential diagnosis is narrowed considerably. Intermittent benign bilateral myalgia of the calves or thighs is one of the more common muscle pain presentations encountered in young children. These pains occur in an active child who has normal physical examination findings without evidence of weakness or systemic illness. Symptoms typically occur in the evening and resolve with massage or mild analgesics such as acetaminophen or ibuprofen, usually within an hour. The frequency of pain can vary and, in some children, may escalate periodically. Additional evaluation or treatment is unnecessary in most children, and eventually the pains resolve completely.

As myalgia may accompany polymyositis and dermatomyositis, every child complaining of muscle pain should undergo careful muscle strength testing. Myalgia may also be seen with vasculitis and SJIA. Many children with acute-onset diffuse myalgia have a transient viral illness, and pain usually resolves within several days; however, infection with influenza can cause an exquisitely painful myositis of the gastrocnemius muscles with resultant difficulty ambulating. This condition is usually distinguished easily from a chronic inflammatory muscle disease by the sudden onset and localization to these specific muscles. The creatine kinase level may be very elevated. Myoglobinuria may ensue and potentially affect renal function; therefore, affected children should undergo urinalysis, in which the presence of myoglobin yields positive results for heme on macroscopic analysis, though no erythrocytes on microscopic examination. The myositis resolves within several days, and treatment is based on symptoms.

Nails Abnormalities

KOILONYCHIA (SPOON NAILS)

The nails will be concave with everted edges more apparent when viewed laterally. Serrated koilonychia is transverse grooves with koilonychia.

CLASSIFICATION OF KOILONYCHIA

- Idiopathic
- Hereditary, congenital, and associated with other ectodermal defects:
  - Palmar hyperkeratoses
  - Steatocystoma multiplex
  - Nail–patella syndrome
- Acquired
- *Cardiovascular:*
  - Anemia
  - Polycythemia vera
  - Coronary disease
- *Infections:* Syphilis, fungus
- *Metabolic:*
  - Acromegaly
  - Hypothyroidism
  - Thyrotoxicosis

TRANSVERSE OVERCURVATURE OF NAIL

It is caused due to repeated nail avulsions, psoriasis, and osteoarthritis of the distal interphalangeal joints leading to repeated infections.

Dolichonychia (Lengthy Nails)

Normally length/width of nail is 1 ± 0.1 cm. Here, >1.9 cm is seen in Marfan syndrome, Ehlers–Danlos syndrome, eunuchoidism, and hypopituitarism.

Brachyonychia (Short and White Nails)

It occurs in habitual nail biters, bone resorption in hyperparathyroidism. Onychotrophia is reduction in size and thickness of the nail plate. Example is lichen planus.

MODIFICATION OF NAIL SURFACE

Longitudinal lines/striations can occur physiologically, pathologically (lichen planus, Darier's disease, etc.), and median nail dystrophy affecting thumbnail in the center.

Beau's Lines

Occurrence of transverse grooves in physiological conditions, zinc deficiencies, Raynaud's disease, eczema, etc.

Trachyonychia (Rough Nail)

It occurs in idiopathic congenital conditions and acquired conditions such as psoriasis, lichen planus, alopecia areata, and ectodermal dysplasia.

Onychoschizia Lamellina (Lamellar Nail Splitting)

The nails splits horizontally similar to scaly skin and seen in repeated soaking of nails, polycythemia vera, lichen planus, and retinoid therapy.

Leukonychia

It is whitish discoloration of the nails due to congenital causes, acquired causes (trauma and severe stress), renal disease, shock, fractures, measles, tuberculosis, syphilis, autoimmune disorders, neoplasias, gout, enteric fever, ulcerative colitis, etc.

CHAPTER 278

Nasal Deformity

The nose is the most prominent part of the face and is easily examined. Observe it for shape, deformity, or deviation to one side. Ask the child to tilt his or her head upward so that you can observe the septum and the presence of nasal discharge. A foul-smelling unilateral discharge indicates that the child may have a foreign body in that nostril or an obstruction due to polyp or other anomaly. Nasal discharge colors are not predictive or viral versus bacterial infections. Develop the habit of observing the alae nasi during quiet breathing.

Flaring of the alae nasi is a subtle sign of respiratory distress and may indicate the presence of pneumonia or congestive cardiac failure. A horizontal crease across the lower part of the nose is frequently seen in children with allergies who rub the tip of the nose by pushing it upward with the palm or heel of their hand, the so-called "allergic salute."

Next, inspect inside the nose. You will need a nasal speculum and light or a regular otoscope with a large nasal speculum. Remember that the anterior septum, little's area, is extremely vascular and sensitive. Any trauma to this area will induce pain and possibly bleeding, as well as an uncooperative child and an upset family.

Insert the speculum slowly, being careful to follow the floor of the cavity that runs toward the occiput. Gentle pressure against the lateral wall will expose the nasal turbinates and mucosa. Observe the presence of edema, pallor, inflammation, bleeding, or secretions. Swollen, pale turbinates that obstruct the nasal airways partly or completely are the hallmarks of nasal allergy. Polyps may be seen as pale boggy masses that occlude posteriorly. Note if the nares are patent and allow equal air determine bilateral patency. Choanal atresia on both sides may lead to cyanotic episodes and apnea in infants who are all obligate nasal breathers.

CHAPTER 279

Nasal Discharge

The causes of nasal discharge are listed in **Box 1**.

INFECTIVE CAUSES

Sometimes, the pus becomes inspissated, giving rise to the so-called "caseous sinusitis" or "rhinitis". This is particularly common with fungal infection. The material is whitish, cheesy, and foul-smelling. Even worse are the crusts and dry discharge of an atrophic rhinitis. In these patients the nasal fossae are unduly wide and the mucosa thin and devoid of mucus cells. The especially disgusting odor is called "ozena".

BOX 1: Conditions causing nasal discharge.

- Choanal atresia
- Acute rhinitis
- Rhinosinusitis
- *Caseous rhinitis:*
  - Syphilis
  - Tuberculosis
  - Leprosy
  - Foreign body
  - Rhinolith
  - Cerebrospinal fluid rhinorrhea
  - Atopy or hypersensitivity
  - Allergic rhinitis
  - Vasomotor rhinitis

Pathogenic fungi and yeasts are a common cause of nasal infection and discharge in tropical countries but, of course, nowadays these infections are occasionally seen in this country in immigrants and travelers returning from exotic places.

FOREIGN BODIES

A unilateral nasal discharge in an infant or child is pathognomonic of a foreign body, often a piece of foam rubber or paper inserted into the nasal fossa. Small hard objects may remain in the nose for some time before symptoms develop. Longstanding foreign bodies calcify to form rhinoliths. These are associated with chronic discharge and halitosis.

TRAUMA

A clear watery discharge following a head injury suggest a fracture of the anterior cranial fossa or cribriform plate and a cerebrospinal fluid (CSF) leak. Such a discharge will increase on leaning the head forward, or on compression of the jugular veins. The presence or sugar in this fluid confirms that it is CSF. This can be further confirmed by serological tests for β-transferrin.

CHAPTER 280

Nasal Obstruction

Nasal obstruction—the inability to breathe through one or both nostrils—is a very common complaint.

Choanal atresia may be membranous or bony, unilateral or bilateral. Nasal respiration is innate and, therefore, in bilateral cases, the obstruction must be bypassed immediately after birth, by placement of an oropharyngeal airway. Surgical correction of the abnormality is undertaken in the first few days of life. Unilateral choanal atresia is sometimes not discovered until later. Babies breathe continuously while feeding; hence, those with choanal atresia are unable to do so when the patent nostril is blocked by their mother's breast. Consequently, they suckle better from one breast rather than the other. The causes of nasal obstruction are mentioned in **Box 1**.

Deviations of the nasal septum are extremely common, and present in up to 30% of normal individuals. It has been speculated that these deviations are caused by birth trauma, but there is little evidence to support this contention.

A subperichondrial hematoma of the nasal septum may develop spontaneously, but is more commonly caused by blunt trauma or inadequate packing after nasal surgery. It may be either unilateral or bilateral, and present as a tender soft tissue swelling within the nose. The hematoma should be evacuated by removal of a patch of mucosa, as the pressure may cause cartilage necrosis and later a saddle nose deformity. Infection sometimes intervenes to produce a septal abscess; this is an extremely painful condition, and is almost always followed by significant cosmetic deformity.

Swelling of the mucosa, sufficient to block the airway, may be caused by acute or chronic infection (rhinitis). The common cold is the most simple and frequent example of this. Chronic rhinitis is most often associated with sinusitis, which needs to be addressed in order to relieve the obstructive symptoms.

In certain parts of the world, specific bacterial infections (rhinosporidiosis and rhinoscleroma) are a relatively common cause of protracted nasal obstruction. These conditions require long-term antimicrobial therapy and, in the case of rhinosporidiosis, surgical resection of the obstructive growth.

Allergic rhinitis is the most common manifestation of type 1 allergy, affecting up to 20% of the population in western countries. Both acute and chronic forms are recognized. In the acute form—hay fever, the patient complains of bouts of sneezing associated with watery rhinorrhea, nasal obstruction, and sometimes conjunctival irritation. In the chronic form, nasal obstruction is the most prominent symptom, while discharge and sneezing are sometimes absent. Possible treatment includes allergen avoidance, specific immunotherapy, mast cell degranulation inhibitors, and antihistamine or steroid preparation.

BOX 1: Causes of nasal obstruction.

Congenital:
- Choanal atresia:
  - Bilateral
  - Unilateral

Acquired:
- Physical obstruction:
  - Adenoids
  - Deviated nasal septum
  - Concha bullosa

Trauma: Hematoma and abscess of septum

Inflammation:
- Viral, bacterial, fungal rhinitis
- Allergic rhinitis
- Nasal polyps
- Rhinitis medicamentosa

Autonomic imbalance: Vasomotor rhinitis

Neoplastic:
- Epithelial:
  - Papilloma
  - Inverted papilloma (Ringertz tumor)
  - Schneiderian polyp
  - Squamous cell carcinoma
  - Transitional carcinoma

Nonepidermoid:
- Adenocarcinoma
- Adenoid cystic carcinoma

Neuroectodermal: Olfactory neuroblastoma

Vascular: Angiofibroma

Connective tissue tumors:
- Fibroma
- Fibrous dysplasia
- Fibrosarcoma
- Chondrosarcoma

Miscellaneous:
- Lymphoma
- Plasmacytoma

Polyps appear as bilateral, glassy swelling which progressively fill the nose and are associated with chronic sinusitis, anosmia, and chronic discharge. The etiology of nasal polyps is unknown, but they are not (as previously thought) due to atopy. In some patients, a dramatic response to systemic steroids may be maintained by the regular use of topical steroid drops. In others, the response is less satisfactory or more short-lived, and for these patients, surgical removal of the polyps is required. However, polyps tend to recur and it is not unusual for patients to have multiple surgical procedures through their lives. Nasal polyposis in a few patients is associated with hypersensitivity to salicylates, and their management may be improved with a special diet.

Rhinitis medicamentosa is an uncommon condition caused by the abuse of nasal vasoconstrictor medication. Some of these patients use ten or more bottles of vasoconstrictor drops per day. Nasal obstruction is the predominant symptom, and is extremely resistant to therapy. Topical steroid nasal drops can be effective, but care must be taken as they are absorbed extremely well by the chronically inflamed mucosa, and significant adrenal suppression can result.

Vasomotor rhinitis or autonomic imbalance is a diagnosis of exclusion made when no other cause for nasal obstruction can be incriminated. The nasal vasculature undergoes cyclical and alternate changes (physiological nasal cycle). In this way, the mucosa of one or other nostril is congested while the other is relatively constricted. Vasomotor rhinitis is thought to be the derangement or exaggeration of this physiological process.

281 CHAPTER

Nasal Polyps

These are considered as end result of recurrent infection and/or inflammation. Polyps originate in the ethmoid or maxillary sinuses and protrude through the sinus ostia into the nasal cavity. This is usual in children younger than 10 years. Symptoms consist of those of progressive nasal obstruction, frequently associated with discharge. Recurrent sinusitis is a common complication as a result of impaired sinus drainage. In some cases, chronic sinusitis may be the cause of polyp formation. Patients may also have intermittent epistaxis. Nasal polyps are seen as moist, glistening and peduculated growth that may have smooth or grape-like appearance are seen. Bilateral opacification of the ethmoid and maxillary sinuses is commonly found on radiography.

CHAPTER 282 Nasolacrimal Duct

The most common developmental anomaly of the nasolacrimal drainage system is nasolacrimal duct obstruction (NLDO), which occurs in up to 20% of infants. A thin mucosal membrane at the distal end of the duct, the valve of Hasner, is the most common cause of obstruction. Typically, the infant has epiphora and a mucopurulent discharge that causes matting of the eyelids beginning at about 1 month of age. Pressure applied to the lacrimal sac with a finger or cotton swab often results in reflux of cloudy fluid from the puncta.

The infection is usually polymicrobial, but a bacteriologic diagnosis is not necessary for clinical management. Eyelash washes with dilute baby shampoo can decrease the frequency of infections. Topical antibiotics can be used to decrease purulence but this likely leads to resistant organisms. Recurrent infections may be considered an indication for early probing. Lacrimal sac massage may push fluid through the mucosal membrane and thereby open the duct, but the pressure applied to the lacrimal sac needs to be forceful. Most NLDOs will spontaneously resolve. If resolution does not occur within the 1st year of life, probing of the duct can be done and is effective in 90% of cases. Effectiveness of nasolacrimal duct probing decreases after the age of 18 months. A silicon stent can be placed to maintain an open duct, which increases the success of long-term patency.

Stenosis or obstruction of the nasolacrimal duct is present in 30% of newborns and is even more common in Down syndrome patients. The obstruction is usually caused by a membranous obstruction of the nasolacrimal duct. Obstruction may also be caused by the inferior turbinate within the nose. Signs include tearing and mucopurulent discharge, which usually begins 3–5 weeks after birth. The absence of conjunctival injection differentiates this condition from conjunctivitis. A helpful diagnostic technique is to apply gentle pressure over the nasolacrimal sac to cause reflux of tears and mucopurulent material from the sac. Spontaneous resolution of the obstruction is common before 6–8 months of age. If the obstruction has not cleared by 8–10 months old, spontaneous resolution is much less likely, and the patient should be referred for probing of the nasolacrimal duct. Beyond 13 months old, the success rate of simple probing begins to decrease due to the recurring infections, which may cause scarring and stenosis of the nasolacrimal duct, increasing the need for more complicated procedures for treatment.

LACRIMAL SAC EXAMINATION

In case of lacrimal duct obstruction, the most important way to eliminate recurrent infections (and, according to some persons, a good way to help spontaneous resolution of the problem) is to know how to empty the lacrimal sac of its mucopurulent secretions. The technique is simple and is actually the best way to examine the lacrimal system to confirm a blockage. Minimal knowledge of the anatomy is required: simply palpate the bony depression behind the insertion of the inner canthal ligament on the medial orbital rim. The best place to start is on yourself, as follows:

- Find the small, hard bump in the inner corner of your eye with the index finger of your hand on the same side.
- Roll your finger posteriorly to feel a small depression where the end of a small cotton tipped swab could fit.

The next step is to do the same in a normal newborn to realize the difference in size. Finally, try it in a patient with a presumed blocked tear duct. You will discover that (1) it is difficult to feel the depression and (2) while you roll your finger, a significant amount of secretion will appear in the child's eye.

The latter finding is proof of a blocked tear duct, whereas the fullness of the tissues on palpation was the dilated lacrimal sac waiting to be drained. All you have to do now is to show the parents how to do the finger roll, which, by the way, is not a message.

The NLDO should be differentiated from infectious conjunctivitis, especially gonococcal, chlamydial, and herpetic infections. Chronic tearing occurs in congenital glaucoma in addition to blepharospasm and photophobia.

A *dacryocystocele* is a variation of congenital NLDO that occurs in newborns. These infants present with a bluish mass in the naso-orbital region below the medial canthal tendon. This mass is a dilated lacrimal sac that has both distal obstruction from a membrane and proximal obstruction from a 1-way valve effect from an incompetent valve of Rosenmüller. A hemangioma or dermoid cyst may have a bluish hue but hemangiomas typically do not present at birth. An encephalocele or dermoid cyst may also appear to be a bluish mass but will lie above the medial canthus.

CHAPTER 283

Natal Teeth

Teeth that are present at birth are called natal teeth, whereas erupting during neonatal period (30 days after the birth) are called neonatal teeth. Although seen in normal infants, it is seen with cleft palate. It is associated with Ellis-van Creveld syndrome, Hallermann-Streiff syndrome, and pachyonychia congenital. 90% of these are true primary teeth but occasionally they are supernumerary. Some are abnormal, with either hypoplastic defects or poor crown or root development. Natal teeth may cause feeding problems for both infant and mother. Ulceration of the ventral surface of the tongue by sharp tooth edges may develop if natal teeth remain. Most normal appearing natal teeth can be retained. Supernumerary, abnormal, and very loose may be removed to reduce the risk of aspiration.

Nausea

The term "nausea" reflects a constellation of unpleasant symptoms including bloating, postprandial fullness, early satiety, and a sensation of an impending need to vomit. Nausea may be an acute or chronic phenomenon that develops from a stimulus anywhere in the gastrointestinal tract or systemically. The majority of cases are trivial, the cause evident, and their resolution spontaneous.

In order to search more widely for a cause of nausea, it is important to consider the potential physiological mechanisms underlying this symptom, namely luminal (noxious stimulus), duct wall (mucosa, muscle, and nerve ending), local feedback pathways (splanchnic nerves), and higher centers.

Nausea is a symptom that easily can be rationally ascribed to a cause in the upper gastrointestinal tract, in particular to pathology of the stomach. It is a noxious symptom, and noxious cause ought to be considered first: dietary (fatty or spicy/hot foods); toxins (alcohol; medications of any type, although especially non-steroidal anti-inflammatory drugs, metronidazole, erythromycin, cholestyramine); peptic ulcer disease (gastritis, duodenitis, reflux esophagitis or peptic ulceration; helicobacter pylori); infections, whether bacterial (food poisoning: *Staphylococcus aureus*, *Bacillus cereus*, giardiasis), viral (Norwalk virus, cytomegalovirus, Epstein–Barr virus, HIV) or fungal (esophageal candida); or cancer (adenocarcinoma, gastric mucosa-associated lymphoid tissue lymphoma, small-bowel lymphoma).

Nausea is a primary symptom of gastrointestinal motility disorders. The best known of these is diabetic gastroparesis, but other systemic conditions involving the gut wall (scleroderma, amyloid, Chagas' disease), muscle (dystrophies), or nerves (HIV, autoimmune disease) may present with nausea.

CHAPTER 285

Neck Webbing

The newborns with webbing of neck have a short neck, with excess skin where neck joins the shoulders. This is seen in Noonan syndrome. The loose skin folds around the neck will form webbed neck.

Webbed neck (Pterygium colli), "Sphinx Neck", is characterized by presence of a thick web of skin which extends from behind the ears to the distal portion of the clavicle and to the acromial process **(Fig. 1)**. It is seen in Turner's syndrome and associated with gonadal dysgenesis.

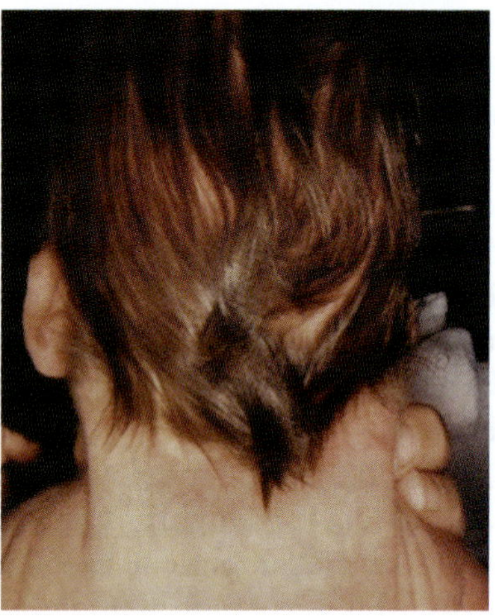

Fig. 1: Webbing of neck.

CHAPTER 286

Neurocysticercosis

It is the most common central nervous system (CNS) parasitic infection present with signs of increased intracranial pressure. Cerebral cysticercosis occurs when larvae of pork tapeworm (Tenia solium) encyst in CNS tissues. Eating contaminated pork carrying the *T. solium* larvae leads to acquisition of the intestinal tapeworm. Cysticercosis results from fecal/oral transmission of the ova shed by the adult intestinal tapeworm, and it is often transmitted to affected children by family household or community contacts who carry adult *T. solium* tapeworm. After transmission, hematogenous spread to neural, ocular, or muscular tissue can occur. Seizures are most common presenting sign and are often accompanied by headache. Patients can develop meningitis as a result of inflammatory reactions of ruptured cysts or they may present with signs and symptoms of raised intracranial pressure due to obstruction of CSF pathways by cysts, resulting in noncommunicating hydrocephalus.

287 CHAPTER

Neurofibroma

These are solitary or multiple growths of neural tissue presenting as soft, skin colored or pink dermal and/or subcutaneous nodules. The central portion of early lesion is soft, and fingertip pressure an illusion of a pressing in a buttonhole. Neurofibromatosis type 1 or von Recklinghausen disease, a syndrome characterized by a presence of multiple neurofibromas, café-au-lait spots, axillary and inguinal freckling. The clinician must remember that the neurofibromas usually appear after puberty, whereas in prepubertal, café-au-lait spots are the most important cutaneous marker of von Recklinghausen disease. Solitary neurofibromas occasionally develop in normal individuals.

CHAPTER 288

Nummular Eczema

It is an acute papulovesicular eruption named for its annular or coin-shaped configuration and probably also represents another clinical pattern found in atopic individuals. Lesions are intensely pruritic, fairly well circumscribed, round or oval red, and scaly patches studded with 1–3-mm vesicles. They are usually located on extensor thighs or abdomen of children. Vigorous scratching causes excoriation and crusting. Although the rash is resistant to therapy, it may respond to therapy for acute dermatitis.

Nystagmus

Nystagmus describes a series of rhythmical oscillations of one or both eyes. The movements may be horizontal, vertical, or rotatory, and the oscillations may be equal in velocity and amplitude to either side (pendular) or may have a slow phase and a fast phase in opposite direction (phasic or jerky nystagmus). By convention, the direction of phasic nystagmus is described by its fast phase and the movements is usually exaggerated on gaze to the side.

GRADING OF NYSTAGMUS

- *Grade 1*: Nystagmus with fast phase to left looking toward the left
- *Grade 2*: Nystagmus with fast phase to left looking straight ahead
- *Grade 3*: Nystagmus with fast phase to left looking toward the right side

SITE OF LESION AND CLINICAL FEATURE

- Cerebellum horizontal nystagmus maximum on gaze to the side of the lesion
- Vestibular apparatus or nerve horizontal or rotatory nystagmus maximal on gaze opposite to the side of lesion (unless irritative lesion in labyrinth)
- Midbrain superior colliculus vertical upbeat nystagmus evoked by upward gaze
- Pons, midbrain, medical, longitudinal, fasciculus ataxic, nystagmus most marked in abducting eye, associated with under nuclear ophthalmoplegia, vertical up beating nystagmus on upward gaze
- Lower medulla down beating nystagmus on downward or lateral gaze

Ataxic nystagmus is seen in lesions of medial longitudinal fasciculus. It causes disconjugation of lateral eye movements, especially during rapid changes of gaze. So that one eye is slow to adduct while the adducting eye shows coarse horizontal nystagmus, commonly it is seen bilaterally.

Ocular nystagmus is often congenital in origin and sometimes associated with head tile and titubation. The nystagmus is pendular in type to central gaze but becomes phasic on lateral gaze, and tends to diminish on convergence.

Positional nystagmus and usually vertigo may occur only in certain head positions. Two types of positional nystagmus are recognized:

1. *Peripheral type*: This is due to abnormalities of the inner ear. If the patient is put into certain position, after a latent period of a few seconds, vertigo is experienced and rotational nystagmus can be observed. If the position is maintained, the vertigo and nystagmus abate usually within a minute. This condition may follow head injury, ear infection, and viral or vascular damage to the inner ear.
2. *Central type*: This is due to the cerebellum or brainstem vestibular connections.

DIFFERENTIAL DIAGNOSIS OF NYSTAGMUS

Congenital:
- Associated with blindness
- Familial
- Idiopathic

Spasmus nutans:
- Idiopathic
- Tumors of optic nerve and chiasm

Acquired nystagmus:
- *Pendular*:
    - Spasmus nutans
    - Multiple sclerosis
    - Brainstem infarction
    - Oculopalatal syndrome:
        - Spinocerebellar degeneration
        - Brainstem infarction
- *Jerk*:
    - Horizontal:
        - Drag induced
        - Vestibular nystagmus
        - Ictal
    - Vertical:
        - Upbeat
        - Downbeat
- *Dissociated*:
    - Monocular
    - Divergence
    - Seesaw
    - Convergence

It is the rhythmic oscillation of eyeball. This may be due to imbalance of eyeball posture in the orbit. The oscillation may be a slow drift in one direction with a fast correction in the opposite direction. Direction of the fast phase is used to categorize the nystagmus.

The oscillating movements may be in horizontal plane or vertical plane.

Horizontal Nystagmus

It may be ataxic, multidirectional gaze evoked, and unidirectional, i.e., peripheral. In ataxic type, the nystagmus of abducting eye is more than adducting eye. It is seen with internuclear ophthalmoplegia or in cerebrovascular accidents.

Vertical Nystagmus

It is rare. It indicates brainstem lesion. It may be upper brain lesion or medullary cervical junctional lesion.

Paralytic squint should be differentiated from concomitant squint. Concomitant squint is characterized by early onset below 3 years, normal eye movements in all direction, identical primary and secondary direction, and defective vision in the deviating eye.

EXAMINATION OF THE PATIENT WITH NYSTAGMUS

The child is asked to look at examiners finger. This is moved slowly horizontally in both directions that are vertically up and down. Position of the eye is noted when the nystagmus occurs. Its character and direction of fast component are noted.

CAUSES OF NYSTAGMUS

- Physiological nystagmus
- Visual defects—optic atrophy
- Labyrinthine nystagmus
- Congenital nystagmus
- Neurological disorders
- Cerebellar ataxia
- Cerebellar tumor
- Friedreich's ataxia
- Hydrocephalus
- Drugs
- Diphenyl hydantoin sodium
- Aspirin
- Colistin sulfate
- Diphenoxylate hydrochloride

CLINICAL TYPES OF NYSTAGMUS

Congenital Motor Nystagmus

This is often idiopathic; in this case, visual acuity is only moderately impaired, and the fundus examination findings and the electroretinogram are normal. Usually an affected individual will have a null point or a preferred position in which the eye movements are minimized. This may affect the head position as the patient tries to keep the eyes in the null point. In patients with congenital motor nystagmus, there is often dampening or quieting of the nystagmus with convergence.

Congenital Sensory Nystagmus

This occurs with disorders that impair normal image formation (bilateral congenital cataracts) or image processing in both eyes (a retinal dystrophy or bilateral optic nerve atrophy or hypoplasia). Eye movements may be searching and there is no null point. Visual acuity is more severely impaired than in idiopathic congenital nystagmus (20/200 or less), and visual loss may be progressive in some instances.

Acquired Childhood Nystagmus

Spasmus nutans is a special form of acquired nystagmus with onset in the first 2 years of life. The usual triad of findings consists of nystagmus (often a shimmering type of nystagmus that is frequently asymmetric or even monocular), head nodding, and torticollis. This form of nystagmus is generally benign and disappears by the age of 3–4 years. In some cases, spasmus nutans can be associated with chiasmal or suprachiasmal or retinal dystrophies. Neuroradiologic investigation is indicated.

Opsoclonus is a special form of eye movement abnormality that is not truly nystagmus in that the bizarre, seemingly random oscillations of the eyes are not rhythmic and are frequently multifactorial. The most common cause of opsoclonus in children is acute cerebellar ataxia. The child presents with "dancing eyes and dancing feet." Opsoclonus can occur also with occult neuroblastoma, as a paraneoplastic phenomenon, viral encephalitis, and hydrocephalus.

CHAPTER 290 Obesity

Obesity is the most common nutritional disorder of children. Here, adipose tissue is enlarged out of proportion to other body organs. It is the term used when the weight exceeds 120% of standard weight. In practice, simple observation of undressed child leaves little doubt about the diagnosis.

The body mass index (BMI) defined as weight/height^2 (in kg per m^2) is most useful index. The term overweight is used when BMI exceeds 95th percentile for that age and sex. Skin fold thickness above 85th percentile for age and sex also suggests obesity. It can be measured at triceps, mid-abdominal, or subscapular sites.

EVALUATING THE OBESE CHILD

When parents of an obese child are asked to tell you their concerns, they often describe a succession of problems, worries, and disappointments related to issues such as the child's eating habits, lack of physical activity, and problems with peer relationships. The self-image of an obsess youngster will not be strengthened by listening to such a recital.

In the overwhelming majority of patients with childhood onset obesity, the principal determinants are genetic, and this supposition is often confirmed by a detailed family history.

Recent evidence suggests that some obese individuals may have inherited disorders in the regulation of energy balance, which may partly explain why, for many obese children, dietary energy intake is not greater than average.

The next important item in history taking is a rough estimate of the child's energy output. An excellent individual indicator is an estimate of the total number of hours of television watching, computer activity, and video games play per day.

PHYSICAL EXAMINATION

A useful way to begin is by examining the child's hands and feet. In obese children, always check the area of skin over the base of the fifth finger and fifth toe. The presence of a small stellate scar is a telltale sign that a skin tag was removed soon after birth with a suture tried tightly around it. In fact, such a skin tag was almost certainly a rudimentary supernumerary digit. This finding, coupled with obesity, raises the likelihood that the child has Laurence-Moon-Biedl syndrome, in which obesity is often associated with polydactyly, retinitis pigmentosa, progressive loss of vision, some developmental delay, and often a progressive nephropathy.

Another uncommon bit important sign to look for in the hands of obese children is the metacarpal sign. Children with pseudohypoparathyroidism (a syndrome associated with obesity) often having strikingly short fourth and fifth metacarpals and metatarsals. Elicit the metacarpal sign by having the youngster make a first. When the fourth and fifth metacarpals are hypoplastic, the relevant knuckles are absent and are often replaced by dimples. Incidentally, this sign also is seen in girls with Turner syndrome (XO anomaly).

Stretch marks often are observed in the skin of the abdomen and thighs of obese children.

Another obesity syndrome that usually can be suspected simply from the history and physical findings is Prader–Willi syndrome. In affected children, obesity typically develops between 6 months and 6 years of age and usually is associated with mild-to-moderate developmental delay, hypotonia, and feeding problems in infancy. The facies is characteristic, with a prominent forehead and rather almond-shaped eyes. The hands and feet are small. Compulsive overeating usually appears by 3 years of age. In boys, the penis and scrotum are often small, and in girls, the labia are poorly formed. The syndrome is usually caused by a defect in the paternal chromosome.

The "metacarpal sign" (unusually short fourth and fifth metacarpals) is seen in pseudohypoparathyroidism and in Turner syndrome.

CLINICAL FEATURES

Many times, diagnosis is made from child's appearance. Obesity or overnutrition is generalized. It is mainly due to excessive intake of the food.

Genetic predisposition may also be present. Lack of activity may be responsible for obesity even though intake of food may not be unusual. Adipocytes appear to increase in number when caloric intake is increased.

Stocky children may have relatively large skeletal frames and have more than average amount of muscular tissue. Appetite may be influenced by various factors. These include psychogenic disturbances, hypothalamus, pituitary, or other brain lesions. Some inherited syndromes such as Laurence–Moon–Biedl, Prader–Willi, and Cushing may also be responsible.

The obesity of the extremities is usually greater in the upper arm and thigh. The hands may be relatively small and fingers are tapering. Genu valgum is common. Psychological disturbance is also common.

Obese children carry a large body weight. This tires them more easily and further reduces physical activity. Clinical features of endocrine, hypothalamic, or various cryptogenic syndrome are obvious. Traumatic inflammation, neoplastic lesion of hypothalamus, and pituitary gland cause increased appetite and, hence, obesity.

Leptin is adipose tissue-secreted hormone with receptors in hypothalamus. Plasma level of leptin correlates with body fat mass and is regulated by feeding, fasting, insulin, and steroid.

Insulin decreases lipolysis and increased fat syntheses and uptake. Genetic studies have shown the relation between leptin, gene, and obesity.

Obesity may be exogenous and endogenous:

Exogenous obesity:

- Constitutional
- Excessive food intake
- Decreased energy expenditure
- Fat cell hyperplasia

Endogenous obesity:

- *Genetic:*
  - Prader–Willi syndrome
  - Laurence–Moon–Biedl syndrome
- *Hormonal:*
  - Hypothyroidism
  - Hypogonadism

    - Pseudohypoparathyroidism
    - Cushing's syndrome
- *Hypothalamic:* Obesity

Those with BMI >85 percentile for the age should be investigated, if they have any of the following:

- Family history of cardiovascular complications of type II diabetes
- Rapid increase in obesity
- Hypertension

Blood sugar, serum cholesterol, lipid profile, CFT, skeletal maturity evaluation, hormonal test, i.e., urine-free cortisol, free thyroxine (FT_4) and thyroid-stimulating hormone (TSH), testosterone, estradiol, and gonadotropin assays are done as suggested by clinical examination.

DIFFERENTIAL DIAGNOSIS

- Overeating
- Endocrine disorders such as hypothyroidism, pseudohypoparathyroidism, and Cushing's syndrome
- Fröhlich's syndrome (adipose genital dysmorphy)
- Prader–Willi syndrome—obesity starts from late infancy, upper slanting of palpable fissure, hypogonadism, mental retardation, strabismus, and short stature

CHAPTER 291

Obturator Test

If the inflammatory process is adjacent to the obturator internus muscle, as in the presence of pelvic abscess or a ruptured appendix, lower abdominal pain may be elicited by flexing the thigh to a 90° angle and rotating it internally and externally. This is known as the obturator test.

Abdominal masses can also have pulsation. Pseudopancreatic cyst, for example, may give rise to transmitted pulsation. Liver, on the other hand, can have expansile pulsation secondary to tricuspid regurgitation or hemangioma.

The "head-raising test" is used to differentiate between an upper intra-abdominal mass from an intra-abdominal one, whereas the "leg-raising test" is used to determine whether a lower abdominal mass is intra-abdominal or extra-abdominal.

Intra-abdominal masses tend to move freely with respiration. Liver, spleen, and stomach have good movement with respiration; kidney, however, moves less with respiration. In a crying child, an extra-abdominal lump will become more prominent compared to an intra-abdominal lump.

This is elicited by flexing the thigh to 90° angle and rotating it internally and externally. This produces pain in the lower abdomen. This occurs as a result of inflammatory process adjacent to obturator internal muscle as in pelvic abscess or a ruptured appendix.

CHAPTER 292

Obstructive Murmurs

All obstructive murmurs are organic. The turbulence caused by obstruction produces eddies of large but varying sized, and the vortex shedding that results in a dissipation of a large amount of energy. Therefore, obstructive murmurs are coarse and loud. Because the turbulence occurs during forward flow, it must wait for the aortic and pulmonary valves to open, and there is a pause between the first heart sound and the beginning of the murmurs.

Obstructive murmurs are caused by mitral or tricuspid stenosis, which are uncommon congenital heart lesions, in areas where rheumatic fever is still endemic, this murmur may be encountered when an older child has mitral stenosis associated with chronic rheumatic carditis, decrescendo-crescendo in shape related to flow velocity. The murmur is low pitched, and it does not begin until the mitral valve opens; therefore, there is a pause between the second sound and the start of the murmur.

With mitral valve stenosis, the murmur occurs in the left ventricle and is loudest at the apex. Frequently, only the late diastolic portion of the murmur is present; in which case, it is presystolic in timing.

CHAPTER 293 Oliguria

CAUSES OF OLIGURIA

- *Renal:*
  - Acute glomerulonephritis
  - Nephrotic syndrome
  - Acute renal failure
  - Chronic renal failure
- *Others:*
  - Mismatched blood transfusion
  - Hypotension
  - Congestive cardiac failure
  - Hypoxia

CHAPTER 294

Optic Disk Atrophy

OPTIC ATROPHY

Optic atrophy represents the permanent loss of retinal ganglion cell axons. Optic atrophy may be due to injury to the optic nerve head. However, because of anterograde or retrograde degeneration, it may reflect upstream injury of the retinal ganglion cells or downstream injury of the posterior optic nerve, optic chiasm, or optic tract. Optic atrophy is of two types, viz., primary and secondary.

PRIMARY OR SIMPLE OPTIC ATROPHY

Primary or simple optic atrophy can be a consequence of any injury of the retinal ganglion cell or its axon in the nerve fiber layer, the optic nerve head, the orbital, intracanalicular or intracranial optic nerve, optic chiasma, optic tract, or lateral geniculate nucleus. Causes of primary optic atrophy are anterior ischemic optic neuropathy, compressive lesions of optic nerve, posterior ischemic optic neuropathy, trauma, granulomatous inflammation of optic nerve, and ophthalmic artery aneurysm.

SECONDARY OPTIC ATROPHY

Secondary optic atrophy reflects the disorganized appearance of the surface of the optic disk due to axonal injury in association with severe edema or inflammation at the optic nerve head. Although secondary optic atrophy most commonly occur in cases of severe papilledema, it may also develop in cases of longstanding severe orbital inflammation. The other causes are Behcet's syndrome, Vogt–Koyanagi–Harada syndrome.

CHAPTER 295 Optic Fundus Abnormalities

FUNDUSCOPIC EXAMINATION

Ask the patient to look straight ahead and to keep the eyes as still as possible. The ophthalmoscope is held a few centimeters from the patients eyes. The ophthalmoscope is then brought as close as possible to the patient's eye and the light directed slightly toward nasal side. By doing this, the optic disk can be found and the light will not fall directly on the macula (which may constrict the pupil). If the optic disk is not in focus, the strength of the lens of the ophthalmoscope should be gradually reduced until the disk is sharply focused. If only blood vessels are seen, they should be followed backwards (i.e., against the angle of any branches that are seen) and the disk will eventually come in view.

LENS

Lens appears clear. Pearly gray, opaque, and round area in the center of the lens is typical of cataracts. The lens may be dislocated upward as in patients with Marfan's syndrome, downward in homocystinuria.

RETINA

Normally, the fundus will be pink and shiny. It may be gray in deeply pigmented or in anemic children. The retina becomes gray and losses its shine whenever it becomes avascular.

- Cataracts
- Retrolental fibroplasia
- Retinal detachment
- Retinoblastoma
- Chorioretinal coloboma
- Coat's disease
- Ocular trauma
- Vitreous hemorrhage

RETINAL VESSELS

Retinal veins are slightly larger than arteries. Narrow retinal arteries are seen in hypertensive retinopathy, especially in nephritis.

The disk appears white in children with optic neuritis or optic atrophy and may be seen in children with meningitis and encephalitis. Unilateral papilledema with contralateral optic atrophy may be due to frontal lobe tumor (Foster Kennedy's syndrome). If the retina appears opalescent, retinal detachment may be present.

Cupping of the disk in which the vessel appears to dip down from the retina toward the disk may be physiologic or may be exaggerated with glaucoma. A white disk may indicate optic nerve atrophy, which occurs with osteopetrosis causing compression of the nerve and with neurofibroma of the optic nerve.

Macula is the most light-sensitive area of the eye, the pupil constricts as the macula is approached. In older children, the macula can be visualized if the child is told to look at the ophthalmoscope light. This area appears to be cherry-red in reticuloendothelial diseases such as Tay-Sachs and Niemann-Pick disease and in other cerebromacular

TABLE 1: Difference between primary and secondary optic atrophy.

Features	***Primary***	***Secondary***
Optic disk	White	Normal
Disk margin	Well defined	Hazy
Arteria	Normal	Attenuated
Veins	Normal	Tortuous and dilated
Hemorrhage	Absent	Present
Exudate	Absent	Present

degenerative diseases. The macula may be brown and appear fragmented in children with the juvenile form macular degeneration. Bruit over the eyeball may occur with congenital arteriovenous fistula in the brain.

The differences between primary and secondary optic atrophy are mentioned in **Table 1**.

CAUSES OF PAPILLEDEMA

- Increased intracranial tension
- Malignant hypertension
- Central retinal vein thrombosis
- Cavernous sinus thrombosis
- Guillain-Barre syndrome
- Pseudotumor cerebri
- Leukemia

CAUSES OF OPTIC NEURITIS

- Multiple sclerosis
- Devic disease
- Tuberculosis
- Encephalitis
- Meningitis
- *Drugs:* Isoniazid (INH), ethambutol, and chloroquine

CAUSES OF OPTIC ATROPHY

- Cerebromacular degeneration
- Retinitis pigmentosa
- Congenital optic atrophy
- Papilledema
- Optic neuritis
- Glaucoma

CHAPTER 296 Orotracheal Intubation

Adequate ventilation and oxygenation by face mask are in progress. Manual immobilization of the neck by an assistant is made if the cervical spine injury is suspected. A folded sheet or towel is kept under the baby's back and neck to allow the extension of the head. Laryngoscope is held in left hand; it is inserted into the right hand side of the mouth displacing tongue to the left. In the infant, it is sometimes useful to hold the laryngoscope with the left thumb, index, and middle finger leaving the little finger free to stretch down to press on the larynx to improve the view of the vocal cords. This is particularly useful if single handed. Endotracheal tube is then inserted into the trachea, concentrating on how far the tip is being placed below the vocal cord. The tip should lie 2–4 cm below the vocal cords depending on the age. The placement of the tube is confirmed by chest movement and auscultating the chest.

297 CHAPTER Otorrhea

Discharge from the ear is called otorrhea. It may arise from the external auditory meatus, middle ear, or, occasionally, intracranial or adjacent structures.

CAUSES OF OTORRHEA

- *External ear:*
  - Foreign bodies
  - *Otitis externa:*
    - Furunculosis
    - Diffuse otitis externa
  - Otomycosis
- *Middle ear:*
  - Acute otitis media:
    - Acute suppurative otitis media
    - Acute necrotizing otitis media
  - Chronic otitis media:
    - Chronic suppurative otitis media
      - Tubotympanic disease
    - Permanent perforation syndrome:
      - Atticoantral disease
      - Cholesteatoma

SECTION 16

CHAPTER 298 Paronychia

Paronychia is a common childhood disorder that presents with redness, swelling, and tenderness of the lateral or proximal nailfold. The acute form presents with a more sudden onset of swelling and marked tenderness.

A paronychia is a relatively superficial abscess that develops under the cuticle or along the nail fold of a finger or a toe. It occurs when staphylococci and occasionally streptococci gain access through a traumatized hangnail or through lesions created by trauma. On occasion, an ingrown toenail is the predisposing condition; in such cases, the nail, which usually was cut improperly, grows laterally into the nailfold, lacerating the soft tissue. In typical cases, erythema, pain, and tenderness develop at the site of injury and are followed rapidly by suppuration. The infection then advances from the portal of entry around the nailfold, and, if treatment is delayed, it can burrow beneath the base of the nail, creating a subungual abscess (onychia). On occasion, secondary lymphangitis may develop. Drainage is accomplished readily by undermining the involved portion of the cuticle and nailfold with a scalpel blade. Unless secondary complications have developed, subsequent soaking is usually sufficient to promote healing, although oral antistaphylococcal agents hasten the process.

Onychomycosis, or fungal infection of the nail plate, is not as common in children as it is in adults. Thus, nail dystrophy should not automatically be treated as a fungal infection unless proven by microscopic examination and/or fungal culture. Dystrophic nails can be the end result of many different types of inflammation of the nail matrix and are seen frequently following discrete or more low-grade repetitive trauma or friction or from an underlying dermatosis, such as psoriasis, atopic dermatitis, or lichen planus.

CHAPTER 299

Parotid Gland Swelling

Mumps are the most common cause of all parotid swelling.

A useful point in this connection is that a generalized parotid swelling tends to lift the auricle away from the head. Inspection of the orifice of Stensen's duct will usually reveal some abnormality. The presence of other enlarged nodes and of a primary lesions should be sought, if the lymph nodes are suspected.

Sialography may prove helpful. Radiopaque contrast is injected into the appropriate orifice (Wharton's submandibular or Stensen's for injection). The branching system of ducts is well visualized in the radiograph. Blockage by a stone or by growth, sialectasia (dilatation and beading of the duct system, especially in the parotid gland), or the presence of a fistula is the lesion most likely to be demonstrated in this way.

In sarcoidosis, asymptomatic enlargement of the parotid, sublingual, and submandibular gland occurs in about 6% of cases. Spontaneous resolution often occurs. The glands are not tender. Facial pals may occur with parotid enlargement. The syndrome of fever, uveitis, and lacrimal and salivary gland enlargement is known as "uveoparotid" fever.

CHAPTER 300

Pectus Carinatum

The sternum is prominent, forming an anterior ridge and the ribs inclined forward causing a greatly increased anteroposterior diameter **(Fig. 1)**. The condition can be acquired (asthma), but if congenital is due to premature obliteration of the sternal sutures during growth or to malattachment of the anterior portion of the diaphragm to the posterior portion of the rectus sheath rather than, as normally, to the xiphoid process, with consequent distorting mechanical effects.

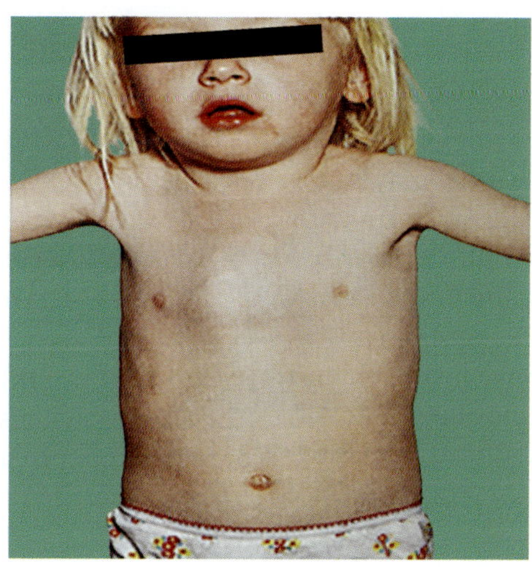

Fig. 1: Pectus carinatum.

Pectus Excavatum

The costal cartilages are prominent, cures inward, and the body of the sternum is depressed backward toward the spine from the manubriosternal joints downward with maximum recession at the xiphoid **(Fig. 1)**.

Deep sternal concavity is present almost touching the spine is present in severe form. The heart is displaced to the left side of the chest. Radiographic displacement of the heart to the left and is rotational.

Changes of the electrocardiogram may be wrongly interpreted as evidence of heart disease. The electrocardiogram may show persistence of the juvenile pattern with T-wave inversion in the right precordial leads, incomplete right bundle branch block and right axis deviation. Because of cardiac rotation, there may be p-wave inversion and a QR pattern in lead V_1. Minor lung function abnormalities occur with reduced total lung, maximum breathing, and vital capacities. The condition does not predispose to cardiac or respiratory disease in later life.

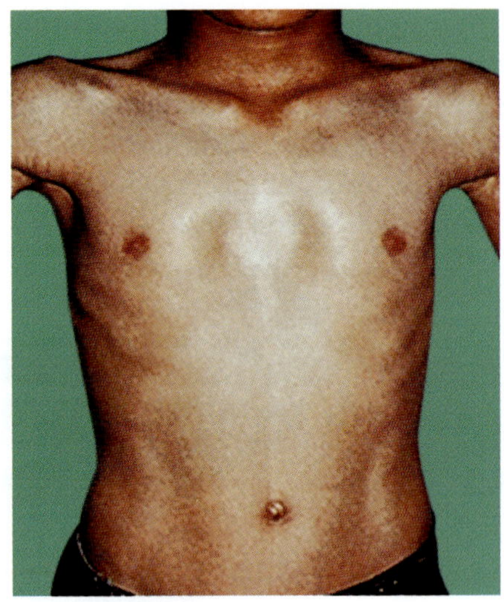

Fig. 1: Pectus excavatum.

CHAPTER 302

Percussion Notes

In 1761, Leopold Auenbrugger introduced percussion as a cornerstone or physical diagnosis and by mid-1800, clinicians were using it as a bedside technique.

PURPOSE OF RESPIRATORY PERCUSSION

- To determine the state of underlying tissues
- To delineate or define the boundaries or border of the lung

Percussion involves striking one object against another, thus producing vibration and subsequent sound waves. The sound waves thus produced are heard as percussion tones (called resonance) that arise from vibration 4–6 cm deep in the body tissue. The percussion sound that is produced reflects the ease with which body wall vibrates, which in turn is influenced by many variables including the strength of stroke, the condition, and state of the body wall and the underlying organs. Prominent dullness or unusual resonance over one side indicates disease in that part.

TECHNIQUE

- *Direct (immediate):* It involves striking the finger or hand directly over the body surface. This is done over clavicle, sternum, and in infant's chest.
- *Indirect (mediate):* The finger of one hand acts as hammer (plexor) and a finger of the other hand acts as the striking surface (pleximeter). The distal phalanx of the middle finger should be placed firmly on the body surface with the other fingers slightly elevated off the surface. Snap the wrist of your other hand downward and with the tip of the middle finger, sharply tap the interphalangeal joint of the finger that is on the body surface.

TYPES OF PERCUSSION NOTES

- Normal percussion notes
- Abnormal percussion notes

Normal Percussion Notes

The normal percussion note of the chest is due to the underlying lung tissue, containing a normal amount of air in the air vesicles, air sacs, and air passages. The percussion note over the healthy lung tissue has a distinctive and clear character with a low pitch.

Normally the *resonant* note is found over the lungs.

Impaired Resonance

- Pleural thickening
- Fibrosis of lung
- Collapse of the lung
- Small pleural effusion
- Bronchopneumonia

Abnormal Types of Percussion Notes

- *Tympany:* A drum-like note, elicited normally over the stomach, intestine,

larynx, or trachea, is referred to as tympanic note. When such a note is heard over a region of the chest wall, it indicates:
  - Pneumothorax
  - Subcutaneous emphysema
  - Superficial cavity
- *Hyperresonant:* A note intermediate in pitch between normal lung resonant, and tympany can be elicited, over normal lung tissue, by keeping the chest in full inspiration during percussion.

Pathologically:
- Bilaterally in case of emphysema
- Unilaterally in case of pneumothorax, lung cyst, large bullae, diaphragmatic hernia, compensatory emphysema, and obstructive emphysema
- *Impaired note:* When a part of a lung becomes comparatively airless, it fails to vibrate sufficiently to the percussion stroke and gives rise to at impairment of note or slight loss of resonance and found in:
  - Consolidation
  - Collapse
  - Fibrosis
- *Dull note:* An impairment of note, of greater degree than the impaired note, is referred to as dullness and is found in:
  - Consolidation
  - Collapse
  - Thickened pleura
  - Extensive tuberculous infiltration of lung

  Basal dullness as a consequence of diaphragm elevation can be confused with pleural fluid, but the diaphragmatic dullness will move downward on deep inspiration (unless muscle is paralyzed).
- *Stony dullness or flatness:* A percussion note completely devoid of resonance or displaying absolute dullness is referred to as flat or stony dull note, it can be elicited normally percussing on the thigh of the patient. It is found in:
  - Pleural effusion (volume >200 mL)
  - *Empyema*: In these conditions, the fluid dampens the vibration of both chest wall and underlying retracted tissue. A feeling of resistance to the percussion blow within the finger used for stroking is also present in solid intrathoracic tumor
  - Fibrosis with pleural thickening

LIVER DULLNESS

Normally, liver dullness lies in the 5th space in the midclavicular line, 7th space in the anterior axillary line, and 9th space in the scapular line.

Liver dullness is present in the 4th space—in amoebic liver abscess, diaphragmatic paralysis, and collapse of the lower lobe of the lung. Liver dullness is pushed to 6th space in emphysema, right-sided pneumothorax, and air in peritoneal cavity.

TIDAL PERCUSSION

It is the percussion on the upper border of the liver dullness on the right side anteriorly, at the peak of deep inspiration and expiration. It serves to determine the extent of diaphragmatic movements. It is restricted in pulmonary fibrosis, empyema, and subdiaphragmatic abscess.

Pericardial Bulge

The anterior part of the chest wall above the heart is called as precordium. Any bulge over the precordium should be looked for and noted. Any bulge will indicate chronic cardiac lesions. Precordium should be viewed tangentially from the side of the bed.

Precordial bulge is associated with:

- Scoliosis
- Kyphosis
- Rickets
- Right ventricular hypertrophy
- Pneumomediastinum
- Pleural effusion
- Mediastinal growth

The other aspect of the bulge, i.e., *flattened precordium* is seen in:

- Old pericarditis
- Fibrosis or collapse of lung

Precordial Pulsations

Any *precordial pulsation* present in second-left intercostal space (ICS) or third-left ICS should be looked for:

Second-left ICS:

- Patent ductus arteriosus (PDA)
- Pulmonary hypertension
- Enlarged left atrial appendage

Third-left ICS:

- Right ventricular hypertrophy (RVH)
- Ventricular septal defect (VSD)

Third and fourth ICS:

- RVH
- VSD

Extra precordial pulsation:

- *Epigastric pulsation:*
  - RVH
  - Aortic pulsation
  - TR
- *Suprasternal:*
  - Coarctation of aorta
  - Aneurysm of aorta
  - Hyperkinetic state
- *Right side:* Dextrocardia
- *Back:*
  - Coarctation of aorta
  - Arteriovenous fistula

CHAPTER 305

Pericardial Puncture

This is occasionally indicated in cardiac tamponade. This is because of pneumopericardium. FG12 cannula is connected via three-way tap to a 10 mL syringe. This is inserted under the ribcage to the left of xiphisternum. It is then advanced upward and to the left at an angle of 45° from the ventricle and 45° from the midline while applying the gentle suction. Pericardium is applied at a depth of about 1 cm. Air is withdrawn, if necessary, it can be left in situ. It is then connected to underseal water drainage **(Figs. 1 and 2)**.

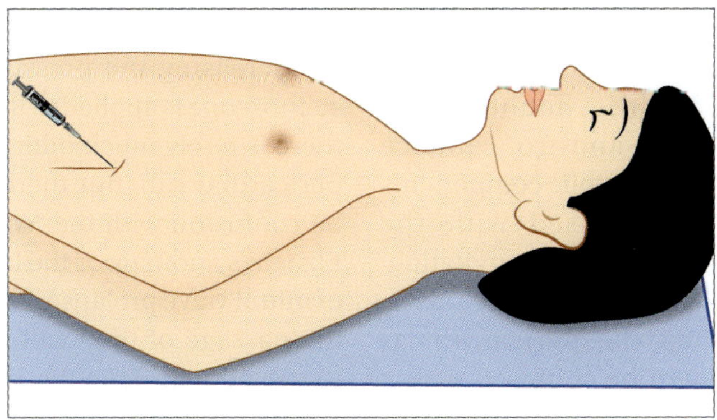

Fig. 1: Needle pericardiocentesis—angle.

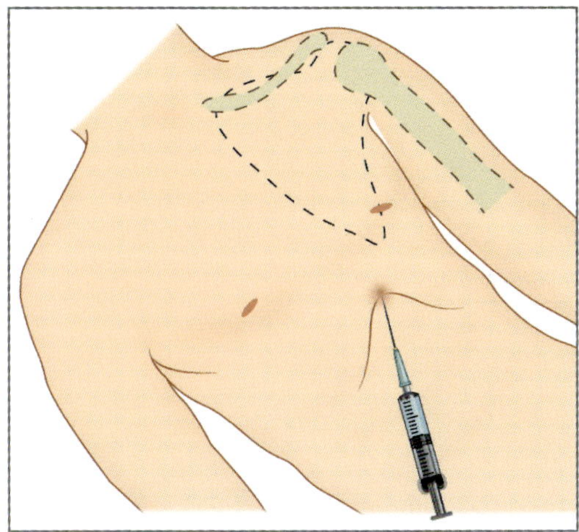

Fig. 2: Needle pericardiocentesis—direct.

CHAPTER 306

Pericardial Rub

A pericardial rub, once identified as such, is pathognomonic of acute pericarditis. A rub has a characteristic "creaking" or "leathery", but this quality does not certainly differentiate it from a cardiac murmur. A typical rub is virtually continuous throughout the cardiac cycle, but three components have been identified—systolic, early diastolic, and, if the patient is in sinus rhythm, late diastolic. If all three components are heard, there is little doubt in the diagnosis, but the to-and-fro cadence of the systolic and early diastolic components can sometimes be confused with the murmurs of aortic stenosis and regurgitation. If the rub is heard in systole only—as is often the case when the pericarditis is resolving—it may often be confused with a murmur.

A rub may be heard anywhere over the precordium. It may be markedly influenced by respiration (increasing on lying and reducing on sitting up) and posture, although the change is not predictable and, to be sure of not missing a rub, it is necessary to auscultate in all phases of deep respiration and with the patient in several postures. Sometimes, it may be possible to increase the intensity of a rub by increasing the pressure with which the stethoscope is applied to the chest. In practice, there is rarely much difficulty in identifying a pericardial rub, but there may occasionally be confusion with the "scratchy" murmur of Ebstein's anomaly or the late systolic murmur of mitral valve prolapse. When doubt remains, the passage of time will usually resolve the issue; pericardial rubs are evanescent and usually disappear within a few days.

307 CHAPTER Peristalsis, Visible

Usually, visible peristalsis is pathological. However, in a number of conditions, the normal movements of the bowel may be visible; these circumstances are divarication of the abdominal recti muscles, an incisional or massive umbilical hernia containing bowel, and extreme thinness of the abdominal parietes—the result of emaciation or rarely, congenital absence of the recti. It is not uncommon to see visible peristalsis within the sac of a very large ventral or inguinoscrotal hernia. In all these circumstances, the diagnosis can be made at inspection, and the patient is otherwise symptomless. In all other situations, visible peristalsis is pathological and may be of two types—gastric and intestinal.

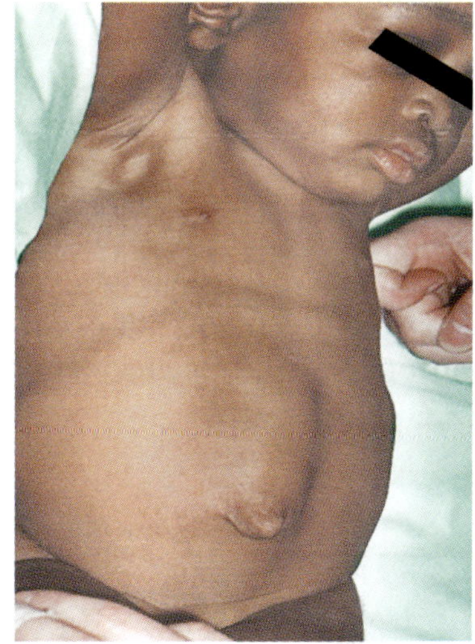

Fig. 1: Visible gastric peristalsis.

GASTRIC PERISTALSIS

Gastric peristalsis takes the form of a comparatively large swelling in the upper abdomen showing slow waves of peristalsis which progress from under the region of the left ribs, slowing downward and to the right **(Fig. 1)**. This swelling indicates obstruction to the gastric outlet. There may be other signs of gastric dilatation and distension, particularly a loud succussion splash. Typically, there is a history of the vomiting of large amounts of liquid in a projectile manner, and which may contain fragments of food ingested 24 hours or more previously. The diagnosis can be confirmed by the passage of a nasogastric tube, which will yield a pint or more of fluid several hours after the last food or drink has been taken. The aspirate has a typical stale, unpleasant smell, and may contain recognizable particles of food eaten even several days before. A barium X-ray examination will clinch the diagnosis by demonstrating the gastric retention and dilatation. An X-ray taken 6–8 hours after the ingestion of the barium is particularly valuable as this will confirm the extent of gastric holdup. In doubtful cases of visible gastric peristalsis, the signs may be accentuated by asking the patient to swallow several glasses of soda water. In the normal subjects, no peristalsis is seen, but in cases of pyloric obstruction, previously invisible peristalsis may now become obvious.

In congenital hypertrophic pyloric stenosis of infancy, not only can gastric peristalsis be seen after a drink from a bottle but the hypertrophied pylorus can often also be felt. This interesting and eminently treatable condition does not become apparent immediately, but some 4 weeks after birth.

VISIBLE INTESTINAL PERISTALSIS

Visible intestinal peristalsis is a feature of advanced intestinal obstruction, with the limitations discussed above. As a pathological entity, it will not occur alone, but is accompanied by colicky abdominal pain, abdominal distension, vomiting, and absolute constipation. The discussion of the differential diagnosis of the different causes of the symptoms will be found elsewhere. If the small intestine alone is involved, the waves are multiple and run more or less transversely across the abdomen—the ladder pattern. When the colon is obstructed, peristalsis takes the form of vertical waves, especially in one or both flanks, but this is much more rarely seen.

Plain radiographs of the abdomen taken in the erect and supine positions are invaluable; the first demonstrate multiple fluid levels, the second the distribution of gas shadows within the dilated loops of bowel which will often enable the clinician to determine whether small or large bowel is obstructed.

CHAPTER 308

Peritonsillar Abscess

A peritonsillar abscess occurs between the tonsil and constrictor muscle. It extends into the soft palate. They typically have a history of sore throat a week or two earlier. There is a sudden onset of high fever and severe throat pain. That is worse on one side. The pain usually radiates to the ipsilateral ear and marked dysphagia.

On examination, the child is toxic and has enlargement of the ipsilateral tender tonsillar lymph node. Many have torticollis. Speech is hoarse and muffled. Trismus or limitation of mouth opening is a result of inflammation of the internal pterygoid muscles. Pharynx is a bright red, smooth bulge is seen in the supratonsillar area projecting forward and medially, obscuring the tonsil, and deviating the uvula to the opposite side. Group A β-hemolytic streptococci and *S. aureus* are mixed infections with gram-positive and gram-negative aerobic, as well as anaerobic, pathogens are common. Treatment includes drainage of peritonsillar abscesses transorally in the office. If examination and cooperation are limited, the abscess may require incision and drainage in the operating room.

CHAPTER 309 Pes Planus (Flat Foot)

Pes planus: Normally where a child stands on a flat surface, the lateral border touches the floor, while the medial border touches the floor only in the region of forefoot and hind foot. This is because of the concavity produced by medial longitudinal arch. In children with pes planus, the surface of the foot is flat and, hence, touches the floor throughout.

ETIOLOGY

- *Mobile flat foot:* This is common in neonates and toddlers. It can persist till 6 years. This is due to laxity of bone-ligament complex that forms the arch and the presence of fat in the medial longitudinal arch.

  In older children, this is due to generalized ligamentous laxity (autosomal dominant trait).

  Children with flexible flat foot are usually asymptomatic.
- *Fixed flat foot:*
  - *Etiology*:
    - Tendo-Achilles contracture
    - Congenital vertical talus
    - Cerebral pals

Pes planus, or physiologic flatfoot, is an extremely common condition to which there is a familial predisposition. It is characterized by laxity of the soft tissues of the foot resulting in loss of the normal longitudinal arch, with pronation or eversion of the forefoot and valgus or lateral orientation of the heel. Secondary tightness of the Achilles tendon may exist. In general, the condition is asymptomatic in children, and evaluation is sought primarily because of parental concern about the appearance of the foot and the possibility of future problems. On occasion, affected patients report discomfort after long walks or running.

On examination, the characteristic appearance is easy to recognize, and laxity of other joints, particularly the thumb, elbow, and knee, may be noted. Weightbearing radiographs reveal loss of the normal longitudinal arch without osseous abnormality. Treatment is unnecessary if the condition is asymptomatic. Corrective shoes with arch supports are of no use unless symptoms of foot strain are present.

CHAPTER 310

Pigmentary Mosaicism

The term *pigmentary mosaicism* refers to a group of conditions in which affected children have genetic mosaicism (i.e., they are born with at least two genetically different cell lines, resulting in the existence of keratinocytes of two different pigment tones). When these different populations of skin cells migrate during development, they create a whorled, fountain-like pattern of alternating hypopigmentation and hyperpigmentation. This pattern is referred to as a *Blaschkoid distribution,* because it occurs along the "lines of Blaschko," which are lines of embryologic ectodermal development. They may be evident at birth and, if not, appear in infancy or early childhood. The bands are macular and are found most commonly over the trunk and respect the midline, but they can also be seen on the extremities, where they tend to be more linear. In contrast to the hyperpigmented macules of incontinentia pigmenti, those of pure pigmentary mosaicism have no antecedent vesicular or verrucous lesions and are not associated with atrophy.

Pigmentary mosaicism most often stems from a postzygotic mutation or an error in cell division early on in the course of embryogenesis, or may be the result of random X chromosome inactivation in X-linked conditions. The phenomenon has been reported in association with a number of different types of chromosomal mosaicism including trisomies 13, 18, and 20, among others. Affected individuals may be completely healthy or conversely can have associated abnormalities of the central nervous system (CNS), the musculoskeletal system, and/or the eye. Although the risk of associated anomalies has probably been overestimated because of reporting bias, children with more extensive cutaneous lesions may be at greater risk for extracutaneous involvement and should receive a careful medical and developmental examination and targeted studies where indicated clinically.

CHAPTER 311 Pinpoint Pupils

Pupils that are abnormally small under normal lighting conditions are called pinpoint pupils. The part of the eye that controls how much gets in. In bright light the pupil constricts:

- Pontine hemorrhage
- Organophosphorus poisoning
- Barbiturates
- Morphine
- Overdosage of neostigmine
- Iritis
- Apneic spell
- Syringomyelia
- Cavernous sinus thrombosis

CHAPTER 312

Pityriasis Alba

The rashes of pityriasis alba are common in patients with atopic dermatitis; inflammatory changes are minimal. Poorly defined, hypopigmented round or oval scaly patches measuring 2–4 cm in diameter are noted most commonly on the face and extremities. They may involve trunk. These patches fail to enhance with Wood lamp examination which distinguishes from vitiligo. Lesions are more prominent in children with dark skin and are more noticeable during spring and summer, because they do not tan like surrounding skin after sun exposure. Because the lesion is usually asymptomatic and spontaneously resolves in several months to few years, treatment is usually unnecessary. Moisturizers may help to reduce surface scaling.

CHAPTER

Pleural Rub

The diagnostic sign of pleurisy is a rub of a creaking superficial nature usually located close to the site of pain.

The pleura is a double serous membrane separating the lung from the chest wall and mediastinum. The pleural surface consists of a uniform layer of mesothelial cells supported on a connective tissue framework which is well supplied with capillary and lymph vessels. The parietal pleura is innervated with pain-sensitive nerve fibers supplied by the intercostal and phrenic nerves, and is exquisitely sensitive to painful stimuli.

In health, the visceral and parietal pleural surfaces are smooth, glistening, and separated by a small amount of fluid, allowing low friction movement of the lungs with respiration.

In contrast, if the pleural surfaces become thickened or roughened by inflammation or neoplastic infiltration, movement with breathing will cause increased friction, which may be heard a stethoscope. Patients commonly complain of thoracic pain on breathing or coughing. On auscultation, sounds of varying intensity may be heard during inspiration and expiration, often described as having a “leathery” or “creaking” quality that may be exaggerated when the stethoscope is applied firmly to the chest wall. Pain associated with a pleural rub may vary in degree from lancinating discomfort during slight inspiratory effort to a less sharp “catch” of pain at the end of maximum inspiration. Pleural pain is often reduced by breath-holding or by exerting firm pressure over the affected thoracic segment. Except when it involves the diaphragm, the affected pleura typically underlies the area in which pain is perceived. The central portion of the diaphragm is innervated from the third and fourth cervical posterior nerve roots running via the phrenic nerve. Pain caused by diaphragmatic pleural irritation is often referred to the neck and shoulders.

A pleural rub may last for as little as a few hours short-lived inflammatory conditions such as pneumonia, but to months or even years in patients with more chronic causes of pleurisy. Typically, as the pleurisy settles the pain and physical signs (including the rub) become less obvious, although in some patients, the rub may persist after the pain has gone and occasionally a loud rub may persist indefinitely.

CHAPTER 314

Polyarteritis Nodosa

Polyarteritis nodosa, the prototype medium-sized vessel vasculitis, is a systemic necrotizing vasculitis with segmental aneurysm formation leading to the classic "beading" of vessels pattern demonstrated in vascular imaging studies. Worldwide, polyarteritis nodosa is associated with hepatitis B and C infections; however, pediatric polyarteritis nodosa is quite rare. The average age of children affected is 9 years old, with a slight predominance in boys. There is an association with the periodic fever syndrome familial Mediterranean fever (FMF). Systemic polyarteritis nodosa can affect any organ system and can be quite devastating. Typical skin findings, which suggest a larger size vessel involvement, include palpable purpura, livedo reticularis, tender nodules, and necrotic lesions. Other findings suggestive of the disease include hypertension, abdominal pain, myalgia, arthritis, neuropathy, weight loss, and fever. Although suspected clinically, the diagnosis requires tissue biopsy, angiography, or magnetic resonance angiography of segmental aneurysms.

Cutaneous polyarteritis nodosa is limited to the skin and musculoskeletal system and is often noted in the setting of poststreptococcal infection. The lower extremities are most commonly affected, with arthritis of knees and ankles and associated skin changes in this distribution. Although this condition is much milder than the systemic form, chronic immunosuppressive agents are often required because of persistence of disease and relapse.

CHAPTER 315

Polydactyly

Polydactyly or duplication of digit can occur either as preaxial deformity (involving thumb) or as a postaxial deformity (involving the small finger). Each has a genetic and inherited component. Transmission is typically in an autosomal dominant pattern and has been linked to defects in genes localized to chromosome 2. The extra fingers are usually small and abnormally developed.

There are more than five fingers in the limbs. It can be congenital or familial. It is associated with Laurence-Moon-Biedl syndrome, Carpenter syndrome, Turner syndrome, and Trisomy 13 **(Figs. 1A and B)**.

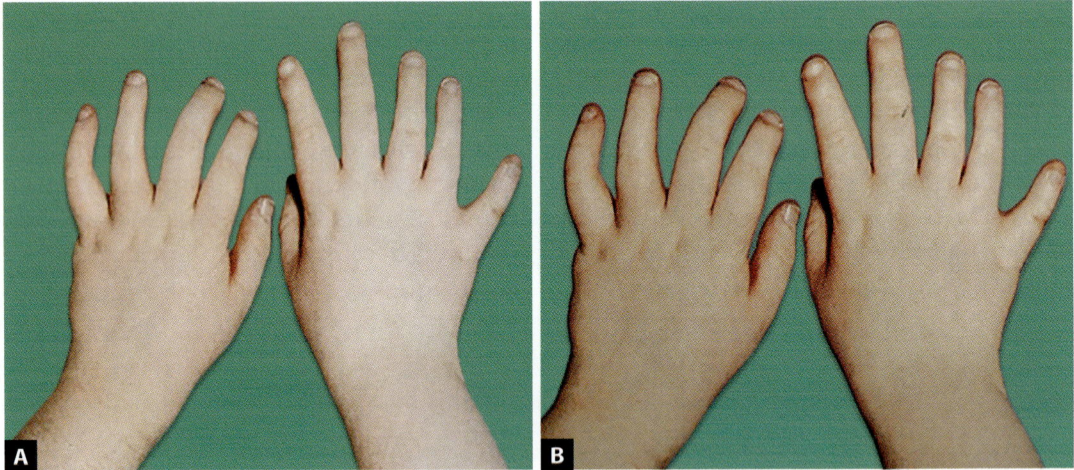

Figs. 1A and B: Polydactyly.

316 CHAPTER

Polydipsia

Polydipsia is defined as excessive or abnormal thirst. The primary stimulus to the sensation of thirst is dehydration, which gives rise to an increase in the plasma osmolality of the blood passing through the thirst center in the hypothalamus. An increase in plasma osmolality can also be achieved by increasing the solute load, e.g., by drinking salt water. The sensation of thirst must be distinguished from a dry mouth caused by Sjogren's syndrome, or mouth breathing or by drugs (in particular antidepressant and antipsychotic medications with pronounced antimuscarinic activity). Apparent thirst may also be due to a psychiatric disorder, when it is called "psychogenic polydipsia".

Polyuria

The term "polyuria" signifies a larger than normal daily volume of urine. There is considerable variation from subject to subject in the amount of urine passed, but a urinary output of >2–3 L per 24 hours is nearly always abnormal. Polyuria must not be confused with frequency of micturition due, e.g., to prostatic hypertrophy or cystitis. Also, although polyuria will almost always lead to a complaint on nocturia, many individuals complaining of the latter have no increase in the total output of urine but show a reversal of the normal diurnal variation in urine flow. This is the cause in most cases of sodium and water retention, as in cardiac failure or the nephrotic syndrome, in suprarenal disorders, and in chronic renal failure. Polyuria may be due either to an increased solute load with obligatory water loss or to a primary water diuresis, and will be discussed under these headings **(Box 1)**.

BOX 1: Causes of polyuria.

Due to increased solute load:
- Diabetes mellitus
- Diuretic therapy
- Chronic failure
- Following relief of obstruction
- During recovery from acute tubular necrosis
- Resolving hematoma

Due to water diuresis:
- Psychogenic polydipsia
- Cranial diabetes insipidus
- Nephrogenic diabetes insipidus:
  - X-linked
  - Potassium depletion
  - Hypercalcemia
  - Drugs
  - Sickle-cell anemia
  - Early chronic pyelonephritis

Other causes:
- Following fevers
- After attacks of migraine, etc.
- Paroxysmal tachycardia

POLYURIA DUE TO INCREASED SOLUTE LOAD

Any osmotically active solute will produce a diuresis if present in excess in the distal tubular fluid. For example, the massive protein breakdown occurring in a large hematoma may be associated with a diuresis, urea itself being the active solute. It is also the mechanism of diuretic therapy in which the solute concerned is sodium. Diabetes mellitus is the most common pathological condition in which this type of polyuria occurs. The daily urine volume is often 4 L or more, and polyuria and excessive thirst are the most common symptoms. In children who were previously dry at night, enuresis may be an early symptom of diabetes. The diagnosis is usually straightforward. In chronic renal failure, the total solute load may be normal, but the reduction in the number of nephrons results in a greater than normal load per nephron and consequent polyuria which is usually only of moderate severity. The polyuria which may follow the relief of chronic urinary tract obstruction is also partly due to this mechanism, but some defect of concentrating power may also be present. Diuresis is also common during recovery from acute tubular necrosis; this is partly due to the elimination of water and electrolytes retained during the phase of oliguria, and partly to incomplete recovery of tubular function.

POLYURIA DUE TO WATER DIURESIS

The simplest cause of this is an increased water intake, which may reach pathological dimensions in the condition known as psychogenic polydipsia or compulsive water-drinking. This is a hysterical manifestation and simulates diabetes insipidus. The differentiation is discussed below but, clinically marked fluctuations in urine output would strongly suggest psychogenic polydipsia. Patients with Sjogren's syndrome may try to relieve the dryness of their mouths by drinking large volumes of water, with a consequent modest polyuria.

The urine is normally concentrated in the distal tubules and collecting ducts. Antidiuretic hormone (ADH) is secreted by the posterior pituitary in response to a rise in plasma osmolality; its action is to increase the permeability of the tubular epithelium to water. The effect of this is to increase the transport of water from the tubular lumen into the hypertonic renal medulla through which these tubules pass. Thus, a pathological water diuresis may be due either to failure of secretion of ADH or to failure of the renal tubules to respond to its action.

Cranial (neurogenic) diabetes insipidus is often caused by an identifiable lesion of the hypothalamus or pituitary (or both), but in about one-third of cases, no such cause can be found. Tumors in that region are a common cause and include craniopharyngioma, pinealoma, glioma, and metastases from distant primary growths. Diabetes insipidus may also follow trauma to the skull (including operative), infections such as exanthemas in childhood, or infiltration with granulomatous lesions such as sarcoidosis histiocytosis X. In such cases, other evidence of hypothalamic pituitary disease may well be present.

Hypercalcemia also can cause a water diuresis, and might be suggested by associated abdominal pain and vomiting. Thus, polyuria may be a feature of primary, hyperparathyroidism, vitamin D intoxication, sarcoidosis, multiple bony metastases, or primary tumors secreting parathyroid hormone-related protein. The renal lesion is reversible unless severe nephrocalcinosis has developed or renal calculi have produced irreversible damage. As in hypokalemia, there is response to ADH. A reversible nephrogenic diabetes insipidus can also be produced by a number of drugs including lithium carbonate, demeclocycline, amphotericin B, glibenclamide, and gentamicin.

Other conditions in which failure of urinary concentration occurs are sickle-cell anemia and chronic pyelonephritis at an early stage. The polyuria due the latter must not be confused with the osmotic diuresis of chronic renal failure discussed above.

TRANSIENT POLYURIA

Polyuria lasting for only a few hours can occur in various circumstances. It is rarely of any great significance, and indeed is often physiological. The diuresis which follows excessive water drinking needs no comment. The same applies to polyuria in the course of diuretic therapy, although the diuretic effect of such substances as tea or coffee may occasionally provoke a complaint from a patient who has not realized the association. Cold weather may also induce polyuria as a result of reduced fluid loss from the skin; travelers returning from a long stay in the tropics and accustomed to a large fluid intake may occasionally complain of polyuria on return to a colder country. It is this contrast with previous oliguria that partly explains the polyuria following fevers; there may also be a temporary impairment of ADH secretion.

Polyuria can also occur following various stressful situations, and has been described after attacks of migraine, asthma, and angina. A more striking polyuria may occur during and after attacks of paroxysmal tachycardia. Any arrhythmia—either supraventricular or ventricular—which lasts for more than half an hour may produce this effect. This is probably due the release of atrial natriuretic peptide.

CHAPTER 318

Popliteal (Baker) Cyst

Popliteal cyst (Morrant Baker's cyst): It is a herniation of the synovial membrane posteriorly through the fibers of the oblique popliteal ligament to form a swelling in the middle of the posterior aspect of the knee. The swelling becomes prominent on extension and disappears on flexion. The condition is often associated with tuberculosis/ osteoarthritis of the joint.

Popliteal cysts occurring in childhood are encountered most commonly in children between 5 and 10 years old and occur significantly more frequently in boys than in girls. They are located in the posteromedial aspect of the knee joint in the region of the semimembranosus tendon and medial gastrocnemius muscle belly. Pathologically, a fibrous tissue or synovial cyst filled with synovial-like fluid is seen. In contrast to those seen in adults, popliteal cysts in childhood generally do not communicate with the joint capsule but originate instead beneath the semimembranosus tendon, presumably as a result of chronic irritation. On occasion, vague pain is noted, but evaluation is usually sought because of a recently noted painless mass.

On examination, a soft, nontender, cystic mass is found in the described location. Range of motion of the joint is normal unless the cyst is particularly large, limiting flexion. The knee is otherwise normal, and radiographs show no osseous abnormality. An MRI clearly delineates the cyst and its position in relation to nearby structures. Popliteal cysts are benign and may resolve over time, although surgical excision is reasonable if desired.

CHAPTER 319

Posterior Urethral Valve

The most common obstructive lesion of the lower urinary tract in male infants is posterior urethral valve. Such folds traverse the urethra from a point just distal to the verumontanum to the proximal limit of the membranous urethra, and obstruct urinary flow with consequent enlargement of the prostatic urethra, hypertrophy of the bladder neck, trabeculation of the bladder, and significant dilation of the upper urinary tract. Infants with posterior urethral valves may experience renal failure and profound electrolyte imbalance. Older children may have abdominal masses, voiding disturbances, or urinary tract infection (UTI). Diagnosis is made radiologically by voiding cystourethrogram (VCUG) and confirmed endoscopically. Although urinary diversion may be required, many children can be treated directly by transurethral valve ablation. Surgery is usually successful in achieving urinary drainage, but in many cases, associated renal dysplasia may lead to chronic kidney disease (CKD) during infancy or childhood.

Post-tussive Crepitus

These crepitations are audible after making the patient to cough as they are not audible during normal respiration. It indicates the cavity filled with thick material which gets dislodged after coughing. Hence, this allows the air bubble through the remaining fluid producing the crepitations. It is present in early pneumonia, early tuberculosis, and lung abscess. Post-tussive auscultation refers to hissing sound caused due to air entering the cavity (during inspiration) which has collapsed due to forceful expiration during coughing.

321 CHAPTER

Precocious Puberty

Before puberty, blood levels of luteinizing hormone (LH) and follicle-stimulating hormone (FSH) are low and are poorly responsive to administered gonadotropin-releasing hormone. At the time of puberty, gonadotropin secretion begins to increase and gonadal stimulation occurs, with a consequent rise of testosterone in boys and of estradiol in girls. In both sexes, puberty is preceded by an increase in the production of the suprarenal of the suprarenal androgens dehydroepiandrosterone and androstenedione.

In 95% of girls, the first sign of puberty, which is either breast but or pubic hair development, appears between the ages of 8.5 and 13 years. Puberty is precocious if these two events occurs before the age of 8 years in a girl. Menarche occurs in 95% of girls between the ages of 11 and 13 years.

In 95% of boys, the testes begin to enlarge between the age of 9.5 and 13.5 years (mean 11.6 years), and reach adult size between the ages of 13 and 17 (mean 14.9 years). Pubic hair growth develops after testicular enlargement has begun, so it is rare before the age of 9.5 years. Testicular growth is stimulated by the action of FSH on germinal epithelium and of LH on Leydig cells. The testosterone produced by the Leydig cells is responsible for the growth of the pains. Puberty is precocious in a boy, if any of the above-mentioned change takes place before the 9th birthday.

Precocious puberty can be either a true puberty or a false pseudopuberty. In true puberty, the changes proceed in the normal physiological manner, albeit at an early age. In false puberty, on the other hand, changes such as secondary sexual growth and enlargement of the phallus occur because of abnormal androgen production, and gonadal function is in fact inhibited. A rare intermediate variety may be produced by nonpituitary, gonadotropin-secreting tumors.

CAUSES OF PUBERTY (BOX 1)

Constitutional Precocious Puberty

This is the most common cause of precocious puberty, especially in girls, where it accounts for 80% of cases. Early puberty in boys is five times less common than in girls, and in boys a pathological cause (especially neurological) is found in 50%. A family history of precocious puberty may be found, though the majority of cases are sporadic. Ovarian cysts may be detected in girls on ultrasound examination. They should not be confused with granulose cell tumors.

Other variants of premature puberty may be present. Premature adrenarche is characterized by the early growth of pubic hair and a slightly advanced bone age. There are no other signs of premature sexual development, and full puberty develops at the normal age. Premature thelarche refers to the early development of breast tissue, often

BOX 1: Causes of puberty.

True (LHRH-dependent):
- Constitutional
- *Cerebral:*
  - Trauma
  - Cranial irradiation
  - Granulomata
  - Brain abscess
  - Hypothyroidism
  - Hydrocephalus
- *Encephalitis:*
  - Meningitis
  - Tuberous sclerosis
  - Neurofibromatosis
  - Cerebral tumor
  - Pineal tumor
  - Craniopharyngioma
  - Hamartoma
  - McCune–Albright syndrome (polyostotic fibrous dysplasia with cutaneous pigmentation)
  - Russell–Silver syndrome

False (LHRH-independent):
- *Gonadotropin-producing tumors*:
  - Hepatoma
  - Hepatoblastoma
  - Teratoma
  - Chorionepithelioma
- *Suprarenal*:
  - Congenital adrenal hyperplasia
  - Tumors
  - Cushing's syndrome
- *Testicular*:
  - Leydig cell tumor
  - Leydig cell hyperplasia
- *Ovarian*:
  - Granulose cell tumor
  - Androblastoma
  - Lipoid cell tumor
  - Chorionepithelioma
  - Benign ovarian cyst
- *Drugs*:
  - Androgens
  - Androgens
  - Estrogens

(LHRH: luteinizing hormone-releasing hormone)

in the second year of life. It usually regresses spontaneously within 2 years but may lead on to a full early puberty.

Normal Variants

Idiopathic Isolated Premature Thelarche

This common condition is the development of breast tissue in females before 8 years of age with no other manifestations of puberty. Elevated serum estrogen levels for age have been difficult to demonstrate, although higher levels than in age-matched normal females have been measured by an ultrasensitive estradiol assay. Development of breast tissue commonly begins between 2 and 3 years of age; it may be present from birth. The observed tissue may be asymmetric, unilateral, or bilateral. When asymmetric or unilateral, parents are typically concerned about the possibility of malignancy, an extremely rare occurrence in childhood. The early breast tissue frequently regresses without intervention, but it may persist. If it persists, the degree of development does not usually exceed Tanner stage 3. The bone age, if determined, is not frequently advanced, and there is no associated growth spurt. If these simple clinical criteria are met, no hormonal studies or additional radiologic procedures are necessary. Physiologic breast enlargement also occurs in neonates from placental transfer of estrogens. Most marked in the 1st weeks of life, it usually regresses by 1–2 months.

Idiopathic Isolated Precocious Adrenarche

This common, normal variant is characterized by the development of pubic hair, axillary hair and odor, and/or a small amount of acne in white females before the age of 8 years and in males before the age of 9 years. It appears to result from early production of adrenal androgens. There is no associated evidence of virilization (no growth spurt, no significant advancement of bone age, no increase in muscle bulk, no voice deepening, and no temporal hair recession). In females, there is no associated clitoromegaly and no evidence of estrogen-mediated components of puberty; in males, there is no phallic or testicular enlargement. If a child presents at a very young age, it is generally presumed that an organic cause (such as congenital adrenal hyperplasia) will be found. However, in infant males with isolated scrotal hair, typically no cause is found, and the hair subsequently falls out. In most cases of idiopathic precocious adrenarche (benign premature adrenarche), serum levels of DHEA and/or DHEAS are consistent with the reference range of Tanner staging of the hair growth, and the 8:00 AM 17-hydroxyprogesterone level is normal. If these criteria are met, no additional laboratory studies are indicated. This pubertal variant was considered benign and self-limited, but data suggest that at least in females with associated low birth weight, it may suggest an increased risk for polycystic ovary disease.

Isosexual Central Precocious Puberty

Central sexual precocity results from activation of the hypothalamic–pituitary–gonadal axis at an earlier-than-normal. Isosexual development refers to pubertal changes appropriate for the sex of the child, such as breast budding in females and testicular enlargement in males. This is to be distinguished from contrasexual development, in which the pubertal features in females are mediated by male hormones (clitoromegaly) and those in males are mediated by female hormones (breast development).

In true male central puberty, testes enlarge and androgen production increases. The size of testes enlargement sufficient to determine puberty is debatable. In general, prepubertal testes are <4 cm^3 in volume and 2 cm in length. If, on examination, both testes are enlarged and androgen signs are present, it is likely puberty is underway and testes-derived testosterone levels are increasing. If basal pituitary gonadotropins are increasing, or if LH levels increase markedly after GnRH stimulation, the diagnosis is central precocious puberty.

The important implication for a child who enters early puberty is that, because bone maturation is advanced, final adult stature may be below that predicated for an offspring of that family.

Incomplete Isosexual Precocity (Precocious Pseudopuberty)

Precocious pseudopuberty refers to gonadal or adrenal sex-steroid secretion *not* resulting from activation of the hypothalamic–pituitary–gonadal axis (pituitary-independent). It is caused by excessive production of or exposure to either androgens or estrogens.

Cerebral

Hypothyroidism is included under cerebral causes of precocious puberty because it seems likely that the mechanism is via the stimulation by thyrotrophin-releasing hormone (TRH) of gonadotrophins in addition to TSH and prolactin.

A wide variety of other cerebral conditions can give rise to precocious puberty, if the area posterior to the median eminence, including the mamillary bodies and the posterior part of the floor of the IIIrd ventricle, is involved.

The McCune–Albright syndrome is only tentatively included under cerebral causes of precocious puberty because it has been postulated that there may be inappropriate secretion of hypothalamic releasing hormones in this condition. The syndrome is rare and is much more common in girls than in boys. Precocious puberty is usual, but other endocrine abnormalities such as thyrotoxicosis, hyperparathyroidism, and Cushing's syndrome may occur. One of the characteristic features is polyostotic fibrous dysplasia, which may be unilateral. There are pigmented areas on the skin roughly corresponding to the underlying bony lesions.

Patients with the Russell–Silver syndrome may develop early puberty. The cause is unknown.

True precocious puberty can develop in children who are adopted from underdeveloped countries. This is thought to be secondary to correction of malnutrition generally after 3 years of age. The correction of a virilizing condition can be followed by true precocious puberty due to activation of the hypothalamic–pituitary–gonadotropin–gonadal axis. This occurs in boys and girls with congenital adrenal hyperplasia who have received treatment with glucocorticoids after the ages of 4–8 years.

Gonadotropin-producing tumors are exceedingly rare, and produce testicular enlargement in boys and vaginal bleeding in girls as the first sign. They are usually malignant.

Suprarenal Causes of False Puberty

Adrenal tumors can be detected with ultrasonography, computed tomography, or MRI. Androgens produced by adrenal tumors are not suppressed by dexamethasone. Excessive adrenal androgens may also be produced as a result of late-onset or nonclassic congenital adrenal hyperplasia, but the androgen production can be suppressed by dexamethasone. The enzymatic deficiency in late-onset congenital adrenal hyperplasia is mild, in as much as it does not cause ambiguity of genitalia at birth; however, it is associated with an accelerated growth rate and advanced bone age and may be clinically recognized any time after birth.

The secretion of excess androgens by the suprarenal causes false puberty. The growth of secondary sexual hair is stimulated and the phallus enlarges. Gonadotropins, however, are suppressed so the testes remain small in a boy, and periods do not develop in a girl. Suprarenal tumors and Cushing's syndrome can be distinguished from congenital adrenal hyperplasia by the presence of raised plasma 17-hydroxyprogesterone and urinary excretion of pregnanetriol in the latter when it is due to a 21-hydroxylase defect, and by normal suppressibility of urinary 17-oxosteroids.

Testicular Causes of False Puberty

If both testes are slightly increased in volume and testosterone levels are increased but LH and FSH levels are low, there are two possibilities: Either the testes are being stimulated by human chorionic gonadotropin (hCG), which acts like LH and does not increase testicular volume, as with FSH, or the testes are functioning autonomously. hCG levels must be determined, and if they are increased, tumors producing hCG must be identified and removed; such tumors may include hepatoma, hepatoblastoma, teratoma, and chorionepithelioma.

Testosterone production and Leydig cell hyperplasia occur in the setting of prepubertal serum LH levels, because of a gain-of-function mutation in the gene for the LH receptor, resulting in its constitutive activation. Affected males are fertile. Females who carry this mutation do not develop precocious puberty.

If one testis is enlarged, a Leydig cell adenoma in that testicle is probably producing excess testosterone; the tumor must be removed. The high levels of testosterone suppress LH and FSH secretion, so the other testicle remains small. Depending on age, a testicular prosthesis may be inserted to replace the removed testicle.

Testicular Leydig cell tumors causing false puberty are exceedingly rare. Occasional cases of Leydig cell hyperplasia have been described. The tumors are usually palpable, but occasionally may be small. However, a useful clue to the presence of a testicular tumor is that the contralateral testis is even smaller because gonadotropins are suppressed. In most cases, the condition is fully established by the age of 6 years.

Precocity is marked: The physique is muscular, body hair growth is considerable, the voice is strikingly gruff and manly, and the penis and prostate are enlarged. In half the cases, there may be grossly overt psychosexual behavior. Because the tumor is secreting testosterone, high levels of 17-oxosteroids are not always found in the urine, but raised plasma testosterone is diagnostic.

Ovarian Causes of False Puberty

Ovarian tumors producing androgens (thecoma) and sometimes also estrogen may be palpable on physical examination and are usually easily seen on a pelvic sonogram. Arrhenoblastoma, a virilizing ovarian tumor, is rare in children. Gonadoblastomas, which are not always virilizing, typically occur in phenotypic females who have a Y chromosome. Granulosa cell tumors usually cause estrogen overproduction but occasionally cause virilization due to excessive androgen production.

Ovarian tumors account for only a few percent of cases of precocious puberty in girls. They usually present at about the age of 4 years with irregular vaginal bleeding, breast development, and pubic and axillary hair growth. There may be abdominal pain and the tumor may be palpable. The usual type of tumor producing endocrine effects is a granulosa cell tumor. This is usually benign, but about one-fifth are malignant.

Androgen-producing tumors of the ovary (androblastomas) cause heterosexual precocious puberty with the development of secondary sexual hair, hirsutism, and virilization.

Estrogen Overproduction

The most common cause of premature progressive breast development is simple premature thelarche. Granulosa cell tumors are usually isolated occurrences but may occur as part of Peutz–Jeghers syndrome (oral melanosis and intestinal polyps). Aromatase is the enzyme that is responsible for conversion of androgen to estrogen; aromatase excess is an autosomal dominant disorder that can lead to increased estradiol levels.

McCune–Albright syndrome: This disorder consists of the clinical triad of polyostotic fibrous dysplasia, hyperpigmented macules (café-au-lait spots) with irregular borders ("coast of Maine"), and multiple autonomous endocrinopathies (most commonly gonadotropin-independent precocious puberty, but also hyperthyroidism, acromegaly, and hypercortisolemia). Precocious puberty occurs much more commonly in females than in males. Precocity in females, often heralded by menstrual bleeding, frequently occurs before 2 years of age. The ovaries are enlarged and have many follicular cysts; the patient has elevated levels of estradiol. Later, when the GnRH pulse generator is activated subsequent to unabated sex steroid exposure, the patient may transition from gonadotropin-independent to central precocious puberty.

Drugs

The accidental or deliberate ingestion of estrogens (commonly mother's contraceptive pills) by girls may lead to vaginal withdrawal bleeding and to some breast development. Androgens and anabolic steroids may cause secondary sexual hair growth and phallic enlargement.

Prehn Sign

This is seen in intravaginal torsion of the spermatic cord. It can occur at any age. Most patients have acute, painful swelling of the scrotum, lower abdominal pain, nausea, and vomiting. On occasion, torsion has much more insidious onset as a dull scrotal pain of subacute nature. Examination may vary depending on the time of acute episode. Scrotum gradually becomes red and swollen, with the testis elevated because of foreshortening of the spermatic cord.

The testis may have an abnormal orientation, with epididymis located in an abnormal position due to torsion of cord. The cremasteric reflex is usually absent, and elevating the testis to pubic symphysis increase pain—negative Prehn sign.

When the inflammation has progressed, the scrotum becomes a firm, homogenous mass. Color Doppler ultrasound may be helpful. When scrotum contains an inflammatory process, blood flow is increased on the involved side, whereas in the presence of an acute torsion, blood flow is diminished. Urgent surgical intervention is warranted.

CHAPTER 323 Premature Pubarche

The development of pubic hair before 8 years old in girls and 9½ years old in boys is considered to be premature. Associated findings may include axillary hair, adult-type body odor, and acne. Diagnostic considerations include premature adrenarche due to premature adrenal pubertal maturation or late-onset congenital adrenal hyperplasia (CAH). Androgen-secreting adrenal or gonadal tumors are extremely rare.

Although advanced skeletal maturation is more common in CAH, adrenocorticotropic hormone (ACTH) stimulation tests are often necessary to distinguish late-onset CAH from premature adrenarche. To diagnose late-onset CAH, the ACTH-stimulated 17-hydroxyprogesterone (17-OHP) value is typically >1,500 ng/dL. In children with premature adrenarche, adrenal steroid hormone concentrations may be elevated for chronologic age but are normal for the degree of pubic hair development. For some girls, premature adrenarche heralds subsequent development of polycystic ovary syndrome (PCOS) in adolescence.

CHAPTER 324

Premature Thelarche

Premature thelarche is a transient and self-limited condition defined by the early onset of isolated breast development. Typically, premature thelarche develops during the first or second year of life without any other signs of puberty. The breast tissue may appear unilaterally or bilaterally and may regress or persist. Other features of pubertal development, including growth acceleration and pubic hair development, are absent. Hence, premature thelarche is a diagnosis of exclusion and cannot be made in the presence or progression of other pubertal signs. The ingestion of exogenous estrogens, such as oral contraceptives, should always be suspected in cases of breast enlargement. One should query regarding exposure to environment factors, such as lavender and tea tree oils.

Premature thelarche must be differentiated from other forms of progressive precocious puberty. Breast enlargement secondary to maternal hormones may occur in either sex in the immediate neonatal period. The etiology of premature thelarche is unclear; in some instances, activating mutations of the *GNAS1* gene encoding the alpha subunit of the GS protein have been described in the absence of other elements of McCune–Albright syndrome.

325 CHAPTER

Premenstrual Syndrome

Premenstrual syndrome (PMS) can be defined as cyclical recurrence of psychological, behavioral, and physical symptoms during the luteal phase of the menstrual cycle. This is essentially the 2 weeks prior to menstruation, and the symptoms resolve by themselves, or should be free of symptoms between the end of menstruation and ovulation. Psychological and somatic disturbances are part of the normal physiology of the menstrual cycle, but when exaggerated they may lead to sever psychological disturbance and behavioral abnormalities. The symptoms include bloating, cramping, pain and tenderness in the breast, temporary gain in weight, and some swelling of the hands and feet. They also include emotional tension, bad-temper, nervousness, irritability and headache, lack of concentration, depression, and insomnia, sufficient to interfere with the normal enjoyment of life. The majority of women (95%) will have some symptoms, only a small precent age (5%) is totally symptom-free. In a small group of women (5%), the symptoms of PMS have a major impact on their lives and have led to suicide, acts of aggression, and even cited as defense in murder trials.

The etiology remains obscure, and consequently presents therapeutic difficulties when dealing with this problem. The underlying cause may be a combination of imbalances/abnormalities of the ovarian steroid production and central nervous transmitters. It has been shown that women with PMS have lowered levels of whole blood serotonin concentrations and platelet serotonin. Several serotonin reuptake inhibitors (SSRIs) have now been shown to improve PMS symptoms. Elimination of the cyclical ovarian function results in the complete suppression of symptoms. Despite cyclical ovarian steroid function being the trigger for PMS, there is no definitive test to distinguish it from other disorders. The nature of the symptoms is less important than the timing, and keeping a diary of symptoms may be useful to distinguish primary PMS from secondary. The latter are a group of patients who have true PMS with underlying psychopathology.

Treatment depends on the severity of symptoms, and may range from a mixture of counseling, education, and reassurance in patients with mild problems. Essential fatty acids and pyridoxine have been used in the past. SSRIs may be used to good effect in moderate cases. In more severe cases, ovulation suppression can be used, and this can start with continuous combined oral contraceptive (OCP) usage, provided that there is no contraindication to OCP use, or continuous progestogens. Danazol and GnRH analogs can be used. If these treatments are successful, then total abdominal hysterectomy and bilateral salpingo-oophorectomy may be indicted. But these patients would need subsequent HRT in the form of continuous estrogen only.

CHAPTER 326 Priapism

Priapism is a persistent, painful erection in which the corporal bodies are firmly erect but the glans is soft. The shaft and preputial skin may become edematous, and the pain of priapism is usually severe. Priapism in children is usually related to an underlying disease state as opposed to the more common idiopathic variety seen in adults.

"Priapism" signifies erection of the penis, which is persistent, of trouble some degree, and not necessarily accompanied by sexual desire. Though generally spoken of in connection with the male sex, a precisely similar affection may occur in the female clitoris. The symptom is not often by itself of diagnostic importance. Although it may be due to a considerable number of different condition, the ultimate cause is usually thrombosis in the vascular space of the cavernous tissue, which are found to contain thick grumous blood.

The important causes are:

- After injury to the upper dorsal region of the spinal cord. The damage may have produced fracture dislocation of the spine with paraplegia, in which cases the diagnosis will be obvious. A minor degree of injury, with contusion and small hemorrhages into the substance of the cord, may be followed by painful priapism, persisting sometimes for weeks before recovery occurs. Cerebrospinal syphilis or tumor may also rarely be responsible.
- In leukemia, apart from obvious in the penis (e.g., cavernous hemorrhage), priapism has been noted in both myelocytic leukemia even before the other symptoms and signs have led to a hematological diagnosis. The cause of the priapism in leukemia is obscure, but the diagnosis is suggested by the concomitant splenomegaly and/or lymphadenopathy, and is confirmed by the hematological findings.
- Sickle-cell anemia
- New growths of the urethra, either primary or secondary to carcinoma of the bladder or testis
- Trauma with hematoma formation

Chronic intermittent priapism is the term used to describe frequently repeated erections which are of long duration but lack the persistence of true priapism. The attacks occur in the night, and may or may not be associated with sexual desire. They are due to nerve irritation arising lesions of the central nervous system or from local lesions in the posterior urethra, prostate, or seminal vesicles. In elderly men, they are frequently associated with enlargement of the prostate. Seldom will priapism be the only symptom in that case; the diagnosis will be made from the history and from the other symptoms and signs.

It is most frequently associated with sickle cell disease but may be seen in relation to pelvic malignancy, leukemia, blunt perineal trauma, or secondary to acute spinal cord injury. Sickle cell-related priapism should initially be treated as a sickle cell crisis, with oxygenation, exchange transfusion, and systemic alkalinization. Surgical therapy may be necessary to irrigate the corpora cavernosa or perform a cavernosal–spongiosal shunt or vascular bypass.

CHAPTER 327

Primitive Reflexes

ASYMMETRIC TONIC NECK RESPONSE

Assess for the asymmetric tonic neck response by turning the baby's head from midline to one side and noting the arm's gradual extension on the side to which the head is turned, along with flexion of the other arm. The position resembles the classic fencing or boxing posture.

Because of this reflex, it is important to ensure that the baby's head is midline before you elicit any of the other responses.

MORO REFLEX

Newborns often demonstrate the Moro, startle, or embrace reflex spontaneously when they are suddenly moved, exposed to a sudden loud noise, given the feeling of falling, or feel unstable on a flat surface. You can most reliably elicit this reflex by allowing the infant's head to drop (while supporting it gently) below the level of the rest of the body while the baby is in a reclining position. The baby extends the arms suddenly and rapidly with the hands open, then brings them back together more slowly in a movement that looks like an embrace. The initial rapid movement may be accompanied by a grimace or cry. Symmetry of movement is important. Weakness of one arm (e.g., in an infant with brachial plexus injury) results in an asymmetric Moro reflex.

Normal:

- *28 weeks:* Only opening hands
- *32 weeks:* Opening hands, extreme abduction, followed by anterior flexion, adduction
- *Less prominent:*
  - Asphyxia
  - Meningitis
  - Septicemia
  - Anesthesia and narcotic effects
  - Kernicterus
  - Hypotonia
  - Hypertonia
- *Asymmetrical:*
  - Erb's palsy
  - Fracture clavicle
  - Humerus
  - Hemiplegia

It disappears by 3–4 months or persists >6 months in spastic CP and other conditions with brain damage.

The Moro reflex evaluates vestibular maturation and the relationship between flexor and extensor tone. Elicitation of the reflex involves a short (10 cm), sudden drop of the head when the infant is supine. The full response involves extension of the arms, "fanning" of the fingers, and then upper extremity flexion followed by a cry. An incomplete but identifiable reflex becomes apparent at approximately 32 weeks' gestation, and by 38 weeks, it is essentially complete. Very immature infants demonstrate extension of the arms and fingers but do not show true flexion or make a sustained cry. Marked asymmetry of response may be associated with focal neurologic impairment.

ROOTING REFLEX

The rooting reflex may be elicited by lightly stimulating the infant's cheek and observing the reflexive attempts to bring the stimulating object to the mouth. The sucking reflex is activated by placing an object in the infant's mouth and observing the sucking movements. In the grasp reflex, transverse stimulation of the midpalm (without touching the back of the hand) or midsole leads to flexion of the digits or toes around the examiner's fingers.

GALANT'S INFANTILE REFLEX

Galant's infantile reflex is a truncal incurvation reflex. It can be elicited by holding the infant in ventral suspension and stroking from shoulder to hip along one side of the spine. The infant will contract the abdominal musculature and laterally flex toward the stimulated side. Lack of the Galant reflex may indicate a spinal cord lesion.

ASYMMETRIC TONIC NECK RESPONSE

Asymmetric tonic neck response is assessed by turning the baby's head from midline to one side and noting the arm's gradual extension on the side to which the head is turned, along with flexion of the other arm. The position resembles the classic fencing or boxing posture. Because of this reflex, it is important to ensure that the baby's head is midline before you elicit any of the other responses.

PALMAR GRASP

The palmar grasp is found by placing your index fingers in each of the baby's open hands; the baby's fingers should close around your fingers with strength enough to lift the baby's body part of the way off the bed or table.

PLACING AND PROPULSIVE (STEPPING AND WALKING) REFLEXES

The baby is held upright. The dorsum of the feet is touched to the bed or a table, and it will seem as if the baby is trying to walk. Parents are invariably fascinated and delighted by the demonstration that their newborn baby can "walk".

If there is any doubt about the integrity of the baby's CNS, either because of the history (difficult labor, delivery, traumatic procedures, or birth asphyxia) or because of associated physical findings, such as an abnormal cry, major deformities, or malformations, a more complete neurologic examination should be conducted.

CHAPTER 328

Proteinuria

Though 24-hour urine collection is the gold standard to quantify the proteinuria, spot urine protein-to-creatinine ratio can be used for initial confirmation after a positive screen with dipstick or to trend proteinuria. In timed collection, protein excretion >100 mg/m^2 in 24 hours or 4 mg/m^2/hour is considered abnormal, and over 40 mg/m^2/hour is considered nephrotic range. The common causes of proteinuria are mentioned in **Box 1**.

BOX 1: Causes of proteinuria.

Transient proteinuria:
- Fever
- Exercise
- Dehydration
- Cold exposure
- Congestive heart failure
- Seizure
- Stress

Orthostatic (postural) proteinuria:

Glomerular diseases characterized by isolated proteinuria:
- Idiopathic (minimal change) nephrotic syndrome
- Focal segmental glomerulosclerosis
- Mesangial proliferative glomerulonephritis
- Membranous nephropathy
- Membranoproliferative glomerulonephritis
- Amyloidosis
- Diabetic nephropathy
- Sickle cell nephropathy

Glomerular diseases with proteinuria as a prominent feature:
- Acute postinfectious glomerulonephritis (e.g., streptococcal, endocarditis, hepatitis B or C virus, and HIV)
- Immunoglobulin A nephropathy
- Henoch–Schonlein purpura nephritis
- Lupus nephritis
- Serum sickness
- Alport syndrome
- Vasculitic disorders
- Reflux nephropathy

Tubular diseases:
- Cystinosis
- Wilson disease
- Lowe syndrome
- Dent disease (X-linked recessive nephrolithiasis)
- Galactosemia
- Tubulointerstitial nephritis
- Acute tubular necrosis
- Renal dysplasia
- Polycystic kidney disease
- Reflux nephropathy
- Drugs (e.g., penicillamine, lithium, and NSAID)
- Heavy metals (e.g., lead, gold, and mercury)

(NSAID: nonsteroidal anti-inflammatory drug)

MINIMAL CHANGE DISEASE

Most cases of nephrotic syndrome in children are caused by minimal change nephrotic syndrome, defined as normal histologic features of the kidney by light microscopy and immune stains. Preschool-aged children constitute the age group in which minimal change nephritic syndrome is most common. Patients often present with asymptomatic edema, which may manifest as swollen or puffy eyes upon awakening in the morning; increasing abdominal girth (increased waist or belt size) from ascites; pedal or leg edema, which causes difficulty in putting on their regular-sized shoes, especially after being upright during the daytime; or swelling in other sites, such as the scrotum, penis, vulva, and scalp. Tense edema or ascites is occasionally painful.

Urinary protein is typically composed of plasma (57%) and histones or tissue proteins (43%). Albumin excretion is by far the most abundant component of proteinuria associated with renal disorders, but the proportion of albumin to low molecular weight (LMW) proteins, such as β-2 microglobulin, is lower in tubulointerstitial than in glomerular disorders. LMW proteins are freely filtered in the glomerulus. Because of very efficient protein binding and endocytosis mediated by unique receptors on megalin and cubilin in proximal tubular cells, healthy individuals have minimal proteinuria.

Isolated proteinuria refers to proteinuria above the normal limits but <1,500 mg/1.73 m^2/day and absence of concurrent systemic illness, hypertension (HTN), hematuria, pyuria, cellular casts or bacteriuria, renal dysfunction, or abnormal renal imaging studies. Such findings usually denote a transient or reversible disorder (such as fever, heart failure, or pancreatitis) or a common benign disorder particularly in tall active children known as *orthostatic proteinuria.* The latter condition is highly suggested by the absence of protein on dipstick of the first morning voided urine specimen, and 1–3+ protein on testing of an afternoon urine specimen. It can then be confirmed by a split 24-hour urine collection showing normal protein excretion during the overnight supine collection and abnormal excretion during the daytime upright collection. This clear distinction permits forgoing biochemical, immunologic, imaging, and renal biopsy evaluation, which may be needed to exclude other potentially serious renal disorders leading to proteinuria.

CHAPTER 329

Prune–Belly Syndrome

Prune–Belly syndrome usually consists of the absence of abdominal musculature, renal and urinary tract abnormalities, and cryptorchidism. Lack of abdominal muscle causes skin on the abdominal area to wrinkle and appear "prune-like". Boys are affected more severely and 20 times more frequently than girls. Although there is generally no ureteral obstruction, the ureters are dilated and tortuous, and 75% exhibit reflux. The bladder is enlarged despite low renal pelvic and intravesical pressures. Urinary tract infection (UTI) is common because of urinary stasis.

The major determinant of prognosis in these patients is the degree of associated cystic renal dysplasia. Intestinal malrotation is a common associated abnormality; anomalies of the limbs and heart may occur, but these are uncommon. Early orchiopexy may improve the chances for fertility and prevent testicular neoplasia.

CHAPTER 330

Pruritus Ani

Infestation with threadworms (*Enterobius vermicularis* or *Oxyuris vermicularis*) will cause pruritus ani or anal itching. The worms migrate at and around anal region at night and produces itching. Child scratches and results in autoinfection. The parasite is white, about 6 mm long, and the thickness of cotton thread. The parasites may be noted at the anal verge. Continued scratching of the anal region by the patient; irritation of the perianal skin by fecal contamination even when no gross soiling is evident; or of psychogenic cause.

Pseudohypertrophy

This is in Duchenne muscular dystrophy. Enlargement of the muscles, particularly in the calves, is a common feature by 5 or 6 years old. The abnormally enlarged muscles have an unusually firm, rubbery consistency on palpation. Early in the clinical course, this increase in muscle volume may result from true hypertrophy, with muscle strength proportional to bulk. Later, infiltration by fat and connective tissue sometimes maintains this bulk despite loss of muscle fibers. This is called as pseudohypertrophy.

CHAPTER 332

Pseudotumor Cerebri

It is the condition associated with raised intracranial pressure. There is no any specific intracranial cause. It may be the complication of otitis media or sinusitis. It may be associated with some drugs such as steroids, growth hormone, tetracycline, oral contraceptives, and vitamin A. Obesity is one of the causes. Other secondary causes include venous sinus thrombosis, jugular vein thrombosis, and hypercoagulable states. Down syndrome, Turner syndrome, renal failure, and Addison disease are medical causes of the condition.

Clinical features include headache, vision changes, nausea, and dizziness. Papilledema and abducent nerve palsy are present. Progressive papilledema leads to optic atrophy.

It is more common in children above 11 years of age. Headache is typically present posteriorly and aggravated in supine. Pain may be experienced in shoulder neck and back. Vomiting and dizziness may be present. A primary criterion for diagnosing pseudotumor cerebri is elevated lumbar puncture opening pressure.

Ptosis

Ptosis, or blepharoptosis, is a unilateral or bilateral decrease in the vertical distance between the upper and lower eyelids (palpebral fissure) because of dysfunction of the levator muscle.

Congenital ptosis is frequently transmitted as an autosomal dominant trait with variable penetrance. Congenital ptosis may be either unilateral or bilateral. Other causes for ptosis include ocular inflammation, chronic irritation of the anterior segment of the eye, chronic use of topical steroid eye drops, third nerve palsy, and trauma. Ptosis may be severe enough to cause visual deprivation and amblyopia if the visual axis is occluded. Children with even mild degrees of congenital ptosis should be referred for evaluation because they have a higher than normal incidence of strabismus and anisometropic amblyopia than the general population. In congenital ptosis, the eyelid position may improve somewhat from that observed early in infancy, but after that, it tends to remain stable or worsens slightly over time.

BOX 1: Causes of ptosis.

- IIIrd cranial nerve palsy
- Homes syndrome
- Myasthenia gravis
- Congenital syphilis
- Progressive ocular myopathy
- Facioscapular humeral dystrophy
- Beriberi
- Botulism

In the congenital condition called "Jaw-winking", movements of the jaw—especially lateral movements—cause the ptotic lid to rise. The patient is thus seen to "wink: while eating or chewing". The cause appears to be a misdirection of nerve fibers resulting in a faulty innervation of the levator muscle.

The causes of ptosis are listed in **Box 1**.

Puddle Sign

Another maneuver allows you to test for fluid pooling (puddle sign). Ask the patient to assume the knee chest position and maintain that position for several minutes to allow any fluid to pool by gravity. Percuss the umbilical area for dullness to determine the presence of fluid. The area will remain tympanic if no fluid is present.

A doughy feel of the abdomen is found in protein energy malnutrition, worm infestation, and tuberculous abdomen. Indentation on pressure is suggestive of fecal mass. Feeling of crepitus while palpation is indicative of trichobezoar. A sensation of gurgle is felt during palpation of colon; round worm mass is felt as a bag of worms (bag of worm feel).

Edema of abdominal wall can be demonstrated either by digital pressure, which leads to the phenomenon of pitting or by picking up a fold of skin and subcutaneous tissues in which case the thickening of tissues through edema becomes obvious. Edema of the abdominal wall may be associated with generalized edema or anasarca, as in cases of nephritis or cardiac failure or with massive ascites.

This is done to know the minimal fluid in the abdomen. The child is asked to lie on the knee elbow position. This position should be maintained for several minutes. This will ensure the gravitation of fluid to mid-abdominal position. The umbilical area is percussed for the dullness to determine the presence of fluid. The area will remain tympanic if no fluid is present.

Chest piece of the stethoscope is placed over the mid-abdomen. Abdomen is gently tapped with index finger. Tapping is done from one flank toward the center, till water puddle sound is audible when the edge of the ascitic fluid is tapped.

Pulse

Assessment of arterial pulse is the important aspect of physical examination. The radial pulse and other peripheral pulses to be examined include brachial, femoral, popliteal, and dorsalis pedis of both sides are palpated **(Fig. 1)**.

TECHNIQUE OF PALPATING THE RADIAL ARTERY

The radial pulse is felt with the index, middle, and the ring finger of examiner. The index finger steadies the artery and the middle finger feels the volume by upstroke of the pulse. The ring finger is used to obliterate the pulse. The middle finger rolls the artery to feel for the condition of vessel.

VOLUME

It signifies the extent of the movement of the vessel wall. It is judged by the degree of the lift of palpating finger during palpation. Volume of pulse is the direct indicator of pulse pressure. These are two types of pulses depending on pulse volume.

1. *Hypokinetic pulse (weak pulse):* This is due to reduced cardiac output. Pulse

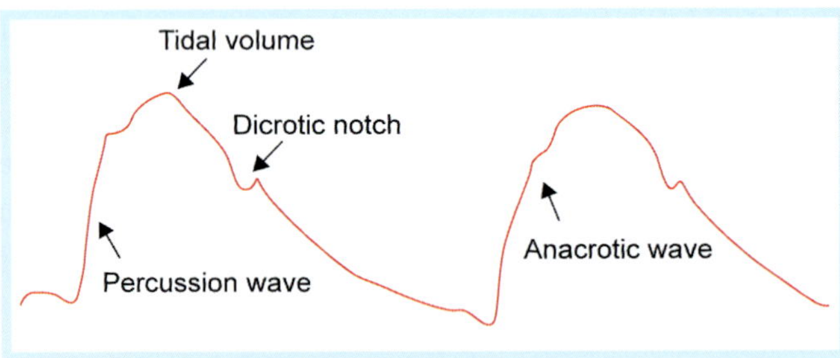

Fig. 1: Normal arterial pulse.

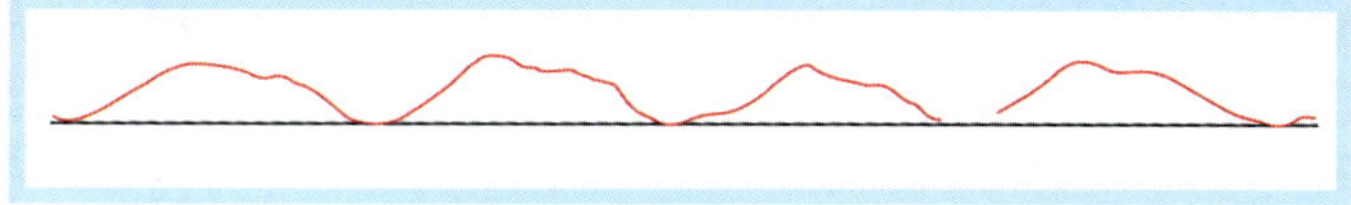

Fig. 2: Small weak pulse.

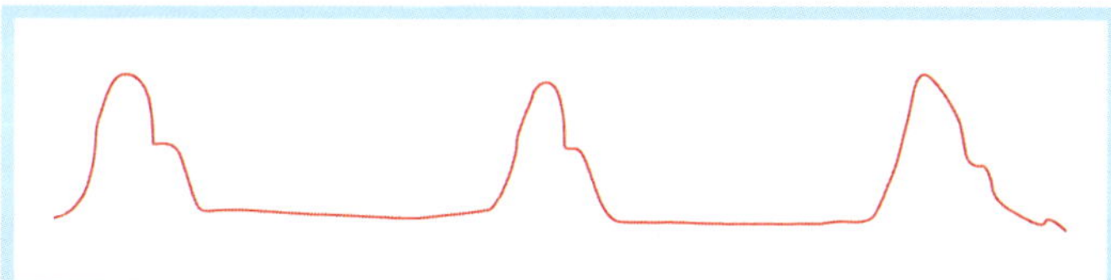

Fig. 3: Large, bounding pulse.

pressure will be in narrow range. The causes include shock, CCF, myocarditis, cardiomyopathy, and mitral stenosis **(Fig. 2)**.

2. *Hyperkinetic pulse (bounding pulse):* This is due to increase in cardiac output and decrease in peripheral resistance. The causes include fever, anemia, thyrotoxicosis, AV fistula, beriberi, and coarctation of aorta **(Fig. 3)**.

336 CHAPTER

Pulse Character

ANACROTIC PULSE

This is a slow rising pulse of smaller amplitude seen in conditions like aortic stenosis. The term anacrotic means an upbeating pulse and refers to the exaggerated anacrotic notch found in aortic stenosis. It is related to a jet effect produced by ejection across the abnormal valve or to decreased velocity of blood flow during early ejection **(Fig. 1)**.

It is a slow rising pulse of small amplitude. It is present in aortic stenosis. It is related to effect produced by ejection across the abnormal valve or the decreased velocity of blood flow during early ejection. The anacrotic is present in the upward slope of pulse wave.

COLLAPSING PULSE (WATER HAMMER PULSE)

It is characterized by a sudden thrust and receding back sensation of the pulse wave. The abrupt upstroke is due to greatly increased stroke volume. The collapsing character is caused by two factors **(Fig. 2)**.

First the diastolic run off into the left ventricle, secondly the rapid run off to the periphery because of low systemic vascular resistance.

Causes

- Physiological exercise, anxiety
- Hyperkinetic circulatory status
- Beriberi anemia
- Hepatic disease, leak in the arterial side of the circulation
- AR, AV fistula, MR
- PDA, large VSD, Truncus arteriosus
- Blalock–Taussig shunt, rupture of coronary sinus

Method of Palpating Collapsing Pulse

Radial artery is palpated above wrist, through the muscles of forearm. Then, the arm is lifted above the level of child's head. Sudden thrust

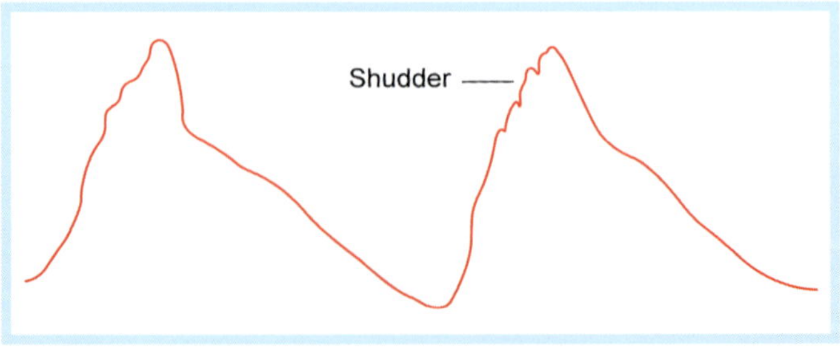

Fig. 1: Anacrotic pulse.

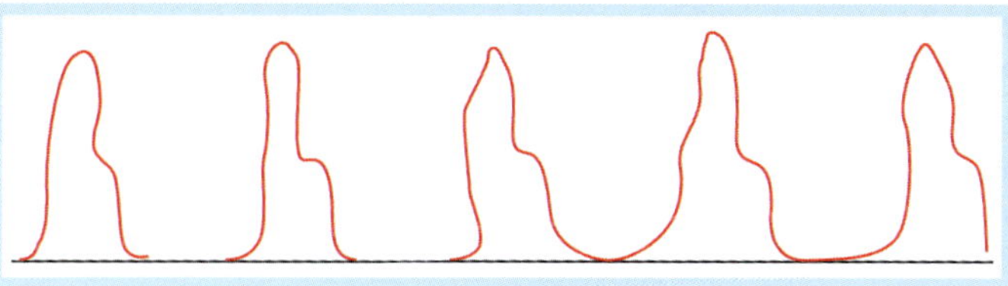

Fig. 2: Collapsing pulse.

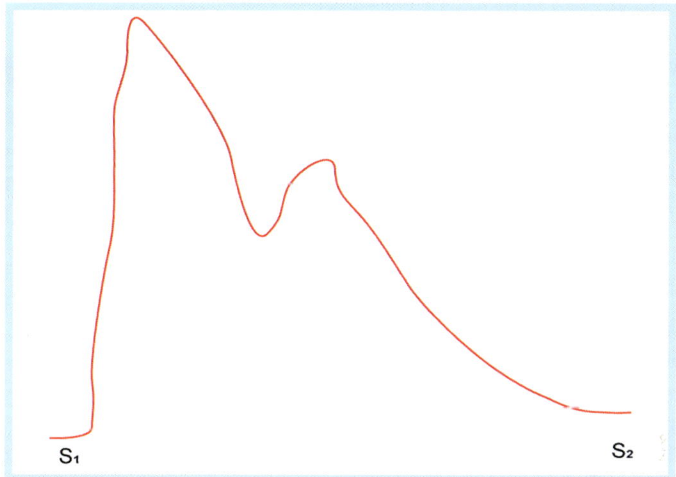

Fig. 3: Dicrotic pulse.

and collapsing sensation are felt if collapsing pulse is present. The raising arm above the level of heart brings the factor of gravity. This exaggerates aortic leak at aortic level. The raising of the arm above the level of the heart brings in factor of gravity, thus exaggerating the leak as aortic level as in AR.

Causes of Water hammer pulse (collapsing pulse):

- Fever
- Anemia
- Beriberi
- AV fistula
- Thyrotoxicosis
- Aortic regurgitation
- Patent ductus arteriosus
- AV window
- Hypertension

DOUBLE BEATING PULSE

Twice beating pulse occurs when there are two palpable arterial pulses per cardiac cycle. It is seen in hypertrophic cardiomyopathy **(Fig. 3)**.

Pulse Rate

Pulse rate varies with age. The rate diminishes with the increasing age **(Table 1)**. The upper and lower limits are standardized at each age. In newborn, the upper limit is 170/min, the lower limit is 70/min.

Tachycardia: This is when heart rate rises above the upper limit for the age and sex:

- *In newborn:* >200/min
- *In infants:* >150/min
- *In older children:* >120/min

Acceptable resting pulse rate/min.

Age	*Awake*	*Asleep*	*Fever*
Newborn	100–180	80–160	<220
1 week to 3 months	100–220	80–200	<220
3 months to 2 years	80–150	70–120	<200
2 years to 10 years	70–110	60–90	<200
>10 years	55–90	50–90	<200

TACHYCARDIA

Causes of tachycardia:

- Fever
- Exercise
- Myocarditis
- Heart failure
- Drugs—atropine, theophylline
- Thyrotoxicosis
- Rheumatic fever
- Diphtheria
- Paroxysmal supraventricular tachycardia
- Atrial fibrillation
- Atrial flutter

TABLE 1: Pulse rate in infants and children.

Age (in years)	*Rate/minute*
Newborn	70–170
Up to 1 year	80–160
2 years	80–130
4 years	80–120
6 years	76–110
6–10 years	70–110

BRADYCARDIA

This is when the heart rate falls below normal lower limit. When it is <100/min in newborn, <80/min in children of 2 years, and <60/min in older children.

Causes of bradycardia:

- Low birth weight babies
- Hypothyroidism
- Congenital complete heart block
- Second-degree heart block
- Sick sinus syndrome
- Drugs—β-blocker
- Jaundice
- Raised intracranial tension
- Digitalis toxicity

Pulse, Rhythm

The lability of the pulse is well-known, hence, it is counted for one full minute to decide if the rhythm is regular or irregular. If irregular, then decide if regularly irregular or irregularly irregular.

Causes of sinus arrhythmias are as follows:

- Many normal children
- Premature infants (normally)
- During convalescence from febrile illness
- Drugs like digitalis

Abolished by exercise or by atropine (sinus arrhythmia is absent in a large ASD and is uncommon in patient over 35 years of age).

Causes of regularly irregular rhythms:

- Heart blocks
- Extrasystoles
- Atrial flutter with varying blocks

Causes of irregularly irregular rhythms: Atrial fibrillation

It may be either regular or irregular. One should decide if the pulse rhythm is irregular, whether it is regularly irregular or irregularly irregular.

Causes of regularly irregular rhythm:

- Heart blocks
- Extrasystole
- Atrial flutter

Causes of irregularly irregular rhythm:

- Atrial fibrillation

Causes of irregular rhythm:

- Normal children
- Premature infant
- Febrile child
- Drugs—digitalis

There are two main mechanisms that can produce an irregular pulse:

1. Disorders of impulse formation
2. Disorders of conduction

DISORDERS OF IMPULSE FORMATION

The rate of discharge of the sinoatrial node can vary, more or less rhythmically, in many normal subjects; this condition, termed sinus arrhythmia, is quite benign and hardly justifies classification as a disorder. The fluctuations in rate are most commonly in phase with respiration, the rate increasing during inspiration and slowing during expiration. This is very common in children and is due to reflex variations in vagal tone.

The absence of respiratory sinus arrhythmia is sometimes of some slight diagnostic significance in a child, as this is a feature of a large atrial septal defect.

Causes of an irregular pulse:

- Sinus arrhythmia
- Ectopic beats (supraventricular or ventricular)
- Atrial fibrillation
- Atrial flutter with varying atrioventricular block
- Sinoatrial block
- Partial atrioventricular block

- Pulsus alternans
- Pulsus paradoxus

Causes of extrasystole:

- Ventricular extrasystole
- Drugs—digoxin
- Sinus arrhythmia
- Atrial flutter
- Second-degree heart block

Causes of atrial fibrillation:

- Rheumatic heart disease—mitral stenosis
- Thyrotoxicosis
- Cardiomyopathy
- Arterial septal defect

DISORDERS OF CONDUCTION

The other mechanism is a disorder of conduction in which a block develops somewhere along the long pathway from the sinoatrial node to the ventricular myocardium; if this block is intermittent, an irregular pulse is likely to result.

Failure of transmission of the impulse from the sinoatrial node to the ventricles causes *"dropped beats"*. The ventricular rhythm will be regular only if every other beat is dropped (as in 2:1 atrioventricular block) or if the beat is complete and a lower pacemaker is driving the ventricles. Any other pattern of failure of conduction will cause an irregular pulse.

Two mechanical causes of a palpably irregular pulse should be mentioned.

PULSUS ALTERNANS

It is characterized by strong and weak beat occurring alternatively **(Fig. 1)**. This can be confirmed by recording the blood pressure. Once the systolic pressure is recorded, the mercury column is lowered. There is abrupt doubling of Korotkoff's sound. It is important sign of left ventricular dysfunction.

Pulsus Paradoxus

Normally during inspiration, due to decrease in intrathoracic pressure, the lung capacity increases and pulmonary vascular bed expands. This reduces the amount of blood reaching the left heart and in turn reduces the systolic pressure by 6–8 mm Hg **(Fig. 2)**. This is considered as normal phenomenon.

In case of cardiac tamponade due to raised intrapericardial pressure, left atrial and left ventricular pressure increases. This further reduces the amount of blood returning to left heart. Hence, it reduces the blood pressure >10 mm Hg during inspiration.

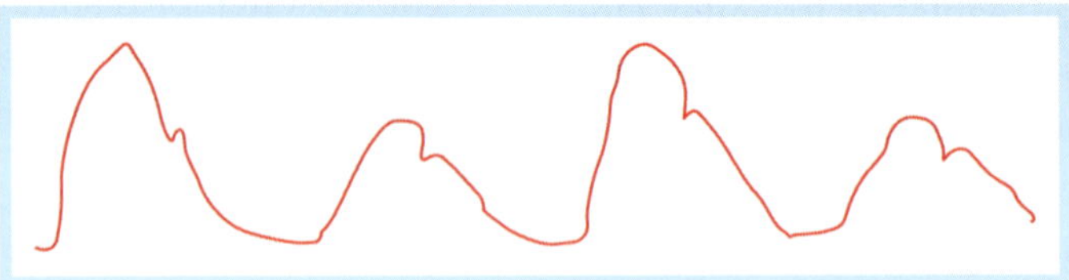

Fig. 1: Pulsus alternans.

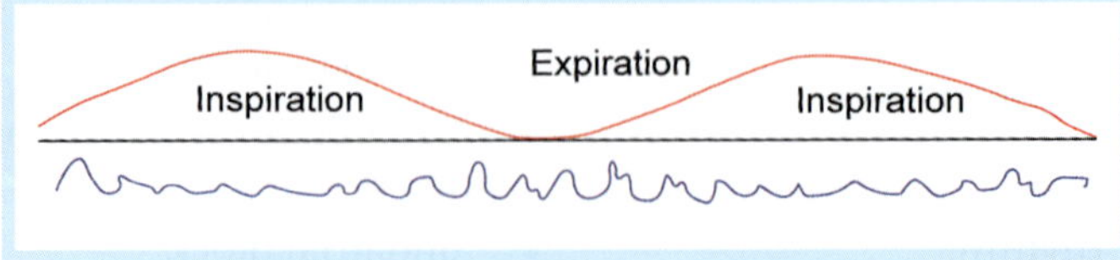

Fig. 2: Pulsus paradoxus.

Sphygmomanometer is applied and inflated until no sounds are audible. Cuff is deflated until the sounds are audible only during expiration. The pressure is noted. Cuff is still deflated until the sounds are audible during inspiration, the difference between the blood pressure is noted. If it is >10 mm, pulsus paradoxus is present.

Cause of pulsus paradoxus:

- Superior vena caval obstruction
- Bronchial asthma
- Emphysema
- Cardiac tamponade
- Congestive cardiac failure
- Airway obstruction

PULSE DEFICIT

This is seen among atrial fibrillation. Here, the auscultated heart rate is faster than palpated pulse rate. This is due to poor contraction of ventricle. The contraction is not strong enough to transmit the arterial pressure through the peripheral artery. Pulse deficit is calculated by counting the heart rate and pulse.

Causes of atrial fibrillation:

- Rheumatic heart disease—mitral stenosis
- Thyrotoxicosis
- Cardiomyopathy
- Arterial septal defect

Causes of extrasystole:

- Ventricular extrasystole
- Hypokalemia
- Drugs—digoxin
- Sinus arrhythmia
- Atrial flutter
- Second-degree heart block

CHAPTER 339

Pulse: Unequal

This type of pulse is seen in:

- Surgical trauma—Blalock operation
- Systemic embolism—mitral stenosis
- Coarctation of aorta
- Congenital absence of radial artery
- Aortal dissection
- Superior vena caval obstruction
- Bronchial asthma
- Emphysema
- Cardiac tamponade
- Congestive cardiac failure
- Airway obstruction

340 CHAPTER Pupils, Abnormalities

SIZE

Size of pupils varies greatly with the intensity of the surrounding illumination. In lighting of average intensity:

- *Normally:* 3–4-mm diameter
- *Neonates:* Pupils are small and react poorly
- *Adolescents:* 4 mm diameter, round
- *Middle age:* 3.5 mm diameter, regular
- *Old age:* 3 mm or less, irregular

MIOSIS

When pupils are small (<2 mm), they are said to be miotic. Miosis is seen in newborns, opium, organophosphorus compound poisoning, pilocarpine, encephalitis, and syringomyelia.

MYDRIASIS

Dilated pupils are seen in mania, atropine poisoning, and damage to cervical sympathetic plexus.

SHAPE

Shape of the pupil is important in neurologic diagnosis. Normal pupil is round and regular in outline. Any irregularity, abnormality in shape, notching, or serration may be significant.

Gross abnormalities in shape of pupils are usually the result of ocular disease (iritis) or eye surgery. There may be:

- Adhesion to the lens (anterior synechiae)
- A gap in the iris (congenital coloboma)

EQUALITY

Comparison of the size of the two pupils has more significance than observation of size alone.

There may be slight difference in the size of the pupils in 15–20% of normal individuals. Gross inequality of pupils is called anisocoria. Sympathetic paralysis on one side will cause a smaller pupil on that side. IIIrd nerve paralysis produces dilatation of the pupil.

- Unequal pupils may be caused by iritis.
- Alternating anisocoria is seen in various CNS diseases.
- The pupil of an amblyopic/blind eye is always larger.
- In inner ear disease—ipsilateral contraction of pupil (since the pupillodilator fibers are in close proximity to the tympanic plexus in inner ear)
- Cerebral vascular accidents/head trauma—unilateral dilation and fixation of one pupil
- Dilated fixed pupil in a comatosed patients may give presumptive localization of a lesion in the ipsilateral cerebral hemisphere.

POSITION

The pupil is usually situated in the center of the iris. Ectopia of pupils or eccentric pupils may be the result of trauma or iritis.

ABNORMALITIES OF PUPIL SHAPE

The normal pupil is circular or slightly oval, with its longer axis horizontal. An irregularly shaped pupil is due to local damage to the iris. The circular shape of the pupil is also lost in coloboma.

PINPOINT PUPIL

- Pontine hemorrhage
- Organophosphorus poisoning
- Barbiturates
- Morphine
- Overdosage of neostigmine
- Iritis
- Apneic spell
- Syringomyelia
- Cavernous sinus thrombosis

DILATED PUPIL

- Raised intracranial tension
- Tentorial herniation
- Cervical rib
- Irritative neck lesion
- Aneurysm of aorta
- Postictal state
- Optic atrophy
- Emotional excitement
- Adrenaline
- Atropine

SMALL NONREACTIVE PUPIL

- Miotics
- Opiates
- ARP
- Pontine hemorrhage

LARGE NONREACTIVE HEMORRHAGE

- Mydriatics
- IIIrd cranial nerve palsy
- Blind eye
- Compression of midbrain

UNEQUAL PUPILS

- Encephalitis
- IIIrd cranial nerve lesion

CHAPTER 341

Purpura

Purpura results from leakage of blood from vessels into the skin or mucous membranes associated with diverse causes **(Fig. 1)**. Purpuric lesions do not blanch when pressure is applied. Small lesions that are pinpoint-sized or a few millimeters in diameter are called petechiae. Large lesions may be referred to as *ecchymoses*.

Nonthrombocytopenic causes of purpura:
Vasculitis:

- Henoch–Schönlein purpura (HSP)
- Systemic lupus erythematosus
- Drugs

Mechanical:

- Coughing
- Orthostatic
- Senile
- *Steroid-induced*
- *Scurvy*
- *Factitious purpura*

Raised or palpable purpura is diagnostic of vasculitis and can be seen in conditions such as Henoch–Schönlein purpura, lupus erythematosus, and Rocky Mountain spotted fever. Inflammation and destruction of blood vessel walls are responsible for the raised quality of these lesions. Nonpalpable purpura can be seen with platelet abnormalities, leukemia, and other thrombocytopenic conditions, capillaritis (pigmented purpuras), scurvy, viral exanthems, and physical exertion. Petechiae on the upper body (above the nipple line) can result from crying, vomiting, or coughing. Careful clinical examination is important for detecting these lesions and establishing a proper diagnosis.

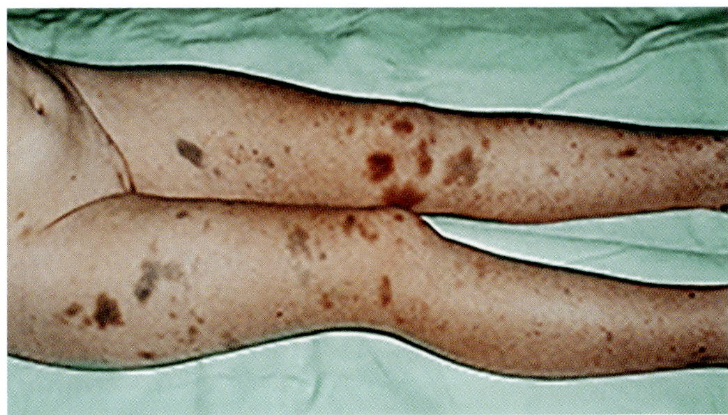

Fig. 1: Purpura.

CHAPTER 342 Pyrexia of Unknown Origin

Pyrexia of unknown origin (PUO) is defined as a temperature higher than 38°C (100.4°F) daily for at least 8–14 days and no diagnosis after an initial evaluation. The initial evaluation recommended varies but always includes a noncontributory history and physical examination, and nondiagnostic initial laboratory and radiologic tests. In accordance with this definition, the differential diagnosis for PUO in children is large.

CAUSES OF PYREXIA OF UNKNOWN ORIGIN

- *Bacterial:*
  - *Abscess*:
    - Dental
    - Perinephric
    - Subdiaphragmatic
  - Bacterial endocarditis
  - Brucellosis
  - Leptospirosis
  - Salmonellosis
  - Tuberculosis
- *Viral:*
  - Hepatitis
  - Infectious mononucleosis
  - Cytomegalovirus infection
- *Parasitosis:*
  - Malaria
  - Toxoplasmosis
  - Visceral larva migrans
- *Fungal:*
  - Blastomycosis
  - Histoplasmosis
- *Collagen vascular disease:*
  - Juvenile rheumatoid arthritis
  - SLE
  - Periarthritis nodosa
- *Malignancies:*
  - Hodgkin's disease
  - Lymphoma
  - Neuroblastoma
- *Miscellaneous:*
  - Drug fever
  - Thyrotoxicosis
  - Serum sickness

DIAGNOSIS

Initial studies should include a complete blood cell count with differential, erythrocyte sedimentation rate (ESR) measurement, CRP, blood cultures, urinalysis, urine culture, tuberculin skin tests with controls (anergy panel) or gamma interferon release assay, and chest radiograph. Because Epstein–Barr virus (EBV) infection is common in childhood, viral-specific antibody titers may also be obtained at the initial evaluation. Further studies should be directed by information obtained from detailed histories and physical examinations.

Complete Blood Count and Other Markers of Inflammation

A WBC count of 5,000–15,000 is generally considered normal for children over 1 month of age. A WBC count <15,000/mm^3 or even leukopenia may be found in children with *N. meningitidis* bacteremia. A minority of children with occult nontyphoidal *Salmonella* bacteremia have been found to have a WBC count exceeding 15,000/mm^3. C-reactive protein (CRP) and procalcitonin combined with a urine dipstick (the laboratory score) can be used to screen for bacterial infection. This combination of tests has been validated for children 7 days to 36 months of age.

The complete blood cell count with differential is neither specific nor diagnostic, except in rare circumstances, such as seeing lymphoblasts on the blood smear. Approximately 30% of patients have abnormal white blood cell counts; 46% may have a left shift, lymphocytosis, atypical lymphocytes, or blasts. An elevated ESR or CRP indicates inflammation. The ESR is usually (70–90% of the time) high in children with PUO caused by infectious pathogens, malignancies, and rheumatic diseases. Of patients with an ESR <10 mm/h, 90% have a self-limited viral disease.

Polymerase chain reaction (PCR) is useful in identifying the cause of fever for common viruses such as respiratory syncytial virus, influenza viruses, parainfluenza viruses, enteroviruses, parechovirus, adenoviruses, or herpes simplex virus.

Rapid multiplex PCR combined with standard blood culture methods may identify a specific pathogen much sooner (~20 hours) than standard blood culture techniques.

Blood Cultures

Blood cultures are the gold standard for determination of bacteremia. Although blood cultures do not provide immediate results, methods allow for continuous and more rapid detection of bacterial growth. Blood cultures are easy to perform and provide essential information in the diagnosis and management of patients with possible bacteremia. Preliminary blood culture results are typically available within 24 hours, with positive identification of most organisms within 48 hours.

URINALYSIS AND URINE CULTURE

Lumbar Puncture

Lumbar puncture is indicated if the patient is younger than 28 days or if a diagnosis of sepsis, meningitis, or encephalitis is considered, regardless of the child's age. Normal cerebrospinal fluid (CSF) findings, including chemistry, cell count with differential, Gram stain, PCR, and culture, help exclude the diagnosis of meningitis.

Chest Radiographs

Chest radiographs are usually normal in children who have PUO. Respiratory signs or symptoms, such as tachypnea, retractions, crackles, wheezing, rhonchi, nasal flaring, grunting, cough, or hypoxia, may predict chest radiograph findings consistent with pneumonia. Chest radiographs may be useful in evaluating for the presence of pleural effusion or other complications of pneumonia.

Stool Cultures

Most acute diarrhea and fever are caused by viral pathogens in developed countries. Obtaining a stool culture is indicated if bacterial enteritis is indicated by the presence of risk factors in the history, such as blood in the stool or certain exposures (petting zoos).

Specific serologic studies aid in the diagnosis of CMV, toxoplasmosis, brucellosis, tularemia, hepatitis A, B, and C, and leptospirosis. Biopsies of lymph nodes, the skin, the liver, or bone marrow may be indicated. Radiologic studies that may be of benefit if directed by the history, physical examination findings, and initial laboratory study results include sinus CT, abdominal imaging, or total body MRI (to evaluate for occult osteomyelitis, malignancy, and histiocytic disorders).

Rebound Tenderness

The principle behind this procedure is the localized mild response in the presence of peritoneal inflammation. If the patient is experiencing abdominal pain, it indicates the peritoneal irritation.

The child is lying in supine position. The examiner's hand is held at 90° angle to the abdomen. The fingers are extended and pressed gently and deeply over the abdomen away from the point of tenderness. Hands and fingers are rapidly withdrawn. The rebound of the structures that were compressed by the fingers causes sharp stabbing pain at the site of peritoneal inflammation, i.e., Blumberg sign. Rebound tenderness at the McBurney point in the lower right quadrant suggests appendicitis, i.e., positive McBurney sign. The maneuver for rebound tenderness should be performed at the end of the examination, because a positive response produces pain and muscle spasm that can interfere with any subsequent examination.

344 CHAPTER

Rectal Prolapse

Rectal prolapse is common in toddlers and is thought to occur in those who have a limited rectal shelf at the level of the puborectalis muscle **(Fig. 1)**. The resulting relatively straight direction between the anal opening and the sigmoid above allows intussusception of both rectal and sigmoid tissues when the infant strains to defecate. Rectal prolapse can occur with relatively little straining. (The very first appearance of a rectal prolapse in an apparently healthy child can be relatively scary event for parents.)

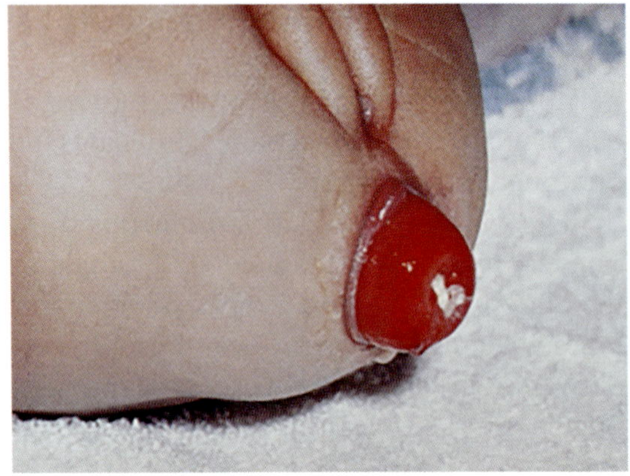

Fig. 1: Rectal prolapse.

Cystic fibrosis, in particular, is associated with an increased incidence of rectal prolapse. One should seek signs or symptoms suggestive of that condition by carefully obtaining a history.

A carefully conducted digital rectal examination is necessary to ensure that the prolapse is not associated with other or pelvic pathology, such as a pelvic mass. When a prolapse in a toddler is unassociated with any other pathology, it usually is a self-limited problem. Measures to minimize straining with bowel movements, patience, and reassurance will allow spontaneous resolution of most cases of rectal prolapse, although resolution may take many months. Children who strain excessively with bowel movements should be treated for constipation. The most important intervention required is strong reassurance of the parents. Most prolapses will reduce spontaneously, but they can be frequent, which can be disconcerting to parents. Occasionally, parents have to manually reduce a prolapse that does not reduce spontaneously.

When rectal prolapse is associated with a neurologic injury or when additional conditions, such as autism, are present, surgery may be a more appropriate option than expectant management.

CHAPTER 345 Reflexes, Abnormalities

A reflex is the most basic form of involuntary response to a stimulus. The anatomical pathway (reflex arc) consists of—(1) a receptor organ, (2) an afferent pathway to the brain or spinal cord, (3) usually interneurons in the central nervous system, and (4) an afferent path which leaves via the lower motor neurons to each a receptor organ, often a muscle. The stimulus may be touch, pinprick, or sudden stretching of a muscle. The response may not only be muscle contraction, but also altered muscle tone or glandular secretion.

GRADING OF DEEP TENDON REFLEXES

- *Grade 0:* Absent
- *Grade I:* Present as a normal ankle jerk
- *Grade II:* Brisk as a normal knee jerk
- *Grade III:* Very brisk
- *Grade IV:* Clonus

THE TENDON REFLEXES

The tendon reflex is reflection of the myotatic reflex, a reflex contraction of a muscle (or a part of a muscle in response to rapid stretch, as caused by tapping with a tendon hammer). It is a monosynaptic reflex; the reflex pathway ascends from the muscle through the posterior roots, passes forward to the anterior horn cells on the same segment, and descends to the muscle or muscles concerned via the motor nerve.

EXAGGERATED DEEP TENDON REFLEXES

- *Pyramidal lesions*:
  - Tetanus
  - Anxiety
  - Hysteria
  - Fear
  - Asphyxia
  - Raised intracranial tension
  - Cerebral palsy
  - Thyrotoxicosis

ABSENT DEEP TENDON REFLEXES

- *Neuronal shock*:
  - Lower motor neuron (LMN) lesion
  - Muscle contractures
  - Down's syndrome
  - Mental retardation
  - Friedreich's ataxia
  - Floppy infant
  - Poliomyelitis

TYPE OF TENDON REFLEXES

Biceps Jerk

The patient's hand is placed on abdomen. The examiner's index finger is placed on tendon of biceps. Gentle tapping is done over the index finger of the examiner. The response includes the contraction of biceps muscle or contraction of elbow **(Fig. 1)**. The spinal cord segments involved are C_5, and C_6.

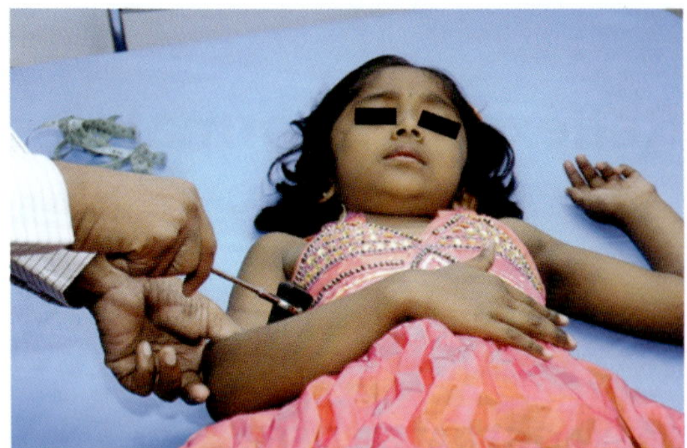

Fig. 1: Biceps jerk.

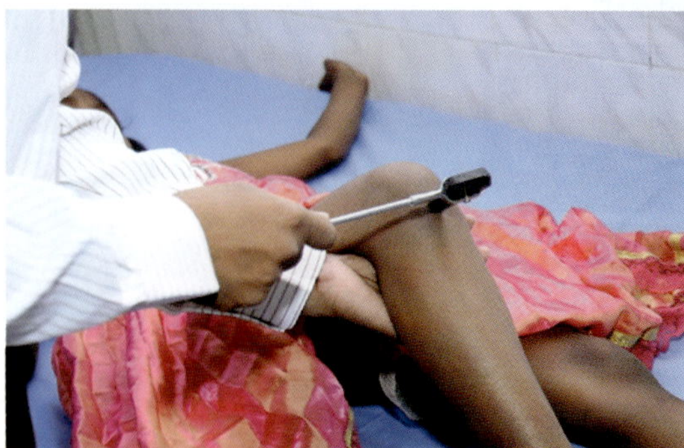

Fig. 3: Knee jerk.

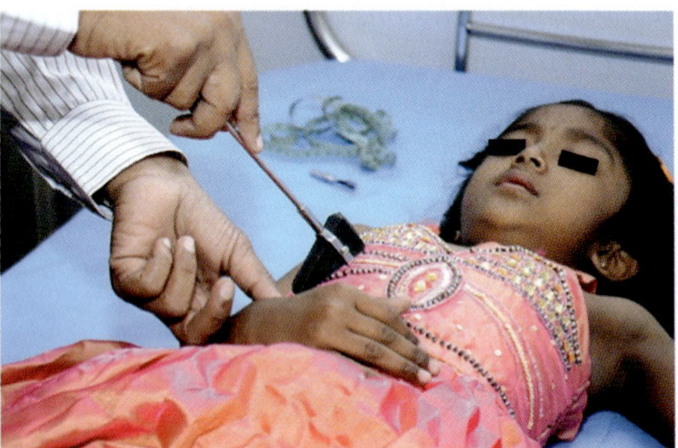

Fig. 2: Supinator jerk or radial reflex.

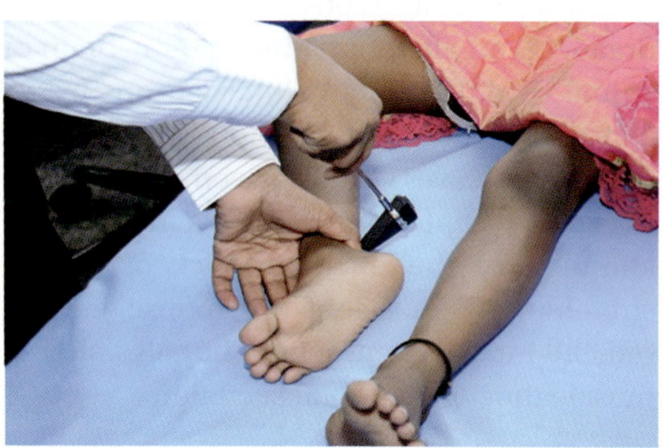

Fig. 4: Ankle jerk.

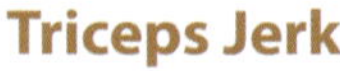

Triceps Jerk

The patient's arm is dragged across the chest. This is done by holding the wrist and elbow at 90°. The triceps tendon reflexes are gently tapped with the hammer. The response is contraction of triceps muscle and extension of elbow. The spinal cord segments involved are C_6, and C_7.

Supinator Jerk or Radial Reflex

Arm is flexed at abdomen. Examiner's finger is placed on radial tuberosity. Sharp tap is given over the examiner's finger, i.e., on brachioradialis tendon insertion. There will be flexion of semipronated elbow and sometimes slight flexion of fingers **(Fig. 2)**. The spinal cord segments involved are C_5, and C_6.

In inversion of radial reflex, brachioradialis contraction is absent. Fingers show flexion movements. It indicates lesion at C_4 and C_3 level.

Knee Jerk

Examiner's arm is placed below the knee so that knee is at 90°. Sharp gentle tap is given **(Fig. 3)**. The response is contraction of quadriceps and extension of knee joint. Spinal cord segments involved are L_3 and L_4.

Ankle Jerk

Foot is held at 90°. The knee joint should be flexed and lying to the side. Sharp tap is given on tendo Achilles **(Fig. 4)**. Response includes contraction of calf muscle and hence plantar flexion of the ankle. The spinal cord segments involved are S_1 and S_2.

CHAPTER 346 Renal Ectopia

CROSSED RENAL ECTOPY

Horseshoe Kidney

Horseshoe kidney results from fusion of the lower renal poles during development. Although generally asymptomatic, patients with horseshoe kidney may have—(1) hematuria after trauma to the pelvic area; (2) midline abdominal mass; or (3) ureteropelvic junction obstruction, a common associated finding in this condition.

Solitary Kidney

There are multiple causes of solitary kidney in children, including congenital renal aplasia, which occurs in about 1 in 1,300 births, involution of a multicystic dysplastic kidney, marked renal hypodysplasia, or acquired disorders, such as removal of kidneys because of tumor, trauma, or severe urologic injury.

Progression to end-stage renal disease (ESRD) may be insidious over decades and is reported to occur in about 20–50% of 30-year-old individuals with solitary kidney in childhood.

Children with good kidney function and no hypertension (HTN) may be monitored every 5 years with a regular physical examination, including BP check, urinalysis to detect proteinuria, glomerular filtration rate (GFR) estimation by serum creatinine, and ultrasonography to assess for compensatory hypertrophy. Children with known additional genitourinary anomalies or renal dysfunction, HTN, proteinuria, or recurrent urinary tract infections (UTIs) are at high risk for progressing to chronic kidney disease (CKD) and need follow-up more frequently.

Anticipatory guidance for preventing blunt renal trauma related to high impact sports injuries, use of nephrotoxic medications including nonsteroidal anti-inflammatory agents, and weight control to prevent obesity may also be provided at regular office visits.

347 CHAPTER Respiratory Distress

INTRODUCTION

The main function of the respiratory system is to supply oxygen to meet the body's demands and remove excess carbon dioxide. Many processes are involved in ensuring that this occurs, including ventilation (gas delivery to and from the lungs), perfusion (blood supply to the lungs), and diffusion (the exchange of gases along the alveoli).

The initial approach to a patient includes determining the severity of illness then determining if immediate treatment is needed by first ensuring that airway, breathing, and circulation are intact.

APGAR SCORE

The traditional way of assessing the newborn is to use the Apgar score. The Apgar score was the first attempt at a systematic assessment of birth asphyxia. This was devised by Virginia Apgar (1953), and grades five clinical features with scores from 0 to 2 at 1 minute of age. In recent years, it is being assessed up to 20 minutes at an interval of 5 minutes each. There has been a tendency to be little with the Apgar score because it is a poor index of asphyxia. If a baby has a poor Apgar score, he has a problem **(Table 1)**. It may well not be asphyxia but sooner the problem is diagnosed and managed better is the outcome.

BRONCHIOLITIS

Bronchiolitis is acute viral infection of the distal lower respiratory tract, and is characterized as lower airway obstruction secondary to airway edema, mucous and cellular debris. Impaired gas exchange can occur as a result of airway obstruction and ventilation-perfusion inequalities. Respiratory syncytial virus (RSV) is the most important respiratory pathogen in infants and young children. The most severe disease occurs in infants younger than 6 months.

STRIDOR

Stridor, a harsh medium-pitched sound typically heard on inspiration, is caused by turbulent airflow in the upper airway.

TABLE 1: Parameters of evaluation using the Apgar score.

Sign	*0 points*	*1 points*	*2 points*
Heart rate (beats/min)	Absent	Slow (<100)	>100
Respiratory effort (breath/min)	Absent	Slow and irregular	Good crying
Muscle tone	Flaccid	Some flexion of extremities	Active motion
Reflex irritability	No response	Grimace	Vigorous cry
Color	Pale	Cyanotic	Completely pink

The phase of respiration in which stridor occurs is helpful in identifying the site of the airway obstruction. The most common cause of stridor of infants and young children is laryngomalacia. Acute inspiratory stridor is most commonly caused by acute inflammation/infection, typically croup; however, an acute foreign body aspiration in the upper airway may also cause acute-onset stridor.

CROUP

Laryngotracheal bronchitis (croup) is generally a slowly progressive, mild, self-limited viral inflammation of the subglottic larynx occurring in infants and young children. The most common causes are parainfluenza virus types 1 and 3, influenza A, respiratory syncytial virus, and adenovirus. The cry or voice may become hoarse. Stridor typically worsens when the patient is upset or active, and improves with warm humidified air. If a patient develops drooling or rapid progression of respiratory distress, epiglottitis or bacterial tracheitis should be considered. The diagnosis is usually apparent from the history and physical examination. If the diagnosis is not clear, obtaining a lateral neck radiograph is indicated and will show the classic "steeple" sign.

BACTERIAL TRACHEITIS

Bacterial tracheitis is a bacterial super-infection of a previous tracheal (croup, influenza virus) viral process and is usually caused by *Staphylococcus aureus*. A variety of other organisms, including *Moraxella catarrhalis*, *Streptococcus pneumoniae*, and non-typeable *H. influenza*, have also been identified as being occasionally involved. There is generally a virus-like mild phase, followed by a rapid deterioration, during which the patient clinically appears more ill with high fever and respiratory distress.

EPIGLOTTITIS

Epiglottitis is an acute, rapidly progressive, potentially lethal infection of the epiglottis, aryepiglottic folds, and false vocal cord area. It is an emergency because of the potential for rapid airway obstruction; evaluation and treatment are directed toward establishing an airway while the physician is confirming the diagnosis and treating the infection.

Typically, there is an abrupt onset, usually without an obvious prodrome, with rapid progression toward airway compromise. Initially, complaints of sore throat and odynophagia are common. Patients are usually febrile, and drooling is present. The typical presentation is an ill-appearing child sitting forward with her or his head hyperextended who does not want to lie down. There is a "hot potato" voice and drooling, the mouth is open, and the tongue is protruding. Mild inspiratory stridor and retractions may be present, but these are usually not obvious, because the patient generally takes short, shallow breaths. An intraoral examination is contraindicated because it may predispose to laryngospasm and airway obstruction.

VIRAL AND BACTERIAL PNEUMONIA

Pneumonia is a significant cause of mortality for children worldwide. Pneumonia is defined as acute inflammation of the lung parenchyma, and can be caused by viruses or bacteria.

Clinically, it is often defined as a lower respiratory tract infection, associated with fever, respiratory symptoms, and evidence of lung parenchyma involvement, either by physical examination or chest radiograph findings. *S. pneumoniae* is the most common bacterial pathogen of community-acquired pneumonia; *H. influenzae* and *S. aureus* are less common causes. Viral pathogens are also a common cause of pneumonia in young children; it can be difficult to discern which pathogen is causing the clinical symptoms.

Atypical pathogens, such as *M. pneumoniae*, are a common cause of pneumonia in school-aged children. Children with immunodeficiency, sickle cell disease, cystic fibrosis, or HIV may present with more atypical pathogens.

Patients will often begin with an upper respiratory infection with rhinitis and cough. They then develop tachypnea and fever and then may develop respiratory distress with subcostal, intercostal, and suprasternal retractions, nasal flaring and use of accessory muscles, and hypoxia. Tachypnea and worsening cough are commonly noted. Patients with lower lobe pneumonias may also present with abdominal pain. Early in the course of illness, crackles, rhonchi, and wheezing are common findings. Later in the course of illness, as lungs consolidate and/or pleural effusions or empyema develop, decreased breath sounds and dullness to percussion may develop. Wheezing is more likely in viral or atypical pneumonia; however, unilateral wheezing may also correlate with a bacterial lobar pneumonia.

348 CHAPTER

Respiratory Rate

Respiratory rate should be counted for 60 seconds, when the child is quite. Increased respiratory rate is called as tachypnea. Normal respiration has inspiration longer than expiration.

- *Newborn to 2 months:* 60 or more
- *2–12 months:* 50 or more
- *1–5 years:* 40 or more

TACHYPNEA

It signifies an increase in rate of breathing. It may occur normally during exercise or abnormally in number of clinical disturbances especially those associated with hypoxia. Tachypnea is associated with the symptoms of breathlessness.

Both rate and depth of respiration are controlled by brainstem respiratory center. This will maintain constant arterial blood oxygen level.

Flaring of the alae nasi exists when there is enlargement of both nares occur during inspiration. This is due to contraction of the anterior and posterior dilators nares muscle. Appearance of flaring indicates accessory muscles are required for inspiration. It is a sign of dyspnea.

Causes of Tachypnea

- *Increased metabolic demands*:
  - Fever
  - Hyperdynamic circulation
  - Circulatory shock
- *Stimulation of central chemoreceptors*:
  - Metabolic acidosis
  - Renal failure
  - Hepatic failure
  - Acute circulatory collapse
  - Salicylate overdose
- *Stimulation lung stretch receptor*:
  - Acute pulmonary emboli
  - Acute pneumonia
  - Bronchial asthma
  - Pulmonary fibrosis
  - Inspiration pneumonia
- *Neurological causes*:
  - Cerebral hemorrhage
  - Meningitis
  - Encephalitis
  - Head injury

Causes of increased rate and depth of respiration:

- Acidosis
- Acute pulmonary disease
- Acute cardiac disease

BIOT'S BREATHING

It is seen in meningitis and is characterized by sudden increase and decrease of respiration during hypercapnic paroxysm. There is irregularly irregular respiration.

KUSSMAUL'S BREATHING

It is characterized by deep and rapid respiration, i.e., air hunger. Deep noisy breathing, i.e., laborers in nature is seen typically in diabetic coma.

PATTERN OF BREATHING

Normally, it is abdominothoracic breathing, i.e., abdominal exertion is predominant compared to thoracic movements. Diaphragmatic movements are more important than intercostal muscle actions. In women, the respiration is thoracoabdominal, wherein chest wall movements are predominant.

In pathological conditions, thoracoabdominal respiration is abnormal. It is seen in ascites, abdominal masses, poliomyelitis, and peritonitis.

PARADOXICAL RESPIRATION

Normally, the diaphragm descends during inspiration and rises during expiration. The reverse occurs in paradoxical respiration; in other words, abdomen goes in during inspiration and bulges during expiration. Paradoxical respiration is seen in following conditions:

- Pneumothorax
- Hydrothorax
- Atelectasis
- Pneumonia
- Phrenic nerve paralysis as in poliomyelitis and diphtheria

Increased rate but decreased depth, i.e., rapid shallow breathing:

- Pleurisy
- Guillain-Barre syndrome
- Interstitial fibrosis
- Miliary tuberculosis

Subcostal, intercostals, and suprasternal indrawing is most definitive sign of inspiratory distress. Prominent suprasternal indrawing is found in upper airway obstruction, i.e., in larynx, trachea or major bronchi, and in pulmonary disease.

Accessory muscles of respiration include that of inspiration and expiration. Accessary muscles of inspiration include sternomastoid, scalene, and trapezius. Accessory muscles of expiration include abdominal wall muscles—rectus abdominus.

GRUNTING

It is expiratory sound due to sudden closure of vocal cords during expiratory phase with an attempt to preserve functional residual capacity. It is a specific sign of hypoxemia. It is heard in newborns and young infants, e.g., pneumonia and hyaline membrane disease.

BRADYPNEA

It is abnormally low slow rate of respiration. It is ominous sign when seen in ill infant or child. Causes include fatigue, hypothermia, and CNS depression.

Causes of decreased rate and depth of respiration are:

- Encephalitis
- Increased intracranial tension
- Barbiturate poisoning

Causes of decreased rate and increased depth are:

- Encephalitis
- Intracranial hemorrhage

HYPERPNEA

There is increased depth of breathing, e.g., acidosis, brainstem lesions, and hysteria.

CHAPTER 349 Retinoblastoma

Retinoblastoma is the most common primary malignant intraocular tumor of childhood. It occurs in approximately 1 in 20,000 infants.

In heritable cases, the first mutation arises during gametogenesis, either spontaneously (90%) or through transmission from parents (10%). This mutation is present in every retinal cell and in all other somatic and germ cells. 90% of persons who carry this germline mutation will develop retinoblastoma. The average age at diagnosis for bilateral tumor is 12 months and for unilateral tumors, it is 21 months.

For tumor formation, loss of second RBI allele within the cell must occur. Loss only is insufficient for tumor formation. The second mutation occurs in somatic (retinal) cell. In heritable cases (60%), both mutations arise in somatic cell after gametogenesis has taken place.

In trilateral retinoblastoma syndrome, pineal tumors develop in approximately 1 in 100 patients with bilateral ocular disease. Characteristically, the diagnosis is made by ophthalmoscopic, radiographic, and ultrasonographic appearance, without pathologic confirmation. The locus is present on chromosome No. 13. It is associated with osteosarcoma, pineal tumor, lung and breast cancer.

The most common presenting sign of retinoblastoma is leukocoria. When a tumor is small and at the macula, the initial sign may be sensory strabismus. When disease is very advanced, presenting symptoms may include pain due to secondary glaucoma, buphthalmos, proptosis, hyphema, or orbital cellulitis.

The differential diagnosis of retinoblastoma includes persistent hyperplastic primary vitreous (PHPV), retinal detachment, Coats disease, glial hamartoma, retinal hemangioma, myelinated nerve fibers, congenital cataract, chorioretinal coloboma, uveitis, larval granulomatosis, congenital retinal folds, retinal dysplasia, and retinopathy of prematurity.

The tumor usually presents with leukocoria, i.e., yellow white reflex in the pupil. Other presenting complaints may be loss of vision reflected as a squint in the affected eye. The other symptoms may be pain, pupillary irregularity, and hyphema. Proptosis may present with advanced tumor. There may be signs of increased intracranial pressure. There may be bone pain associated with metastatic disease.

Retinal Detachment

Trauma is the most common cause of retinal detachment in children. Large retinal detachments may produce loss of the red reflex, and leukocoria occurs when the detached retina is in apposition to the lens or when significant scarring (proliferative vitreoretinopathy) is present.

Symptoms of retinal detachment include photopsias (flashing lights), floaters (caused by vitreous hemorrhage), and changes in vision, including blurring of vision or the sensation of a veil or curtain blocking vision. Patients with blunt trauma to the eye should be advised of these symptoms and should be seen immediately if they are present or develop.

Retinitis Pigmentosa

The clinical manifestation includes visual loss and night blindness. Visual loss will be present in childhood, but it becomes apparent in second and third decade of life. Earliest symptom is poor night vision. This will lead to the extent of visual loss. There will be pigment deposition in midperipheral retina. This leads retinal pigment epithelial changes. In due course, there will be pallor in optic nerve and retinal vessels may be attenuated.

Retinopathy of Prematurity

Preterm newborns born at <34 weeks of gestation and/or weighing <1,750 grams should undergo screening for retinopathy of prematurity (ROP). Recent guidelines include all babies <34 weeks and/or weighing <2 kg, babies >2 kg with risk factors should undergo screening.

Risk factors include sepsis, respiratory distress, apnea, and severe jaundice undergone exchange transfusion.

The retina is divided into zones I, II, and III. Zone I is centered on the optic nerve, from which the retinal arterioles emerge, and zone III exists as a crescent of retina on the temporal side; zone II occupies the midportion of the retina in all four quadrants. The severity is indicated by stages 1-5 with stage 1 representing mild ROP and stage 5 representing a total retinal detachment.

There will be abnormal retinal vascular system. This includes fibrovascular proliferation involving vitreous. This causes poor macular development and retinal detachment. White fibrovascular mass may occupy retrolental space producing retrolental fibroplasia and leukocoria.

353 CHAPTER

Rumination

Rumination is not typically considered reflux, it is the voluntary contraction of abdominal musculature that leads to the episodes that manifests similar to the reflux. It is generally regarded as self-stimulating disorder and is more common in adolescence and in various behavioral disorders.

CHAPTER 354 Salivary Glands Pain

Pain in one or other of the major salivary glands is associated with enlargement of the affected organ itself. Painful enlargement of the sublingual gland is seen as a manifestation of mumps, together with painful enlargement of the other glands.

The painful salivary swellings may be classified as follows:

- *Parotid gland:*
  - Mumps (epidemic parotitis)
  - Acute bacterial suppurative parotitis—postoperative dehydration, following radiotherapy
  - Parotitis association with duct obstruction (calculus and trauma)
  - Carcinoma (primary or spread from another focus)
- *Submandibular gland:*
  - Mumps (rare)
  - Inflammation associated with duct obstruction
  - Carcinoma

MUMPS

Mumps is transmitted by droplet infection and has an incubation period of 17–21 days. It is the most common cause of a painful parotid swelling. There is prodromal fever with malaise. Only one gland may be involved, or both may be affected simultaneously. The swelling progresses for several days with a marked tenderness of the gland and thickening of the overlying skin. There is characteristic uplifting of the lobe of the ear and stiffness of the jaw.

PAROTITIS ASSOCIATED WITH DUCT OBSTRUCTION

Obstruction of a salivary duct, from any cause, results in a typical syndrome in which the gland becomes painful and swollen at meal times, due to the increased secretion of saliva being unable to discharge through the duct. Between meals, as the saliva gradually escapes, the swelling and pain subside. Frequently, inflammation of the obstructed gland occurs as a result of ascending infection from mouth organisms. Under these circumstances, there may be the associated features of infection and there may be a discharge of pus from the mouth of the duct.

Other causes of parotid duct stenosis are trauma from the irritation of an adjacent tooth stump or, occasionally, from traumatic division of the duct.

355 CHAPTER

Salivary Gland Swelling

Bacterial parotid sialadenitis is frequent in young children and presents with painful unilateral parotid swelling. Purulent material can be expressed intraorally from the parotid duct upon parotid massage. Management involves oral antibiotics, hydration, sialogogues, parotid glands massage, and warm compresses **(Fig. 1)**.

Mumps: Patients usually present with bilateral painful parotid enlargement and mild fever, and, rarely, with acute unilateral hearing loss or vestibular weakness.

Therapy comprises adequate hydration and analgesics.

Tuberculosis may affect the parotid or other salivary glands with or without lung involvement; sarcoidosis may present with unilateral or bilateral parotid swelling, along with systemic symptoms and peripheral lymphadenopathy. HIV infection commonly involves the parotid glands, presenting as bilateral intraglandular cysts that recur after needle aspiration.

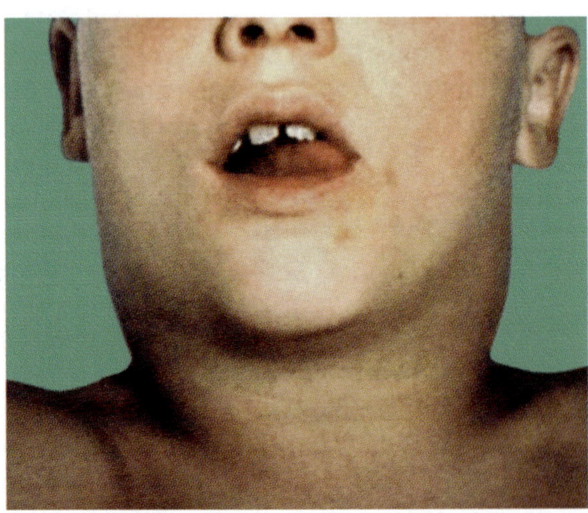

Fig. 1: Salivary gland swelling.

Scabies

Scabies is an extremely common eruption. It occurs in persons of all ages and results from infestation of the superficial layers of skin by the human mite *Sarcoptes scabiei*. The infestation is highly contagious and is, therefore, seen frequently among individuals living in crowded conditions. Humans are the only source of the mite, which can be passed from one person to another. Fomites can also play an important role in transmission. In previously unexposed individuals, the incubation period varies from 2 to 6 weeks. The incubation period is significantly shortened in individuals who have been previously exposed to the mite.

Although the morphologic appearance of scabies can vary dramatically, the hallmark lesion is the burrow. A burrow is a serpiginous or linear papule caused by movement of the mite through the epidermis. Although considered to be characteristic of scabies, the burrow is apparent in only a minority of patients.

Other typical lesions include papules, vesicles, and pustules, the distribution of which is age dependent. Nodules may appear during active infection and may persist for several weeks to months after treatment; these are common in infantile scabies and on the penis and scrotum of affected males. These persistent nodules are referred to as postscabetic nodules and may be a manifestation of an ongoing hypersensitivity response. In infants, the distribution is generalized and involves the trunk, scalp, face, neck, axillae, palms, and soles. Because the eruption is extremely pruritic, secondary infection and eczematization are common, leading to misdiagnoses of impetigo and atopic dermatitis. In affected older children, adolescents, and adults, the lesions characteristically involve the volar aspects of the wrists, ankles, interdigital web spaces, buttocks, genitalia, groin, abdomen, and axillae. Unlike infantile scabies, the lesions always spare the head.

The diagnosis can be confirmed by scraping the newer lesions, ideally a burrow, with a blade after the application of mineral oil. The scraping may be viewed microscopically, and the presence of mites, ova, or feces is considered diagnostic. Although the yield may be low, suspect lesions should be scraped and an attempt to identify evidence of the mite should be made. In prolonged cases of scabies, which have been appropriately treated, the diagnosis of acropustulosis of infancy needs to be considered.

CHAPTER 357 Scleroderma

Scleroderma is classified into systemic sclerosis (SSc) and localized scleroderma. Localized scleroderma (LS), which includes morphea and linear scleroderma, is limited to the skin and subcutaneous tissues, is much more common in childhood, and rarely progresses to involve internal organs. SSc can be life-threatening, as it has the potential to involve internal organs and cause severe and widespread skin disease.

MORPHEA

Morphea is a patch of hardened skin that appears spontaneously on any part of the body. The skin becomes firm, stiff, atrophic, and discolored. Hair is absent. Initially, the lesion appears violaceous, but then it fades to a yellowish-brown or dusky appearance in most individuals. The patches are nontender, and children are otherwise asymptomatic. The natural history of morphea lesions is to gradually fade and soften after an initial period of expansion. Biopsy reveals excessive amounts of collagen in the dermis with absent hair follicles and diminished vascular structures.

LINEAR SCLERODERMA

Linear scleroderma is histologically similar to morphea, though lesions consist not of isolated patches, but rather narrow bands that may extend through an entire limb, part of the limb, or across the scalp and face, a finding termed a coup de sabre lesion. Cosmetically and functionally, linear scleroderma is much more severe than morphea, as the impacted areas may involve the face or limit limb use. Growth of the limb may be affected, and involvement of the digits can cause significant functional difficulty. Coup de sabre lesions, particularly with craniofacial involvement, may be associated with neurologic abnormalities and seizures, and these children should have a careful neurologic examination and brain MRI as part of their evaluation.

SYSTEMIC SCLEROSIS

Systemic sclerosis typically begins with severe Raynaud phenomenon, followed by thickening and tightening of the skin over the digits and hands and then the face, and then by varying degrees of progressive skin changes over the extremities and trunk. Difficulty opening the mouth and decreased facial expression are signs of facial involvement. As the skin over the hands tightens and hardens, pigment changes may occur, and flexion contractures of the small joints may develop. Renal disease, pulmonary fibrosis, pulmonary hypertension, esophageal and gut dysmotility, and cardiac disease may all occur.

The scleroderma disorders in children encompass both SSc and LS, also termed *morphea*. In childhood-onset scleroderma,

SSc is much less common than LS and comprises <10% of all SSc cases. Both share the general features of an earlier inflammatory state followed by collagen deposition and atrophy of the affected tissue. Skin biopsies of these subjects are typically indistinguishable, and they may share some common pathophysiology. However, their clinical manifestations are markedly different with unique morbidities and prognoses. LS is typically confined to the skin and underlying tissue, and although not fatal like SSc, up to a quarter of the patients may have extracutaneous disease manifestations, such as joint contractures and uveitis. Although any organ may be affected in SSc, vascular (Raynaud phenomenon), cutaneous (skin thickening), gastrointestinal, pulmonary, and musculoskeletal involvements are most commonly seen in children. Both SSc and LS can be further classified by subtype.

CHAPTER 358 Scrofuloderma

It is quite common. It constitutes about 20% of tuberculosis; cervical glands are more frequently involved. This is followed by axillary lymph node. Supraclavicular, tonsillar, submandibular, periauricular, axillary, and inguinal lymph nodes are commonly involved. They are less severe form of extrapulmonary tuberculosis.

The gland may caseate and discharge its necrotic material into the skin. This results in exudative skin lesions. This is called scrofuloderma. Fine-needle aspiration cytology or gland biopsy is done to confirm the diagnosis.

359 CHAPTER

Scrotal Swelling

Swelling of the scrotum in the neonate is relatively common, especially in breech deliveries **(Fig. 1)**. Although the differential diagnosis includes hematomas, infections, testicular torsion, and tumors, the majority of cases are attributable to hydroceles or fluid accumulation in the tunica vaginalis. Palpation reveals an extremely smooth, firm, egg-shaped mass that brightly transilluminates. When the hydrocele is noncommunicating, the clinician can often palpate above the mass with the thumb and finger and feel a normal spermatic cord. The testicle may be difficult to palpate but is usually visible on transillumination. With inguinal hernias, the prolapsed intestine may transilluminate as well, but it usually presents visible septa under high-intensity light. Furthermore, on palpation, there is significant thickening of the spermatic cord. Although a hydrocele may persist for months, the majority resolve spontaneously. There is a high association with inguinal hernias, especially in hydroceles that persist. In such cases, the spermatic cord is often noticeably thickened. Given the association with hernias, the possibility of bowel incarceration should be kept in mind. Surgical repair is indicated when a hydrocele persists for >6 months or when as a communicating hydrocele. These hydroceles will randomly appear to become smaller and larger over time.

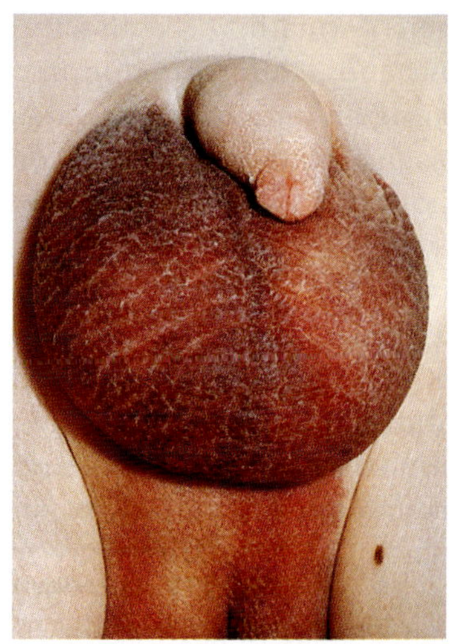

Fig. 1: Scrotal swelling.

A swollen and tender or bruised scrotum may be a sign of testicular torsion and should be investigated with urgency to salvage the testicle if possible. Testicular torsion may occur in utero and may present with scrotal ecchymosis, but there may be no swelling or tenderness, if the torsion was not recent.

360 CHAPTER Seborrhea: Cradle Cap

Seborrheic dermatitis is characterized by erythema and scaling predominantly on hair-bearing and intertriginous areas, such as the scalp; eyebrows; eyelashes; perinasal, presternal, and postauricular areas; and the neck, axillae, and groin **(Fig. 1)**. Lesions often involve the intertriginous areas of the arms, legs, neck, and trunk, and occasionally become generalized. In affected infants, scalp lesions consist of a thick, tenacious, scaly dermatitis that is often salmon colored and is commonly known as *cradle cap*. In adolescents, the dermatitis may manifest as dandruff or flaking of the eyebrows, postauricular areas, or flexural areas.

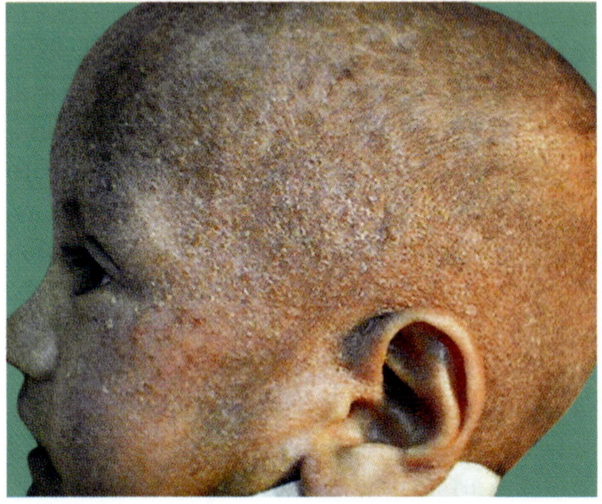

Fig. 1: Cradle cap.

Although the pathogenesis of seborrheic dermatitis is unknown, *Pityrosporum* and *Candida* species have been implicated as causative agents. A role for neurologic dysfunction is suggested by the increased incidence and severity in neurologically impaired individuals.

The dermatitis of seborrhea is usually nonpruritic and mild in nature. Most cases respond to topical steroids, and many clear spontaneously, although residual postinflammatory hypopigmentation may persist for weeks or months thereafter.

Some practitioners find that use of a topical antifungal cream or wash, in addition to a low-potency topical steroid, hastens resolution, but the topical steroid should not be part of long-term management. In infants and young children, atopic dermatitis can have a greasy, scaly appearance and can have overlapping features with seborrhea. However, infantile atopic dermatitis produces intense pruritus and invariably spares moist sites, such as the diaper area and axillae. The two are often present simultaneously in the same patient. The differential diagnosis of seborrhea includes Langerhans cell histiocytosis (in which the rash is more generalized, in part petechial, and can be associated with chronic draining ears and hepatosplenomegaly) and tinea corporis (in which lesions usually are more circumscribed, with an active border and central clearing). Scalp lesions may be difficult to differentiate from psoriasis, and, in fact, there seems to be a spectrum of presentation from mild scaling in seborrhea to moderate scaling in what is termed *sebopsoriasis* to much more thick and resistant scaling in full-fledged psoriasis.

CHAPTER 361 Sensation Abnormalities

TERMINOLOGY

Anesthesia means "without feeling", but neurologists use it for loss of sensibility to light touch; and partial reduction of such sensibility is called "hypoesthesia" or "hyperesthesia". Analgesia (loss of pain) and hypoalgesia or hyperalgesia (reduction of pain sensibility) are useful terms, free from ambiguity. These cutaneous sensibilities, together with those derived from the special senses, are called "exteroceptive". "Proprioceptive" sensibility is concerned with information received from the labyrinths and from muscle and joint receptors. Vibration sense is difficult to classify and is of no apparent value to humans (but it did warn our ancestors of the herd of animals; they could not see but their naked feet could feel by vibration), but its loss may help to localize a lesion, especially of the spinal cord.

Hyperesthesia, hyperalgesia, and hyperthermesthesia refer to increased sensibility to touch, pain, and temperature, respectively. Increased sensibility to proprioceptive stimulation has not been described.

ANATOMY AND PHYSIOLOGY

The four common cutaneous sensations—touch, pain, heat, and cold—together with the deep sensations of pressure and proprioception are referred to as the "somatic sensation". These are consciously appreciated in all parts of the body, and they have a common pathway within the nervous system.

The pathways for somatic sensation are subserved by three orders of neurons: the first-order neuron is concerned with transmitting information from the periphery to the spinal cord; the second-order neuron transmits information from the spinal cord to the thalamus; and the third-order neuron transmits information from the thalamus to the cerebral cortex.

RECEPTORS

Information to the first-order neurons comes from a variety of receptors. Every sensation depends on impulses excited by the adequate stimulation of these receptors, which comprise two main groups—those in skin and those in the deeper somatic structure. Although individual cutaneous sensory receptors are most sensitive to a particular form of natural stimulation. This specificity is not absolute and other forms of stimulation may also excite the receptors.

TRANSMISSION OF INFORMATION FROM RECEPTORS

The simulation of a sensory ending gives rise to a receptor potential which appears at the specialized end of an afferent nerve fiber. Impulses from the receptors travel centrally through the first-order neurons, the cell bodies of which are in the dorsal root ganglia.

AFFERENT PATHWAYS TO THE SPINAL CORD

The afferent sensory fibers from the various receptors pass up the differing peripheral nerves and enter the spinal cord via the dorsal roots. It should be emphasized that there is considerable overlap in the peripheral nerve distributions and in the dermatomes distributions.

There is some evidence to suggest that a number of afferent fibers pass the cord in ventral roots. The significance of these is uncertain, but their presence may be responsible for the persistence of pain in some patients after dorsal rhizotomy.

All of the somatic sensory pathways are crossed and terminate in the opposite sensory cortex in the cerebral hemisphere. Anatomically separate pathways may be recognized there.

DORSAL COLUMN MEDIAL LEMNISCUS PATHWAY

Input to this pathway within the spinal cord is via large, thickly myelinated fibers which pass through the medial division of the dorsal spinal nerve root to enter the dorsal white column of their own side, dividing into ascending and descending branches. The descending branches establish reflex connection by sending collateral branches into the dorsal gray column; the ascending branches are the first link in the sensory pathway. At their entrance, these ascending fibers are situated immediately medial to the dorsal horn, but during their course up the spinal cord they are steadily pushed to a more medial position because the fibers entering at succeeding rostral levels intrude between the ascending fibers and the dorsal horn. As a consequence of this, the fibers occupying the most medial part of the dorsal column in the upper cervical region will belong to the sacral roots, while the fibers from the upper extremity are found most laterally. The fibers terminate at the cervicomedullary junction in the nucleus gracilis and nucleus cuneatus. The fibers terminate synaptically on to the second-order neurons in the gracile and cuneate nuclei and the axons of these neurons curve ventrally and medially, crossing the midline, and then turn upward to form a prominent bundle of fibers, the medial lemniscus.

The classical view is that the impulses ascending in the fibers of the dorsal columns mediate the sensations of touch, deep pressure, vibratory sense and sense of position of joint, and are particularly important for sensory discrimination.

The segmental somatotopic organization presents as the dorsal columns and their nuclei are maintained in the medial lemniscus as it ascends to the thalamic where the fibers enter the ventroposterior lateral nucleus which contains the cell bodies of the third-order sensory neurons.

CLASSIFICATION OF SENSORY SYSTEM

- *Superficial sensory system:*
    - Touch
    - Pain
    - Temperature—cold/hot
- *Deep sensory system:*
    - Pressure
    - Joint sensation
    - Vibration
- *Cortical:*
    - Stereognosis
    - Discrimination
    - Extinction

- *Special sensory system:*
    - Smell
    - Taste
    - Hearing
    - Vision

LATERAL SPINOTHALAMIC PATHWAY

This transmits impulses which are concerned with the appreciation of heat, cold, and pain. It also provides an alternative pathway for touch sensibility, the so-called "crude" or "coarse" touch. The first-order neurons have their cell bodies in the dorsal root ganglia, and their fibers are thinner than those of the dorsal column medial lemniscus pathways; some, indeed (the C fibers), have no myelin at all. They enter the spinal cord in the lateral part of the dorsal root and divide into short descending and ascending branches. The ascending branches run for one or two segments in the posterolateral column before synapsing with second-order sensory neurons which lie deep in the dorsal column. The axons then cross the midline, the so-called "ventral white commissure", and ascend in the ventrolateral white column as the spinothalamic tract. Some of the spinothalamic fibers give off collaterals to certain nuclear regions such as the reticular formation.

In the brainstem, the spinothalamic tract lies lateral to the medial lemniscus, which it accompanies to terminate in the thalamus in the ventroposterior lateral nucleus.

The second-order neuron fibers cross the midline only one or two segments above the level of the dorsal root fibers.

The site of decussation of the fibers in the cord exposes them to damage by expanding ventral cord lesions.

Fibers concerned with pain and temperature sensibility are situated dorsally to those involved with touch and pressure.

The spinothalamic tract is less compactly organized than the medical lemniscus, being intermingled with other ascending pathways giving off collaterals to the brainstem reticular formation.

TRIGEMINOTHALAMIC PATHWAY

This pathway carries information from the distribution of the trigeminal nerve which serves most of the skin of the face, the forehead as far as the vertex, the mucous membranes of the nasal cavities, paranasal sinuses, mouth, tongue and parts of the pharynx, the teeth and gums, and part of the dura mater.

About half of the fibers entering in the trigeminal nerve divide into a branch which terminates in the chief nucleus of the trigeminal nerve, while the other half descend in the spinal tract to end in the spinal nucleus. The chief nucleus, which is in the lateral part of the pons, contains the second-order neurons concerned with tactile and postural sensibility; it gives rise to fibers which cross the midline to ascend near the medial lemniscus. The nucleus of the spinal tract, which extends downward in the lateral part of the medulla to about the level of C2, contains the second-order neurons concerned with pain and temperature sensibility. Second-order neurons cross to the quintothalamic tract, which ascends close to the spinothalamic tract. Both sets of second-order neuron fibers terminate in the ventroposterior medial nucleus of the thalamus.

THALAMUS AND THALAMOCORTICAL PROJECTIONS

The third neuronal link in the ascending somatic sensory fiber system is made up of neurons; the nuclei of which are in the thalamus. The axons of these neurons transmit impulses to the cerebral cortex.

SOMATOSENSORY CORTICAL AREAS

From clinical and physiological observations, it has been known for many years that, in man, the postcentral gyrus is the main (primary) somatosensory area. Another area beneath the lower end of the postcentral gyms is known as the secondary somatosensory area. The first sensory area appears principally to reflect activity in the dorsal column medial lemniscus system and also in the associated trigeminal system. The thalamic relay for these impulses passes through the internal capsule.

However inadequate our understanding of the sensory cortex, one thing is clear: provided that the subcortical structures—especially the thalamus—are intact; certain sensations such as pain, touch, pressure, and extremes of temperature can reach consciousness.

The accurate localization, however, as well as the patient's ability to make sensory discriminations depends on the integrity of the sensory cortex. This is a fundamental distinction and will be discussed further when considering individual sensory syndromes.

MONONEUROPATHY

Changes in this instance will vary, depending on whether the nerve involved is predominantly motor, sensory, or mixed. In sensory nerves, the area of touch loss is usually more extensive than the area of pain loss. Because of overlap from adjacent nerves, the area of sensory loss following damage to a cutaneous nerve is always less than its anatomical distribution. Deep pressure and joint position senses remain intact because they are mediated by nerve fibers from the subcutaneous structures and joints. Particular types of pathological lesion may differentially affect the fibers in a sensory nerve. Compression typically disturbs large touch and pressure fibers and leaves intact small pain, thermal and autonomic fibers. Lesions of the brachial or lumbosacral plexus may be differentiated from multiple peripheral nerve involvement by the distribution of the sensory and motor loss.

POLYNEUROPATHY

In most instances of polyneuropathy, the longest and largest fibers tend to be involved. The sensory loss is most severe over the feet and legs and less severe over the hands, and the trunk and face are usually spared except in the most severe cases. Typically, the sensory loss involves all the modalities, although this varies depending on the type of neuropathy. The term "glove and stocking" sensory loss draws attention to the distal pattern of involvement. However, it is an inaccurate term as the border between normal and abnormal sensation is not sharp, and the sensory loss shades off gradually.

RADICULOPATHY

Irritative symptoms may be present when the dorsal roots are the subject of traction or compression. This shows itself as pain which is often limited to the dermatome belonging to the affected root. In some root disorders, pain is absent and paresthesias in the dermatome distribution are present. Damage to a dorsal root will result in a loss of sensory modalities of all types within the distribution of the dermatome. Because of overlap between dermatomes, interruption of one single dorsal root will often give no definite sensory loss. When two or more roots have been completely divided, the zone of sensory loss is usually greater for pain than for touch. Surrounding the area of complete loss will be a zone of partial loss.

CHAPTER 362 Shifting Dullness

SHIFTING DULLNESS

Shifting dullness and fluid thrill (wave) are clinical signs that confirm ascites. Free fluid will flow to the dependent part of the abdominal cavity, while the gut filled with air will float in the middle. If the child is supine, the fluid collects posteriorly and in the flanks. The percussion note, therefore, will be resonant in the center and dull in the flanks. Starting in the middle, the percussion is carried laterally toward the flanks, where the note will become dull. Ask the child to roll over to the opposite side. The previous area of flank dullness now becomes resonant as the fluid moves to the dependent part of the abdominal cavity. The same technique can be used for either flank.

In ascites, the border of the dullness shifts to the dependent side as fluid resettles with gravity. As fluid accumulates in the flank in supine position, there will be dull to percuss. This resembles horseshoe. Hence, the dullness is called horseshoe dullness.

CHAPTER 363

Short Neck

Short neck: In infants, the neck is usually short but certain conditions have an obvious short neck as their distinguishing feature. They are:

- Morquio disease
- Gargoylism
- Cretinism
- Klippel-Feil syndrome
- Pterygium coli (web neck)
- Bilateral Sprengel's deformity

Short neck is associated with a host of musculoskeletal abnormalities of the neck and skull. Torticollis is a frequent association, wherein the odontoid process is eccentrically poised. Abnormal bone fusions of the cervical spine include assimilation of atlas, C2-3 fusion, and Klippel-Feil abnormalities.

Short Stature

Short stature is defined as height >2 SD below the mean for age, which is at the 2.3 percentile. On growth charts (and in clinical practice), it is more common to define short stature as height below the 3rd percentile for age, which is –1.88 SD. Implicit in this definition is the understanding that height is a normally distributed characteristic; therefore, a proportion of normal individuals have heights >2 SD from the mean.

Growth failure is defined as a subnormal rate of growth, or a height velocity that is below the norm for that age. Since sustained height velocity below the 25th percentile is insufficient to maintain a child's position on the growth chart, growth failure is sometimes defined as a height velocity below the 25th percentile for age.

Growth delay is often associated with delayed puberty. There is often family history of both. The bone age assessed from a radiograph of wrist and hand will usually be delayed by 3 years or more.

Children with short stature can be classified in two groups depending on their skeletal maturation: (1) those with short stature and concordant bone age, and (2) those with short stature and delayed bone age. In turn, each one of these two groups can be divided into those growing at a normal rate and those growing at a decreased rate. Therefore, four groups result from this classification. Those with adequate growth velocity likely have one of the normal variants of short stature: familial short stature (concordant bone age) and constitutional delay of growth (delayed bone age). The genetic height potential of a child is heavily influenced by the growth achieved by both parents and their relatives. The heritability of height has been estimated to be 0.7–0.8, rising to as much as 0.9 between identical twins.

On the other hand, children with decreased growth velocity (e.g., growth failure by definition) are more likely to have a pathological reason for their abnormal growth pattern. Endocrine disorders [e.g., growth hormone (GH) deficiency, GH insensitivity, hypothyroidism, and Cushing syndrome] and nonendocrine causes (e.g., malnutrition, chronic illness, and psychosocial) are likely associated with growth failure accompanied by delayed skeletal maturation, whereas dysgenetic (e.g., chromosomal disorders, some specific genetic syndromes, and chondrodysplasias) are more likely to be associated with growth failure and concordant skeletal maturation.

Although this algorithm is useful in the assessment of short stature, two caveats need to be emphasized: (1) this approach is not fool proof because exceptions may apply, and (2) a short child does not necessarily fall into one single category but may have components of two or more categories. An example of the first caveat is the short stature associated with pseudohypoparathyroidism type 1a (Albright hereditary osteodystrophy). These individuals have both a dysgenetic and an endocrine component to their short stature, yet their skeletal maturation is frequently described as advanced. Another example involves girls with Turner syndrome, a dysgenetic cause of short stature, who may have a delay in skeletal maturation at the usual time of puberty due to low estrogen production and gonadal dysgenesis. The finding of abnormal body proportions in a child with short stature should elicit suspicion for chondrodysplasias and rickets. Body proportions are usually preserved in other causes of short stature.

CAUSES OF SHORT STATURE

- Constitutional
- Nutritional
- Primordial
- Hypothyroidism
- Hypopituitarism
- Down's syndrome
- Renal tubular acidosis
- Achondroplasia
- Rickets
- Emotional deprivation

Normal Variants

The two most frequent causes of short stature in children are familial short stature and constitutional delay of growth and puberty. These are considered normal variants and their recognition can help avoid expensive and unnecessary testing and interventions.

Most short children have small parents. The short child whose centile within parents normal range should be seen in 6 months time to make sure that the growth velocity is normal.

Familial Short Stature

The term "familial short stature" is usually reserved for familial forms of mild-to-moderate short stature that do not have a specific identifiable genetic defect; since hundreds of genes play a role in growth, this height potential likely reflects the influence of multiple loci of small effect or a few loci of relatively moderate effect.

Laboratory studies are not mandatory, but if done are all normal. The bone age is also normal, and this suggests that the short child's "room for growth" is not greater than that of other children of the same age. Prediction of adult height can be made on the basis of bone age, but the accuracy is variable; the predicted height is within 9 cm of the midparental height (MPH).

Constitutional Delay of Growth and Puberty

These children often begin to show moderate short stature (height, –1.5 to –2.5 SD) during early-to-middle childhood but are otherwise healthy. They have delayed onset of puberty and, therefore, a delayed growth spurt. One or both parents (or other family members) may have a history of delayed puberty and a late adolescent growth spurt, with eventual cessation of growth during late adolescence or even into the 3rd decade of life. The affected parent usually is of normal adult stature. Otherwise, the history and review of systems are negative. The physical examination findings are normal except for delayed onset of puberty in children of an appropriate age.

Laboratory tests are not mandatory but are normal if performed, with the important exception of a delayed bone age (bone age <chronologic age).

Idiopathic Short Stature

Idiopathic short stature (ISS) is a clinical description rather than a disease. ISS is generally considered a normal variant of growth (since pathologic causes are excluded by definition). The exact definition varies from country to country; ISS is defined as height >2.25 SD below the age mean (which is the 1st percentile for height) for children in whom no specific cause of short stature has been identified after a thorough evaluation. This corresponds to an adult height <160 cm (5 feet 3 inches) for males and <150 cm (4 feet 11 inches) for females.

Idiopathic short stature is a diagnosis of exclusion; history, physical examination, laboratory studies, and imaging studies do not reveal any specific cause of short stature in an otherwise normal child.

Small for Gestational Age

Children who are born small for gestational age (SGA) usually catch up with their peers by 2–3 years of age, but 10–20% of children born SGA will fail to catch up and will continue to be below the 3rd percentile. This is more likely in children who are born premature as well as SGA and in those most severely affected at birth. The mechanism underlying this failure of catch-up growth is not well understood. Children with intrauterine growth restriction (IUGR) also have an increased future risk of metabolic disorders such as type 2 diabetes. Children who were SGA typically have normal proportions and no other physical findings; in some cases, the IUGR is one component of a genetic syndrome and other features of the syndrome are present.

Children who were born SGA with poor postnatal growth typically have normal or even elevated GH levels, but lower average values of insulin-like growth factor-1 (IGF-1) and insulin-like growth factor binding protein-3 (IGFBP-3) (though most are still in the normal range) indicate some degree of GH resistance in at least some of these children.

Fetal Alcohol Syndrome

The effect of exposure to significant levels of serum alcohol during gestation results in a pattern of microcephaly, prenatal and postnatal growth deficiency, short palpebral fissures, long smooth philtrum, and a thin upper lip. Other features include a short nose and hypoplasia of the nails and distal phalanges (particularly the fifth toes). On occasion, affected infants have eyelid ptosis, epicanthal folds, strabismus, small raised hemangiomas, cervical vertebral abnormalities, and congenital heart disease.

Newborns with fetal alcohol syndrome are SGA and have poor catch-up growth postnatally. They may have increased or decreased muscle tone and can be irritable and tremulous. Most older children tend to be thin and hyperactive, and >80% have some delay in development, especially fine motor function.

The diagnosis of fetal alcohol syndrome should be reserved for those infants who have a history of in utero exposure to large amounts of alcohol and who have the characteristic physical features of the disorder. The past practice of labeling children with developmental disorders who do not have the clinical stigmata as having fetal alcohol effects should be abandoned.

Nonendocrine causes of pathologic short stature include chronic illness (e.g., renal tubular acidosis, celiac disease, cystic fibrosis, inflammatory bowel disease, and so on), adverse psychosocial milieu, undernutrition, and genetic disorders.

Head trauma, brain tumors, encephalitis, pneumonia, and some drugs are associated with overproduction of arginine vasopressin (AVP). This can lead to inappropriate water retention and hyponatremia, known as the *syndrome of inappropriate antidiuretic hormone secretion (SIADH)*. The symptoms of SIADH include headache, apathy, nausea, vomiting, and impaired consciousness. Underproduction of AVP results in central diabetes insipidus. Diabetes insipidus can result from pituitary tumors, head trauma, infiltrative disease processes (such as Langerhans cell histiocytosis, sarcoidosis, hemochromatosis, and autoimmune hypophysitis), or from any surgery that damages the pituitary gland and hypothalamus. Familial central diabetes insipidus, which is inherited in both recessive and dominant patterns, is rare and has its onset in infancy. Wolfram syndrome is an autosomal dominant form of central diabetes insipidus often associated with diabetes mellitus, optic atrophy, and deafness (DIDMOAD).

Endocrine Disorders

Endocrine causes of short stature including GH deficiency, GH insensitivity, GH receptor mutations or defects in the GH post-receptor cascade leading to deficient IGF-1, hypothyroidism, or sustained hypercortisolism (Cushing syndrome) either from endogenous or exogenous sources are characterized by linear growth deceleration, whereas weight gain is either not affected or even increased. This is a useful distinguishing feature of endocrine disorders in comparison to the other three causes of short stature in the last category of the algorithm (malnutrition, chronic illness, and psychosocial) where the weight is usually more affected than the height.

Growth Hormone Deficiency

Growth hormone is essential for postnatal growth, and children who lack it are extremely stunted. GH deficiency may be congenital or acquired. The congenital form may be associated with other pituitary hormone deficiencies [multiple pituitary hormone deficiency (MPHD)] and may be associated with midline craniofacial defects [absence of the septum pellucidum and optic nerve hypoplasia (septo-optic dysplasia), cleft palate, holoprosencephaly, and single central incisor]. Genetic testing has revealed underlying genetic mutations in transcription factors involved in the development of the anterior pituitary in many (but not all) of these cases. Isolated congenital GH deficiency is relatively rare.

Growth hormone deficiency may also be acquired secondary to birth injury, head injury, midline tumors (most commonly craniopharyngioma), and cranial irradiation.

Growth Hormone Insensitivity

Growth hormone action may be impaired due to mutations of the GH receptor (Laron syndrome), defects in postreceptor signaling, mutations in the IGF-1 gene, deficiency of the ALS protein, and defects in IGF-1 action. All of these conditions are very rare and constitute only a tiny fraction of the cases of short stature and growth failure seen in clinical practice.

Other clinical features of Laron syndrome include small head circumference, characteristic facies with saddle nose and prominent forehead, delayed skeletal maturation, small genitalia and testes, short limb length compared to trunk length, and abnormal body composition with osteopenia and obesity. Intellectual development is normal or only modestly impaired. Prenatal growth is near normal, but postnatal growth is profoundly affected, with heights as low as –10 SD.

Hypothyroidism

Hypothyroidism impairs linear growth. Thyroid deficiency may be congenital or acquired. In view of the usefulness of neonatal

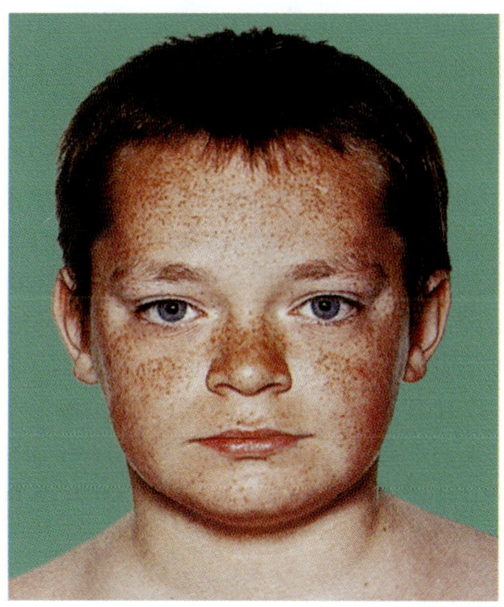

Fig. 1: Hypothyroidism.

thyroid screening programs, it is very uncommon for congenital hypothyroidism to go untreated and cause short stature **(Fig. 1)**.

Acquired hypothyroidism in children usually results from autoimmune thyroiditis. Children with Turner syndrome, Down syndrome, Klinefelter syndrome, celiac disease, or diabetes mellitus are at increased risk for autoimmune hypothyroidism, as are children with a family history of autoimmune disease. Acquired hypothyroidism tends to manifest most commonly in older children and teenagers. Often there are few complaints except for slow growth (after previously normal growth), weight gain, a goiter, or a combination of these. Other symptoms (dry hair or skin, constipation, and cold intolerance) are less common.

Glucocorticoid Excess (Cushing Syndrome)

Cushing syndrome results from excessive levels of glucocorticoids. Whether endogenous or exogenous, glucocorticoids markedly stunt growth. In general, because such conditions are acquired, the history reveals a child previously growing well whose growth velocity slows. The child typically continues to gain weight at a rapid rate, even though linear growth is attenuated. This is in contrast to exogenous obesity, in which affected children tend to grow at normal or rapid rates. The history may indicate that the child was treated with oral, topical (especially with occlusive dressings), or intradermal glucocorticoids at high doses or for long durations. Alternate-day oral glucocorticoids are much less likely to attenuate growth than are daily doses. Cushing syndrome is very unlikely with inhaled corticosteroids (ICS), but a small effect on linear growth may be seen with the use of high-potency ICS.

Physical findings in endogenous Cushing syndrome may include acne, virilization, and increased appetite. Hyperpigmentation may occur when Cushing syndrome is secondary to excessive adrenocorticotropic hormone (ACTH) levels. This may be caused by ACTH from a pituitary tumor (Cushing disease) or (less commonly) from a nonpituitary source (ectopic ACTH syndrome).

The physical examination usually reveals short stature with relative obesity. Many affected children have the moon face and plethora characteristic of Cushing syndrome. A buffalo hump, large purple striae, acne, and hypertension may also be present. Marked virilization is worrisome because it may indicate an adrenal tumor.

Other Endocrine Disorders

Diabetes mellitus, when poorly controlled, can lead to slow linear growth. The diagnosis should be apparent from the history. However, because of the risk of autoimmune thyroiditis and celiac disease, slow-growing children with diabetes should also be checked for hypothyroidism and celiac disease.

Diabetes insipidus, when poorly controlled or untreated, may lead to slow growth. High fluid intake in central diabetes insipidus is dramatically decreased with vasopressin; treatment of nephrogenic diabetes insipidus is more challenging.

Vitamin D deficiency rickets, hypophosphatemic rickets, and pseudohypoparathyroidism are also associated with short stature, but bony abnormalities and disorders of calcium and phosphate metabolism, rather than short stature, are the usual presenting features of these disorders.

GENETIC CAUSES OF SHORT STATURE

Turner Syndrome

Turner syndrome is relatively common, with an incidence of 1/2,500 liveborn females, and is caused by the absence or abnormality of an X chromosome. Short stature is the *single most common physical finding* in Turner syndrome and may occur in the absence of any other physical finding **(Fig. 2)**. The mechanism by which short stature occurs in Turner syndrome is multifactorial, but haploinsufficiency (absence of 1 copy) of the *S*hort *S*tature *H*omeobo*X* gene *(SHOX)* is believed to play a major role. This gene is located within the pseudoautosomal region of the X chromosome, which escapes X-inactivation and is, therefore, normally expressed from both copies of the X chromosome. It is highly active in skeletal tissues, and its absence in Turner syndrome (where only 1 X chromosome is present, or if present, the 2nd X chromosome is abnormal) leads to haploinsufficiency and causes severe short stature.

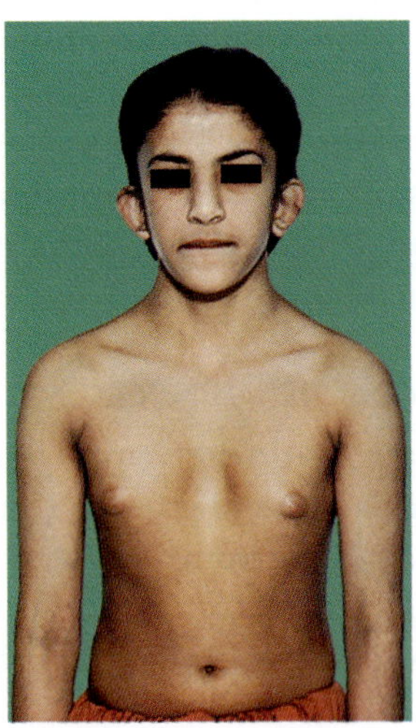

Fig. 2: Turner syndrome.

Down Syndrome

Short stature is a prominent feature in Down syndrome, but the mechanism by which trisomy 21 causes impaired growth is not known. It is independent of the hypothyroidism that may also occur in this condition. Specific treatment for short stature is typically not recommended in this condition.

Prader–Willi Syndrome

Prader–Willi syndrome (PWS) is characterized by hypotonia, failure to thrive with poor sucking during infancy, hypogonadism (manifested as cryptorchidism in males), short stature with small hands and feet, hyperphagia leading to morbid obesity beginning in early childhood, developmental delay/intellectual disability, and behavioral concerns including obsessive-compulsive disorder. The average adult height is 147 cm (4 feet 9 inches) in females and 155 cm (5 feet 1 inch) in males. PWS is caused by the absence or inactivity of a segment of the paternally inherited chromosome 15 (15q11.2-13), whereas deletion of the same chromosomal segment in the maternally inherited chromosome causes Angelman syndrome.

Noonan Syndrome

Noonan syndrome has an incidence of 1 in 1,000–2,500 live births. Approximately 50% of children with Noonan syndrome have a pathogenic variant in the *PTPN11* gene. There are currently 12 genes that have been identified in which pathogenic variants result in Noonan syndrome; these are much less common than *PTPN11* and include the genes: *SOS1, RAF1, KRAS, SHOC2, BRAF,NRAS, RIT1, CBL, KATB6, LZTR1,* and *SOS2*. The syndrome is characterized by minor facial dysmorphism (hypertelorism, downward eye slant, and low-set ears), proportionate short stature, and right-sided heart disease, most often pulmonic stenosis and hypertrophic cardiomyopathy.

Malnutrition

Worldwide, malnutrition resulting from poverty is still the most common cause of short stature. In North America, malnutrition may arise from inadequate intake secondary to poverty or deprivation, poor intake secondary to overt or occult chronic illness (e.g., inflammatory bowel disease, renal failure), or inability to utilize food intake (malabsorption). In all these conditions, weight tends to be depressed to a greater degree than height.

Chronic Illness

Chronic illnesses, such as inflammatory bowel disease, celiac disease, renal dysfunction, and chronic inflammation, can lead to short stature. The mechanisms of impaired growth include poor appetite or poor intake (e.g., inflammatory bowel disease, renal dysfunction), malabsorption (e.g., celiac disease), medications (e.g., chronic glucocorticoids for severe asthma), chronic acidosis (e.g., renal tubular acidosis), and secondary endocrine dysfunction (e.g., GH resistance associated with systemic inflammation). Although the primary disorder is evident in many cases, short stature is sometimes the presenting feature of the chronic disease. This occurs notably in inflammatory bowel disease, celiac disease, and renal dysfunction.

Bone Dysplasias

Achondroplasia

Achondroplasia is the classic example of an autosomal dominant chondrodysplasia. The incidence is approximately 1/20,000. This condition is relatively unique in that near all affected individuals have a gain of function mutation in the fibroblast growth factor receptor 3 *(FGFR3)* gene at position 1138, which results in a glycine to arginine amino acid substitution in the protein (p.Gly380Arg). An estimated 80% of the cases are due to de novo mutations (i.e., the parents do not have the mutation). Short stature, body disproportion with short limbs, hypotonia, and a relatively large head with midface hypoplasia are often noted at birth. A progressive deceleration of growth rate begins in infancy, and the humerus and femur are particularly shortened (rhizomelia; i.e., proximal shortening of the limbs). The hands may show a 3-pronged configuration (trident hand).

Hypochondroplasia

Hypochondroplasia is an allelic variant of achondroplasia and manifests with short stature and dysmorphic features that are often milder than in achondroplasia. In particular, there are few craniofacial abnormalities, and body disproportion may be subtle. Newborns may be slightly small, but short stature generally becomes apparent by age 3 years. The short stature is minimally disproportionate with relatively short limbs. The hands and feet are usually noted to show brachydactyly (shortening of the tubular bones). Genu varum may occur. Radiologic hallmarks include metaphyseal indentation and flaring as well as hypoplasia of the ilia with small greater sciatic notches. Some reports suggested a beneficial effect of GH, but this remains a nonstandard indication for GH treatment.

Spondyloepiphyseal Dysplasias

These are a heterogeneous group of dysplasias that primarily affect the epiphyses and the vertebral bodies. Most forms are characterized by a shortened trunk and vertebral anomalies. These conditions may lead to spinal cord compression due to subluxation of the cervical spine. GH therapy is not recommended.

Osteogenesis Imperfecta

Moderate and severe forms of osteogenesis imperfecta are associated with proportional short stature. The diagnosis is usually evident and short stature is not a presenting feature.

CHAPTER 365 Signs of Meningeal Irritation

NECK STIFFNESS

The patient lies supine on the flat surface. Examiner's hand is placed behind the head. Head is gently lifted off the bed and try to make the patient's chin touch the sternum. Tone or stiffness at the neck is felt. During the process, the legs are watched for hip and knee flexion. Normally, neck easily moves in both the planes and comfortably touches the chin.

KERNIG SIGN

Patient lies supine on the flat surface. The leg is flexed at hip with the knee flexed. Then knee is extended. Resistance to this indicates meningeal irritation.

BRUDZINSKI'S SIGN

Leg sign: It is done a Kernig sign. Leg on other side also flexes at the hip due to meningeal irritation.

Neck sign: Neck flexion produces the flexion at hip and knee.

Symphysis sign: Pressure over the pubic causes flexion of both lower limbs.

366 CHAPTER

Simian Crease

Simian crease: A single palmar crease is present in 5% of normal newborn and 45% of Down syndrome. It refers to single crease across the palm of the hand **(Figs. 1A and B)**. Hypoplasia of the middle phalanx in the fifth finger is present. This produces clinodactyly, i.e., deflection of the finger. Hands are short and broad. Gap between first and second toe is wide.

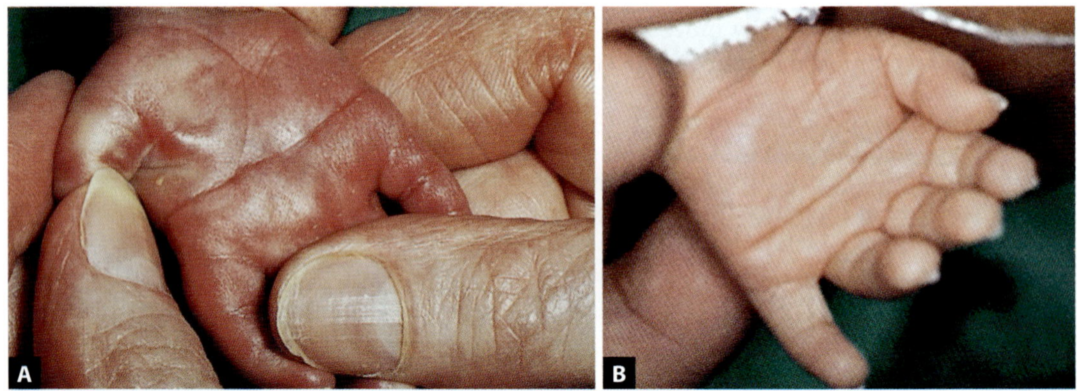

Figs. 1A and B: Simian crease.

CHAPTER 367

Sjögren Syndrome

A syndrome commonly associated with systemic lupus erythematosus (SLE) in children is Sjögren syndrome, characterized by keratoconjunctivitis and xerostomia due to decreased tear production and saliva production (complaints of "dry eye and dry mouth"). Sjögren syndrome may also present as recurring noninfectious parotiditis from recurrent infiltrate with lymphocytes of the parotid gland during times of active disease. The xerostomia can lead to abnormal taste, difficulty swallowing, and severe dental cavities. Other mucosal surfaces are dry, such as nose, pharynx, and vagina. The keratoconjunctivitis causes photophobia and irritation of the eyes described as "sand grinding in the eye." An additional recognizable cutaneous is photosensitivity with an erythematous rash appearing at sun-exposed areas. Only rarely in children, other systemic manifestations develop, such as interstitial nephritis or central nervous system (CNS) vasculitis.

Serologically, this syndrome typically features a positive result for antinuclear antibody (ANA), with specific extractable nuclear antigen antibodies to Ro (SS-A) and La (SS-B). Additionally, polyclonal hypergammaglobulinemia with high-titer RF and hypocomplementemia (low C3 and C4) are commonly demonstrated. Diagnosis is supported by objective ophthalmologic evidence of decreased tear flow, using Schirmer test for tear production and rose bengal stain to detect corneal erosions. Lip biopsy demonstrating a periductal lymphocytic infiltrate confirms the diagnosis, although uncommonly performed in children. Adults with Sjögren syndrome are at a higher risk to develop lymphoma.

CHAPTER 368

Skinfold Thickness

It is useful in the estimation of muscle mass or body fat content. The subcutaneous tissue mass will be maximum by 9 months. It decreases gradually till about 6 years. Later again, there will be increase in subcutaneous tissue. In clinical practice, measurement of triceps and subscapular skin fold thickness is done.

It is taken by measuring the fold of the skin running parallel to the length of the arm over the triceps muscle midway between acromion and olecranon.

Child's arm is flexed at 90°. Midpoint is marked on the posterior aspect of the arm. Skinfold is grasped 1 cm above the midpoint. Skinfold is gently pulled away from the underlying muscle and measured. It is measured to nearest 1.0 mm. It is measured by special calipers (i.e., Scofield's/Herpendis). The normal measurement is 10 mm in children.

CHAPTER 369

Skin Pigmentation

The main component of normal skin pigment is the amount of melanin produced by the melanocytes situated at the dermoepidermal junction. A genetic defect in the ability to produce melanin may cause albinism, while an acquired localized loss of pigment arises from destruction of melanocytes in vitiligo. The pigment loss in vitiligo is usually patchy and often symmetrical; autoimmune disorders may be seen. In red-haired subjects, the melanocytes do not produce melanin, but a related pigment, phaeomelanin, which although present in abundant quantities, does not provide photoprotection, and this accounts for the high incidence of skin cancers in red-haired people.

Excessive pigmentation may arise from localized or generalized abnormal or excessive prediction of melanin, from deposition of hemosiderin, or from exogenous pigmenting agents.

CAUSES OF ERYTHEMA NODOSUM

- *Infection:*
  - Bacterial
  - Streptococcal
  - Meningococcemia
  - Tuberculosis
- *Viral:*
  - *Chlamydia*
  - Cat scratch disease
- *Fungal:*
  - Coccidioidomycosis
  - Histoplasmosis
- *Drugs:*
  - Sulfonamide
  - Penicillin
- *Miscellaneous:*
  - Sarcoidosis
  - Ulcerative colitis
  - Hemolytic-uremic syndrome

CAUSES OF ERYTHEMA MARGINATUM

- *Infection*
- *Bacterial:*
  - Group A and B hemolytic *Streptococcus*
  - Typhoid
  - Pneumococci
- *Viral:*
  - Herpes simplex
  - Glandular fever
  - *Chlamydia*
- *Drugs:*
  - Sulfonamide
  - Penicillin

GENERALIZED HYPERPIGMENTATION

Diffuse hyperpigmentation, including pigmentation of the buccal mucosae, gingival margins, palmar creases, and nail beds, is a feature of Addison's disease. In fact, this disorder is rare in clinical practice, and a more likely cause is the presence of an ectopic hormone-secreting tumor; for example, various lung carcinomas secrete peptides, some of which have MSH-like (melanocyte-stimulating hormone) properties.

LOCALIZED HYPERPIGMENTATION

Many skin disorders appear able to cause a nonspecific post-inflammatory hyperpigmentation. This is particularly seen following lichen planus and in a fixed drug eruption, where the condition can be diagnosed retrospectively from the distribution of the pigmentation. Dark-skinned races seem more susceptible to the phenomenon of postinflammatory changes in pigment, and in lichen planus in south.

A common cause of a symmetrical hyperpigmentation on the forehead and cheeks in middle-aged ladies is chloasma (melasma). This condition is of unknown cause, but may be exacerbated by pregnancy or the oral contraceptive pill and by sunlight. Less common causes of localized hyperpigmentation include lichen amyloid and nevus of Ota.

HYPERPIGMENTATION OF EXPOSED AREAS

Ultraviolet (sunlight) exposure will tan the skin in those with appropriate skin types, but tanning may be accentuated by certain drugs, including thiazides, sulfonamides, amiodarone, nalidixic acid, tetracyclines, and chlorpromazine. A similar phenomenon may arise in metabolic disorders such as pellagra and porphyria cutanea tarda.

HEMOSIDERIN

Hemosiderin is a breakdown of hemoglobin, and will be precipitated in the skin leaving a persistent, localized orange-brown discoloration in situations where there has been chronic extravasation of blood, as in stasis ulceration of the legs, and in some cutaneous vasculitic disorders (pigmented purpuric eruption, Majocchi-Schamberg disease).

BENIGN CUTANEOUS SKIN TUMORS

Sebaceous cysts, which occur most commonly on the back, face, scalp, and scrotum, are of variable size, cysts on palpation, and with a minute orifice (punctum) and can be found somewhere on their surface. Lipomas are usually multiple subcutaneous nodules which may be lobulated and found on any part of the body. They occur as a familial trait, but can often not be discerned until adulthood. Seborrheic keratosis (basal-cell papillomas) is extremely common and starts as papules in middle age, growing into larger, flat, greasy, warty pigmented neoplasms. They are sometimes unkindly called "senile keratoses".

A cutaneous horn is a cutaneous neoplasm surmounted by a spectacular horny overgrowth. The nature of the underlying neoplasm can only be safely diagnosed by examining the histopathology, for example, actinic keratosis, squamous-cell carcinoma, viral wart, keratoacanthoma, and seborrheic wart (basal cell papilloma).

A pyogenic (granuloma telangiectaticum) is a fairly common skin lesion. It often develops at the site of a recent injury, and is composed of proliferating capillaries in a loose stroma. This produces a rapidly growing vascular nodule which bleeds easily when traumatized. It is distinctive, being bright red, 0.5–1 cm in diameter, often pedunculated, and surrounded by a collar of thickened epidermis. The most common sites are the fingers, upper chest, lips, and toes. It must be differentiated from amelanotic melanoma and glomus tumors. Kaposi's sarcoma in HIV-infected patients can accurately mimic pyogenic granuloma, and for this reason, histological analysis after curettage or excision is advisable.

The superficial dermis contains many specialized tissues, some of ectodermal and some of mesodermal origin, forming the various adnexal structures (e.g., hair, sebaceous glands, and sweat glands). Benign, or rarely malignant, neoplasms of all these specialized tissues can occur, for example, leiomyoma, hidradenoma, neurofibroma, sebaceous adenoma, trichoepithelioma, and glomus tumor. The diagnosis of these uncommon adnexal lesions requires many years' experience, and is often first made by the pathologist.

CAUSES OF ABNORMAL PIGMENTATION

- *Endocrine:*
    - Addison
    - Cushing
    - Thyrotoxicosis
- *Deficiency disorders:*
    - Kwashiorkor
    - Pellagra
- *Infections:*
    - Kala azar
    - Chronic malaria
    - Secondary syphilis
    - Tuberculosis
    - Leprosy
- *Skin diseases:*
    - Neurofibromatosis
    - Lichen planus
    - Acanthosis nigricans
- *Miscellaneous:*
    - Malignancy
    - Pernicious anemia

CHAPTER 370

Sneezing

It is caused by irritation of the nasal mucosa of the anterior part of nasal septum or turbinates. Sneeze reflex is protective in nature. It is sudden and involuntary expulsion of air through the nose and mouth. It is controlled by reflex stimulated by Vth and Xth cranial nerves.

Common cold and bacterial secondary infection are the most common cause of sneezing.

When the nasal mucosa encounters an allergen to which the individual is sensitive, the inflammatory mediators are released from mast cells and basophils and they may cause sneezing.

CAUSES OF SNEEZING

- Common cold
- Allergic rhinitis
- Foreign body in nostril
- Postencephalitis

371 CHAPTER

Soft Neurologic Signs

Neurological soft signs are defined as subtle neurological impairments in sensory integration, motor coordination, balance, and sequencing of complex motor acts. They have poor localizing value. A soft neurologic sign may be defined as a particular from of deviant performance on a motor or sensory test in the neurologic examination that is abnormal for a particular age. The tests include repetitive and successive finger movements, hand pats, arm pronation–supination movements, foot taps, hopping, and tandem walking. Although intellectually normal children may demonstrate a soft neurologic signs, the finding of two or more persistent soft signs correlates significantly with neurologic dysfunction, including attention-deficit disorder, learning disorders, and cerebral palsy.

CHAPTER 372 Speech

Speech disorders involve abnormal production or comprehension of written or spoken language.

LANGUAGE FUNCTIONS

- *Dysphonias:* In this, there are mechanical disturbances in speech production due to lesions of vagus nerve and vocal cords. They may sound hoarse or speak with a low volume.
- *Dysarthrias:* They typically result from cranial nerve lesions or muscle diseases and present as difficulties with resonation or articulation. They are not associated with lesions involving cortical associated neurons.

CAUSES OF RETARDED SPEECH

- Deprivation
- Deafness
- Developmental delay
- Delayed mental development
- Degenerative disease
- Dumb

APHASIA

It is the disturbance of the ability to use the language. This may be in speaking, writing, or comprehensing. It is an important neurological sign. Very slight deficit implies disease in limited parts of the dominant hemisphere, i.e., left hemisphere.

There are two types of aphasia:

1. *Expressive aphasia:* Here, the child is unable to speak. Speech is sparse and labored. It is telegraphic style. Understanding the verbal command is preserved.
2. *Receptive aphasia:* It is characterized by loss of comprehension of speech. There are two types:
   a. *Auditory receptive aphasia*: Child is unable to carry out simple verbal commands in the absence of loss of hearing. Here, the lesion is posterior part of superior temporal gyrus.
   b. *Visual receptive aphasia:* Here, the child is unable to read in the absence of loss of vision. Here, the lesion is in medial occipitotemporal gyrus.

In Werneck's aphasia, there is poor comprehension meaningless, fluent speech. In Broca's aphasia, comprehension is preserved and nonfluent speech. In conductive aphasia, comprehension is preserved with loss of repetition. In global aphasia, both the features of Werneck and Broca are present.

Broca's Aphasia (Motor Aphasia, Anterior Aphasia, and Expressive Aphasia)

Lesions involving left inferior frontal gyrus or areas 44 and 45 of Brodman in right-handed people result in dysfluency.

These patients have an articulatory struggle and use predominantly nouns and verbs. Speech lacks normal complement of preposition and grammar as a result of which it is nonfluent.

- *Stuttering:* It is the difficulty in uttering the first phoneme or sound at the beginning of a conversation. The jaw and mouth may move, but no meaningful sound comes out.
- *Stammering:* Repetition of phonemes at the beginning or during the course of the speech that interferes with its normal flow and rhythm.

373 CHAPTER

Spermatocele

Spermatoceles or epididymal cysts are common in adolescents. They are painless cystic masses located in the epididymis (commonly in the upper pole). They contain sperm and are attached to upper pole of the sexually mature testis. They vary in size but are usually <1 cm in diameter. They are mobile, transilluminate, and do not vacillate in size, although gradual enlargement may occur. Ultrasound examination may be helpful if the diagnosis is in doubt. Spermatoceles contain sperm and are essentially retention cysts of the epididymis or tubules of the rete testis. Excision is not usually recommended in routine symptomatic cases but may be appropriate for painful or enlarging cysts.

Spine

SCOLIOSIS

It is a lateral curve. It is designated as left or right according to the direction of the convexity of the curve. It will be always associated with rotational deformity of spine. The bodies rotate toward the convexity and the spines and neural tubes rotate into the concavity.

POSTURAL SCOLIOSIS

This is secondary to other conditions. For example, a short lower limb will produce compensatory scoliosis convex to the side of the short leg. The scoliosis, therefore, disappears and spine reverts to its straight position when the patient is examined sitting. If it is secondary to poor stance, then scoliosis disappears on forward to touch the toes.

STRUCTURAL SCOLIOSIS

It is always associated with rotation. This produces characteristic rib hump and is most noticeable on forward flexion on the concave side. The scapula is usually elevated and hip is prominent.

CAUSES OF SCOLIOSIS

- *Primary:*
  - Postural
- *Idiopathic:*
  - Infantile
  - Adolescent
- *Secondary:*
  - Bone—hemivertebrae
  - Ligaments—Marfan's syndrome
  - Muscle—muscular dystrophy
  - Neurogenic spine bifida
  - Poliomyelitis
  - Cerebral palsy
  - Friedreich's ataxia

INFANTILE SCOLIOSIS

It develops below the age of 3 years. There are no vertebral bony deformities. The curve improves and even dissolves spontaneously. There is an association with plagiocephaly, postural adduction contracture of hip.

LORDOSIS

There is a smooth extension curve. Normal cervical or lumbar lordosis describes the standing posture of these two areas of the spine. Compensatory lordosis indicates an increased curve secondary to a structural kyphosis of the thoracic spine. An increased structural lordosis does not fully correct on forward flexion and is associated with underlying bony abnormalities, for example, spondylolisthesis.

375 CHAPTER

Spina Bifida

Disorders of neural tube formation can involve defects in primary neurulation, closure of the anterior or posterior neuropore, or failure in the development of the lower spinal cord, which may be present before 28 days of gestation. This leads to defects in the spinal cord, dura, meninges, cranium, and vertebrae as well as the dermal coverings. Open neural tube defects, the most common being the myelomeningocele **(Fig. 1)**, are characterized by failure of the surface ectoderm to close over the neural elements leaving meninges and spinal cord exposed.

However, disorders in neural tube formation include a wide array of disorders including cranioschisis (total failure of neurulation), anencephaly (defects in cranial neural tissue development), and encephalocele (herniation of brain or meninges through a cranial defect), as well as occult spinal dysraphisms (skin-covered defects of vertebrae and dermal structures with subtle or absent neural abnormalities).

The defect is usually covered by transparent membrane. This may have neural tissue attached to the inner surface. Cerebrospinal fluid leaks from this membrane initially. But soon after the birth, drying of the membrane prevents it. As the CSF accumulates membrane bulges. This eventually forms large sac.

Neural tube defects result from a combination of environmental risk factors in addition to genetic causes. 70–80% of all cases are the result of environmental/gene interactions, with the rest being related to aneuploidies, duplications, or deletions. The most common risk factors include folic acid deficiency, fetal exposure to drugs such as valproic acid, and gestational diabetes.

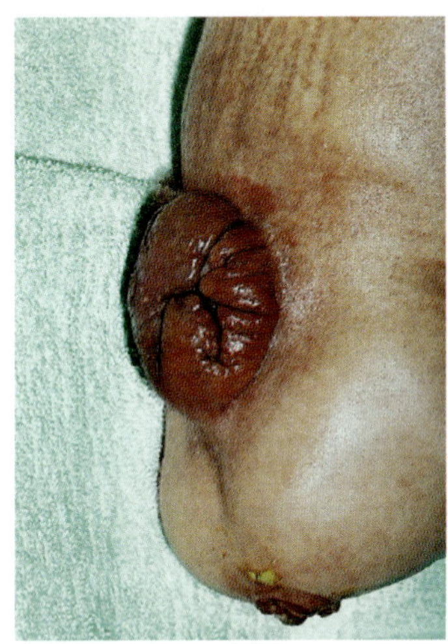

Fig. 1: Myelomeningocele.

In most (80%) of the cases, meningomyelocele is associated with a type II Arnold–Chiari malformation. There will be maldevelopment and downward displacement of the cerebellum, 4th ventricle, and medulla oblongata. Hydrocephalus occurs as a result of aqueductal stenosis. The associated deformities of the meningomyelocele include dislocated hips, talipes equinovarus, and atrophy of the tongue.

Neurological assessment should be done. This is to determine the severity of the functional defect. Pinprick over the legs and trunk will help to know the upper level of the spinal cord dysfunction. Defective innervation of the bladder is indicated by urinary dribbling. Patulous anal sphincter and lack of anal reflex indicate defective perianal region. The denervated limbs are patulous.

Diagnosis of open neural tube defects is suspected early in the second trimester of pregnancy if elevated serum levels of alpha-fetoprotein are detected. Open neural tube defects are also diagnosed prenatally through the routine use of fetal ultrasonography. Changes in the head shape (lemon sign) and cerebellum (banana sign) are often the presenting findings on fetal ultrasound. Early prenatal diagnosis is crucial in order to allow families the opportunity to plan the pregnancy, including considering the option of fetal surgery, which can be performed between 19 and 26 weeks of gestation. Prenatal diagnosis is also beneficial in order to plan for delivery at an institution.

376 CHAPTER

Splenomegaly

The spleen tip is palpable in about 10% of healthy children and often is palpable in newborns. In infants, the spleen enlarges downward toward the left lower quadrant, whereas in order children enlargement is toward the right lower quadrant. Palpation should begin in the right iliac fossa so as not to miss a very large spleen. Be gentle, because an enlarged spleen could rupture if too must force is applied. Size should be recorded in centimeters below the left costal margin.

If the spleen is not palpation with the child supine, turn the child into the right lateral decubitus position. With your left hand lowermost portion of the left rib cage and flank anteriorly, your right should be used to feel the spleen tip on inspiration. In subclinical splenomegaly, other provocative maneuvers may be tried. Castel sign involves percussing the lower intercostal space in the left anterior axillary line. Normally, this area is resonant and should stay so during inspiration. An older child can be asked to take a deep breath while percussion is continued. A change from resonance to dullness suggests splenic enlargement.

Occasionally, it may be difficult to differentiate splenomegaly from a massively enlarged kidney. With an enlarged spleen, one cannot get above it, a notch may be felt along its medical border, and the percussion note over it will be dull.

Is a palpable spleen abnormal in a child? It depends on the clinical context. An enlarged spleen is present in many patients with chronic hemolytic disorders. Sickle cell anemia is an exception because the spleen atrophies over time as a result of repeated infarctions. Splenomegaly is an important finding in portal hypertension from any cause. If an enlarged spleen is present along with hepatomegaly, consider infections, infiltrative disorders, or storage disorders.

CAUSES OF SPLENOMEGALY

- *Infection and infestation:*
  - Malaria
  - Enteric fever
  - Tuberculosis
  - Infective endocarditis
  - Brucellosis
  - Kala azar
  - IMN
  - Intrauterine infection
- *Hematogenous:*
  - Hemolytic anemia
  - Hypersplenism
  - ITP
  - Congestive splenomegaly
- *Storage disorders:*
  - Gaucher
  - Meimann pick
  - Hemosiderosis
  - Amyloidosis
- *Malignancies:*
  - Leukemia
  - Lymphoma
- *Miscellaneous:*
  - Splenic cyst
  - Hemangioma
  - Abscess
  - SLE
  - Still disease

377 CHAPTER

Staphylococcal Scalded Skin Syndrome

A disorder seen most commonly in infants and young children, staphylococcal scalded skin syndrome is caused by exfoliative toxin-producing strains of *S. aureus*. The primary infection is usually mild, with purulent nasopharyngitis, conjunctivitis, impetigo, and infections of the umbilicus and circumcision sites seen most commonly. Rarely, sepsis, pneumonia, or other severe invasive staphylococcal infections may precede the onset of the exanthem.

After infection, exfoliative toxin is spread hematogenously and causes cleavage of the skin between the epidermis and the dermis. This process may begin within hours or days of the appearance of signs of the primary infection, and typically its onset is heralded by fever and irritability, often accompanied by vomiting. These symptoms are followed by the development of a diffuse, sunburn-like erythroderma that spreads rapidly from head to toe. In contrast to streptococcal scarlet fever, the involved skin is tender, even to light touch **(Fig. 1)**. Within 1–3 days, thin-walled, flaccid, bullous lesions appear and rupture soon after formation. Simultaneously, larger portions of the epidermis begin to slough in sheets. During this phase, application of light traction on the skin pulls epidermis away from dermis, leaving a raw, weeping surface. This separation of the skin in response to stroking is called the Nikolsky sign. After exfoliation, the surface gradually dries, forming large, thick flakes.

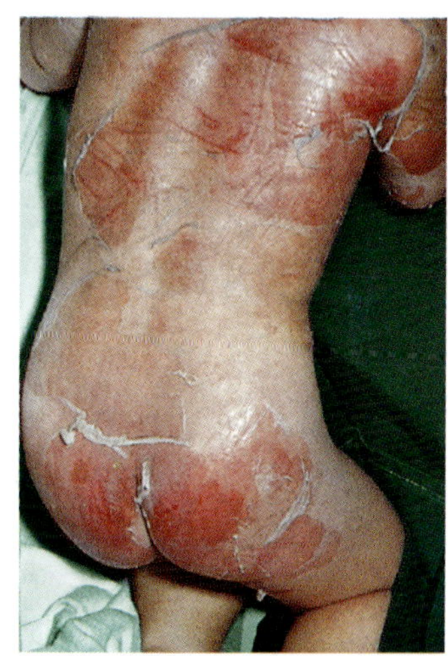

Fig. 1: Staphylococcal scalded skin syndrome.

CHAPTER 378

Startle Response

A startle response is a largely unconscious defensive response to sudden or threatening stimuli (auditory, tactile, visual, or vestibular) that readily habituates (e.g., diminishes with repeated exposure). It is implicated in the formation of specific phobias.

The acoustic startle reflex is thought to be caused by auditory stimulus >80 decibels. This reflex is typically measured by electromyography, brain imaging, or sometimes positron electron tomography.

Stiff Neck

NECK STIFFNESS (NUCHAL RIGIDITY)

The patient lying supine on a flat surface.

Place your hand behind the patient's head and:

- Gently rotate the head as if patient was indicating "no"-feel for the stiffness or resistance to movement.
- Gently lift the head off the bed; try to make the patient's chin touch the sternum feel for the tone in the neck.
- Watch the legs for hip and knee flexion.

Normally: The neck moves easily in both planes, with the chin easily reaching the chest on neck flexion.

COMMON CAUSES

- Meningitis (bacterial/viral)
- Subarachnoid hemorrhage
- Muscles posteriorly.
- Any cause of raised ICP
- Severe cervical spondylosis
- Cervical lymphadenopathy
- Severe pharyngitis/retropharyngeal abscess
- Phenothiazine reaction
- Kernicterus
- Strychnine poisoning

CHAPTER 380

Straight Leg Test

This test is done during a physical examination to determine whether a patient with low backpain has an underlying nerve root sensitivity, often located at L5 (fifth lumbar spinal nerve). This is useful for the diagnosis of sciatica and lumbar disk hernia.

Straight leg raising test: With the patient supine, the limb to be tested is grasped behind the ankle and elevated into hip flexion with the knee in full extension. If pain is produced well before 90° of flexion is achieved, the test is positive, indicating irritation of a sciatic nerve root.

CHAPTER 381

Strabismus

Strabismus occurs when the two eyes fail to move in a coordinated fashion, diplopia usually results, unless one eye has very poor vision or the defect so has been of long-standing since childhood, when information from one eye becomes suppressed at cortical level. Squint may be paralytic or nonparalytic (concomitant).

- *Paralytic squint:* This is due to weakness of one or more external ocular muscles.
- *Nonparalytic or concomitant squint:* This occurs in childhood and is due to failure of development of normal fixation reflexes.

CLINICAL EXAMINATION OF STRABISMUS

- The eyes should be parallel when the child stands in any direction. If there is less parallelism when the eye moves in one direction, a mild paralysis should be suspected. If the deviation from parallelism is equal when the eyes move in all directions, the squint is nonparalytic or concomitant.
- Another easy method for observing squints is to look at the eyes when the child is looking toward a light about 3 feet away. The reflection of the light should come from approximately the same part of each pupil.
- *Degree of strabismus estimation:* Deviation is approximately—
  - 15° if the reflection appears at the edge of the pupil
  - 30° if the reflection is halfway between the edge of the pupil and the limbus (outer edge of the cornea)
  - 45° if the reflection is at the edge of the limbus
- *Cover test:* Hold a light about 2–3 feet from the eyes and sit directly in front of the child. Ask the child to focus on the light. Then cover one eye. The opposite eye is noted for motion.

Stridor

Stridor is a harsh, vibratory, high-pitched, sometimes shrill, crowing noise caused by obstructed air flow.

Stridor may be inspiratory or expiratory or both. A purely inspiratory stridor is less likely to be of serious than one which is both inspiratory and expiratory, or expiratory alone. On the other hand a purely inspiratory stridor can be due to a serious condition demanding surgical treatment. Stridor, which is entirely inspiratory, is usually of supraglottic origin. Biphasic stridor may arise in the cervical trachea. Stridor, which is largely expiratory, usually arises from the trachea.

Inspiratory stridor is usually associated with upper airway obstruction, expiratory stridor with lower airway obstruction, and biphasic stridor with midtracheal disorders.

CAUSES OF ACUTE STRIDOR

Main Causes

- Epiglottis, laryngotracheobronchitis (croup)
- Trauma, corrosives
- Foreign body
- Diphtheria, rabies
- Retropharyngeal abscess
- Laryngeal spasm, tetany
- Angioneurotic edema
- Allergy to cow's milk protein

Main Causes of Chronic Stridor

Supraglottic Causes

- Congenital laryngeal stridor
- Micrognathia, macroglossia
- Down's syndrome
- Gross enlargement of tonsils and adenoids
- Lingual, aryepiglottic, thyroglossal, or laryngeal cysts (rare)
- Supraglottic web (rare)

Glottic Causes

- Laryngeal web, polyp, and papilloma
- Vocal cord paralysis
- Hydrocephalus
- Foreign body
- Dislocation of the cricothyroid or cricoarytenoid articulations

Infraglottic Causes

- Congenital subglottic stenosis
- Tracheal obstruction or stenosis, hemangioma, and neurofibroma
- Tracheomalacia
- Vascular ring
- Mediastinal tumor or thyroid (rare)
- Foreign body

383 CHAPTER

Sturge–Weber Syndrome

The cardinal manifestations of Sturge–Weber syndrome are as follows:

- A vascular malformation or portwine stain over the face that involves the cutaneous distribution of the ophthalmic division of the trigeminal nerve
- Ipsilateral leptomeningeal angiomatosis with associated intracranial calcifications
- A high incidence of mental retardation and ipsilateral ocular complications

The portwine stain is usually present at birth and consists of a pink-to-purple macular cutaneous vascular malformation. Only patients with lesions involving the cutaneous distribution of the ophthalmic division of the trigeminal nerve (i.e., forehead and upper eyelid) are at risk for associated neuro-ocular complications. Repeated ophthalmologic and CT or MRI examinations are indicated only in this high-risk group, which has a 10–20% incidence of associated intracranial angiomas.

The coincidence of seizures and a facial vascular nevus should suggest the diagnosis of Sturge–Weber syndrome, which can be confirmed by CT scan or MRI. These scans may be normal at birth but subsequently show areas of gyriform contrast enhancement corresponding to the leptomeningeal angiomatosis. Serial examinations often demonstrate progressive ipsilateral cerebral atrophy. Additional findings may include serpiginous calcifications of brain parenchyma underlying vascular malformations of the pia. These intracranial calcifications are first seen on CT scan but become evident on plain skull films by the end of the second decade.

Associated ocular abnormalities are often encountered. Buphthalmos (corneal enlargement) or colobomata may be present at birth, and glaucoma frequently develops in infancy or later childhood. Dilated vessels in the sclera, conjunctiva, and retina are common, and angiomatous malformations of the choroid occasionally occur.

The estimated incidence of facial cutaneous angioma is 1 in 5,000, and the estimated frequency of the complete syndrome is 1 in 30,000. Among patients with the complete syndrome, seizures occur in 90%, and contralateral hemiparesis eventually develops in one-third. Early developmental milestones are often normal, but about 50% develop cognitive difficulties ranging from mild to severe. Behavioral problems are common. Patients with refractory epilepsy are more likely to be more severely delayed. Although most cases are sporadic, genetic determination has not been ruled out. However, no cases of direct transmission from parent to child have been reported.

Subcutaneous Nodules

They appear as early as 6 weeks after the onset of fever. These lesions are vary infrequent and are present in 1–10% of patients with rheumatic fever. Nodules are better seen than felt. They are firm nontender, pea-sized nodules approximately 0.5–1 cm in diameter seen over the extensor aspects of tendons near bony prominences of forearm, elbows, wrist, knees, ankles, spine, scalp, and along tendons. The presence of rheumatic nodules indicates presence of activity in 100% of cases and underlying carditis in 70% of cases.

CHAPTER 385

Subdural Tap

These are rarely indicated. That is useful in the diagnosis of subdural hematomas located along the cerebral convexities. It is sometimes used to reduce sign of increased intracranial pressure and to prevent the development of craniocerebral disproportion.

Lumbar puncture needle is entered in the same spot as for ventricular puncture. Once the Dura mater is entered, a giveaway sensation is felt. Then stellate should be withdrawn. If nothing comes out, there is no point in advancing further and in changing posture. If the procedure is indicated, it should be done bilaterally.

386 CHAPTER

Succession Sounds/ Succession Splash

Air and fluid in the pleural cavity simultaneously or in large cavities within the lungs are suspected if one listens over the possible involved area and gently shakes the patient from side to side. This can be achieved with patient sitting. First place a hand on the patients shoulder and then with your hand, move the patient from side to side, not briskly but with a bit of vigor. The fluid will splash, and in the presence of air, a succussion splash will be heard.

It may be elicited by palpation and also on auscultation. It may be heard in pyloric stenosis, advanced intestinal obstruction with grossly distended loops of bowel and in paralytic ileus.

These sounds are heard when a viscus or a cavity contains both liquid and air or gas. This is heard by keeping stethoscope on the part and shaken. The sounds may be loud enough to be audible without stethoscope.

Gastric succession sounds are not necessarily evidence of abnormality. They merely indicate that the viscus contains gas and liquid. Succession sounds may be heard in the chest in cases of hypopneumothorax, when the patient moves the chest to and fro.

Hydropneumothorax may result from paracentesis thoracis. If bleeding occurs during puncture, hemopneumothorax will be produced. It may become infected with pyogenic organism and converted into pyopneumothorax. Fluid often collects in the pleural cavity when an artificial, i.e., therapeutic pneumothorax has been induced giving succession sounds.

This may be present in fallowing conditions:

- Pyloric stenosis
- Intestinal obstruction
- Paralytic ileus
- Normal stomach after food intake

CHAPTER 387

Sunsetting Sign

Wherein upper corneal margin is not covered by lids and is seen in hydrocephalus, kernicterus, and raised intracranial pressure.

Cornea: The cornea forms the anterior sixth of the globe and is continuous with sclera. It transmits light to retina through the lens **(Fig. 1)**.

The cornea should be normally crystal clear and is best examined in good light. The cornea is about 10 mm in diameter at birth and 12 mm in adulthood. Any inflammation, opacity, and ulceration are abnormal. The cornea is clear in a child with conjunctivitis.

Here, upper corneal margin is not covered by lids. It is seen in hydrocephalus, kernicterus, and raised intracranial pressure.

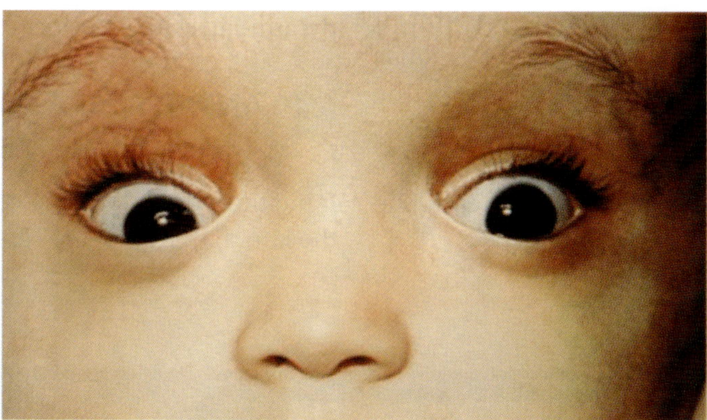

Fig. 1: Sunsetting sign.

CHAPTER 388 Superficial Reflexes

These are polysynaptic reflexes. Afferent impulses originate from the skin. These reach the cerebral cortex. They descend through the motor tract or reach the peripheral nerve via spinal segment. The response occurs due to the muscular contraction involving concerned segment.

ABDOMINAL REFLEX

Abdominal wall, i.e., skin of the anterior abdominal wall is scratched with blunt object from medial to lateral side. Response is the contraction of abdominal wall due to the contraction of rectus abdominis **(Fig. 1)**. Segmental roots involved are above the umbilicus—T_8, T_9 and below the umbilicus—T_3, T_4.

Absent abdominal reflex is seen in obesity, pyramidal involving above that level and in peripheral nerve abnormalities.

CREMASTERIC REFLEX

It involves the scratching gently over the skin of the upper part of the inner part of the thigh. There will be contraction cremasteric muscle with the elevation of testicle. Segment involved is L1. The reflex is absent tin pyramidal lesion, hydrocele, and hernia.

PLANTAR RESPONSE

Normal Response

It includes the scratching with the key end on the lateral border of the sole, extending to the

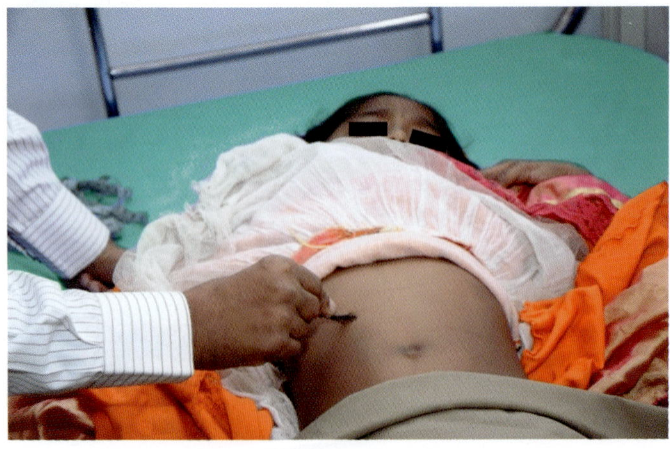

Fig. 1: Abdominal reflex.

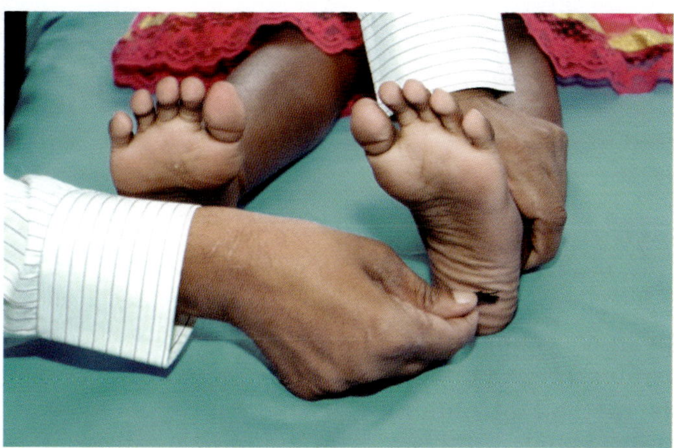

Fig. 2: Plantar response.

balls of toes. The response is plantar flexion of the great toe and flexion and adduction of other toes. Segments involved are S_1 and S_2. This is absent in coma, neurogenic shock, LMN lesion involving concerned muscles **(Fig. 2)**.

Babinski Reflex

There will be dorsiflexion of great toe, fanning out, i.e., abduction and dorsiflexion of other toes. This indicates UMN lesion. It may be normally seen till the age of 2 years when the myelination has not taken place. Positive Babinski reflex is seen in coma, UMN lesion, day sleep following epileptic attack.

Other methods of eliciting plantar response:

- *Chaddock reflex:* It involves scratching lightly the skin below the lateral malleolus.
- *Oppenheim sign:* It includes pressing and stroking skin over anterior border of tibia.
- *Gordon reflex:* It includes the pinching the tendo-Achilles or squeezing the calf muscle.

ANAL REFLEX

This is elicited by stroking or pricking the skin or mucous membrane in the perianal region. The response is contraction of the external anal sphincter. These are absent in pyramidal lesion and lesion of local reflex S_4 and S_5.

CHAPTER 389

Suprapubic Aspiration

This method helps in collecting the urine directly from bladder **(Fig. 1)**. This is the most reliable method of obtaining noncontaminated urine sample.

Baby's lower abdominal wall is cleaned with antiseptic solutions and area is dried. The baby is made to lie on his back on a firm surface. The bladder is an abdominal organ in newborn. Hence, entry into the peritoneal cavity is not possible. Hence, it is safe. However, it should not be done in infants over the age of 6 months.

Needle is inserted 1 cm above the symphysis pubis in the midline. 21 number needle attached to 10 mL syringe is used. Syringe should be aspirated creating the negative pressure. Urine will be aspirated into the syringe. If this method is not used, there is a risk of hitting the intestine through the bladder. Usually, the depth will be 1–2 cm. It will never be more than 2 cm. Local pressure is applied over the puncture site after withdrawing syringe and needle. Elastoplast is put over the puncture site.

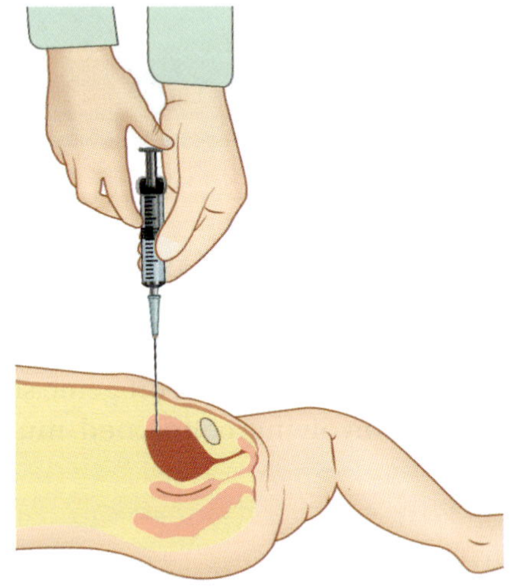

Fig. 1: Suprapubic aspiration.

CHAPTER 390 Sydenham's Chorea

It is one of the major criteria of the diagnosis of the rheumatic fever. One-third of these patients develop rheumatic valvular heart disease. The usual age of onset of the disease is 5–15 years.

It is an autoimmune response to CNS to Group A streptococcal organism. Antineural antibodies cross-react with cytoplasm of the subthalamic and caudate nuclei. The primary pathological changes include vasculitis of the cortical arterioles, round cell infiltration of the gray and white matter. Chorea is the functional overactivity of the dopaminergic system. Classically, the movements are described as irregular, nonrepetitive, quasi-purpose, and involuntary. They are usually proximal but may affect fingers, hands, extremities, and face. The child may appear clumsy. Movements may be limited to one side of the body as in hemiballismus. The movements are aggravated by attention, stress, or excitement. But they disappear during sleep.

The relaxing hand grip on and off as if she is milking the cow—milkmaid sign. The child cannot maintain the tongue in protruded position—darting tongue. The knee reflex may snow sustained contractions resulting in a hung-up reflex. Antistreptolysin O (ASLO) titer may not be elevated as onset of the chorea is late.

CHAPTER 391

Syndactyly

It is common congenital anomaly involving failure of the digits of the hands or feet to separate **(Figs. 1A and B)**. It may be associated with other congenital anomalies, particularly Apert syndrome and Streeter dysplasia. Great variation in the degree of fusion exists. In mild cases, only the skin is joined, making reconstructive surgery simple. In more severe cases, the nails, deeper structures, and bones may be conjoined, contributing to deformity and growth abnormalities and making reconstructive treatment more difficult.

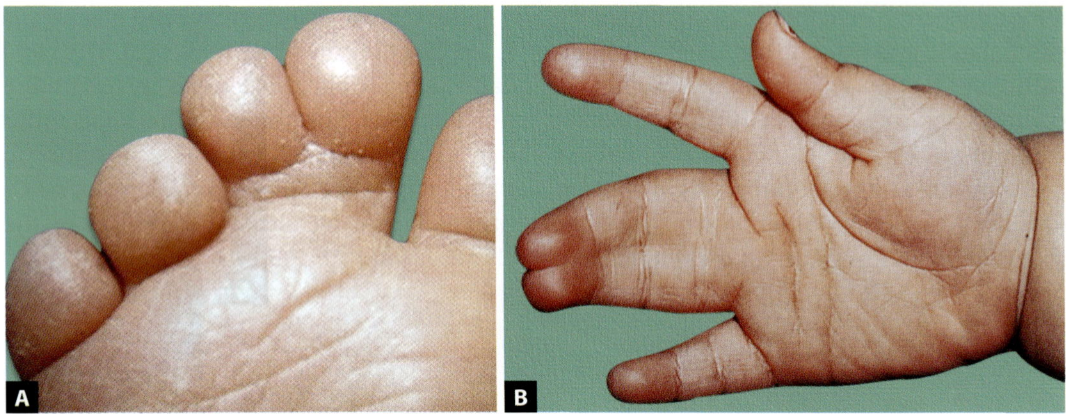

Figs. 1A and B: Syndactyly.

CHAPTER 392

Sweat Chloride Test

The method used is pilocarpine iontophoresis, where a 3-mA current is used and a minimum of 50 mg of sweat is collected on a filter paper. The chloride values are elevated in cystic fibrosis and a value above 60 mEq/L strongly suggests the diagnosis. Newer methods such as linkage analysis or DNA studies, using polymerase chain reaction (PCR), are now used for molecular diagnosis of cystic fibrosis. PCR can be set up to detect common mutations.

SECTION 19

Tachycardia

This is when heart rate rises above the upper limit for the age and sex.

- *In newborn:* >200/min
- *In infants:* >150/min
- *In older children:* >120/min

Acceptable resting pulse rate/minute:			
Age	***Awake***	***Asleep***	***Fever***
Newborn	100–180	80–160	<220
1 week to 3 months	100–220	80–200	<220
3 months to 2 years	80–150	70–120	<200
2 years to 10 years	70–110	60–90	<200
>10 years	55–90	50–90	<200

Causes of tachycardia:

- Fever
- Exercise
- Myocarditis
- Heart failure
- Drugs—atropine, theophylline
- Thyrotoxicosis
- Rheumatic fever
- Diphtheria
- Paroxysmal supraventricular tachycardia
- Atrial fibrillation
- Atrial flutter

Tachycardia may be due to an increased frequency of discharge of the sino-atrial node (sinus tachycardia).

Sinus tachycardia is present in most febrile conditions due to a direct effect of the pyrexia on the sinoatrial node. The sino-atrial node is affected directly in a number of other situations in which tachycardia is prominent.

394 CHAPTER

Tachypnea

It refers to fast breathing with respect to the age of a child. The physiological respiratory rate varies with age of the child.

CAUSES

- *Increased metabolic demands*
  - Fever
  - Hyper dynamic circulation
  - Circulatory shock
- *Stimulation of central chemoreceptors*
  - Metabolic acidosis
  - Renal failure
  - Hepatic failure
  - Acute circulatory collapse
  - Salicylate overdose
- *Stimulation lung stretch receptor*
  - Acute pulmonary emboli
  - Acute pneumonia
  - Bronchial asthma
  - Pulmonary fibrosis
  - Inspiration pneumonia
- *Neurological causes*
  - Cerebral hemorrhage
  - Meningitis
  - Encephalitis
  - Head injury

CHAPTER 395

Tactile Vocal Fremitus

Vocal fremitus (VF) is palpation of vibration of chest wall produced by asking the patient to say one-one-one and in small children this can be done during crying. The medial side of the hand is used to palpate VF symmetrically on either side.

Proceed symmetrically downward from apices to the bases.

Mechanism of TVF: Tactile vocal fremitus (TVF) occurs when sounds vibrations from larynx pass down the bronchi and cause the lungs and the chest wall to vibrate. Intensity of fremitus tends to parallel the breath sound intensity.

Variation of TVF: Even in normal healthy subjects marked variation of VF are common. Degree of fremitus depends upon age, sex, thickness of chest wall, volume, and pitch of voice. Normally, fremitus is less marked in children than adults.

The intensity of tactile fremitus varies considerably from front (strong) to back and from apex (stronger) to lung base in normal persons. Thus, the key comparison is between symmetric points.

Increased tactile vocal fremitus is seen in consolidation and cavity. Decreased vocal fremitus is seen in pleural effusion, pneumothorax, fibrosis, bronchial obstruction, and pneumothorax.

396 CHAPTER

Tall Stature

Tall stature is defined as if the height is >97th centile for the normal population.

Constitutional tall stature can be identified by plotting the patient's height relative to age on growth development chart.

CAUSES OF TALL STATURE

- Familial
- Marfan's syndrome
- Klinefelter syndrome
- Primordial gigantism
- Congenital adrenal hyperplasia
- Thyrotoxicosis
- Hydrocephalus
- Homocystinuria

CHAPTER 397

Telescopic Test

It is used to check for hip dislocation. This test looks for possible hip dislocation, that head of the femur moves out of the socket where it normally sits.

The pelvis is fixed with one hand touching the greater trochanter. The hip is now flexed to 90° and the knee is grasped with the other hand of the clinician who pushes the thigh downward along the axis of the thigh with this hand, while the other hand notes whether the greater trochanter is moving downward. This positive telescopic test is seen in developmental dysplasia of the hip (DDH) as well as pathological dislocation of the hip and also in Charcot's joint.

CHAPTER 398 Tinea Cruris

Tinea cruris, uncommon before adolescence, is an erythematous, scaly eruption involving the inguinal creases and medial thighs. The eruption is usually symmetric, and sometimes the margins are papular. This infection may resemble candidiasis, in which there is also scrotal erythema. *Erythrasma,* an uncommon superficial bacterial infection caused by *Corynebacterium minutissimum* may also mimic tinea cruris. The coral red fluorescence seen on Wood lamp examination is diagnostic of erythrasma, which can be further differentiated from tinea cruris by a negative KOH (potassium hydroxide) preparation and fungal culture.

CHAPTER 399 Tinea Versicolor

Occurring more frequently in adolescents and adults, tinea versicolor is a superficial fungal infection characterized by multiple slightly scaly macules and patches located on the upper trunk, neck, proximal extremities, and on occasion, the face **(Fig. 1)**. The macular lesions vary in hue (pink, tan, brown, and white), hence the name "versicolor." In darkly pigmented or tanned individuals, the macules appear hypopigmented; in fair-skinned persons or during winter months, the lesions usually appear tan-brown. Tinea versicolor is caused by *Pityrosporum orbiculare*, also called *Malassezia furfur*, a dimorphic fungus that is a skin saprophyte. It is generally present in its yeast form, which does not produce a rash. When proliferation of the filamentous form occurs, the organism produces the characteristic lesions of tinea versicolor. Usually asymptomatic or only slightly pruritic, tinea versicolor is primarily a cosmetic disturbance that occurs most commonly in warm and humid environments.

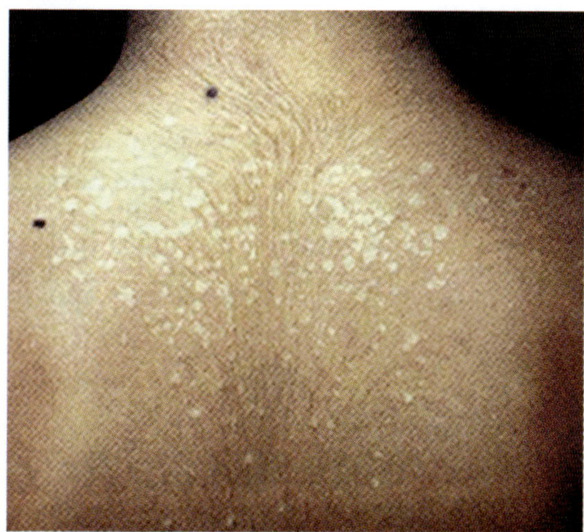

Fig. 1: Tinea versicolor.

Testes

UNDESCENDED TESTES (CRYPTORCHIDISM AND HIDDEN TESTES)

Testes found along normal path of descent and processes vaginalis are usually present.

Incidence

- Percent in full term babies
- 17% in preterm babies (2–2.5 kg)
- 100% <900 g

Examination

Make the patient stand and feel the testes in the scrotal sac. In case of undescended testes, it will be absent in the scrotum. Feel for the testes along the inguinal canal. The testes are recognized by its shape, feel, and testicular sensation. This can be differentiated from ectopic testes, undescended testes are always smaller and well developed.

ECTOPIC TESTES

Completed its descent through the inguinal canal but ends up in a subcutaneous fascia.

Examination

Make the patient stand and look for testes in the scrotal sac. Testes will be absent in the sac. Look for testes above and lateral to the superficial inguinal ring and superficial to the external oblique aponeurosis, at the route of the penis, at the perineum. Ectopic testes are well developed than undescended testes.

RETRACTILE TESTES

Testes retract into the inguinal canal in response to an exaggerated cremasteric reflex. Testes are palpable at birth.

Examination

When a child is relaxed in a warm room, scrotal examination is done in a squatting position along the inguinal canal.

In difficult cases, the child is asked to sit on a chair keeping both feet on its seat and the knees are flexed at the extreme and brought toward its chest. This puts pressure on the inguinal canal downward and brings the retractile testes into the scrotum. This is known as chair test.

VARICOCELE

It is a dilatation of the pampiniform venous plexus predominantly on the left side. Probably because of:

- Left spermatic vein is longer than the right.
- Left spermatic vein enters the left renal vein at a right angle.
- At times, the left testicular artery arches over the left renal vein to compress it.
- The left colon when loaded may press on the left testicular vein.

TORSION OF TESTES

It is mainly a cause of swelling of scrotum, but an undescended testis may frequently undergo torsion. This condition mimics a strangulated hernia. It will give rise to a tense and tender swelling without an impulse on coughing. Absence of testes in the scrotum should arouse suspicion of this condition. Slight fever, no constipation, and dullness on percussion will go in favor of torsion.

EPIDIDYMITIS

Acute Inflammation of Epididymis

It will give rise to a tense and tender swelling without an impulse on coughing. Absence of testes in the scrotum should arouse suspicion of this condition. Slight fever, no constipation and dullness on percussion will go in favor of torsion.

- *Examination:* On palpation, of epididymis, it is swollen and tender.
- *Scrotal swelling:* Although most children with swelling of the scrotum have either a hernia or hydrocele, other conditions must be considered. A thorough history and physical examination can often point to a specific diagnosis prior to or obviating the need for surgical exploration.

HYDROCELE

It is an accumulation of fluid in the tunica vaginalis.

Examination: On inspection, swelling of the scrotum is seen.

On palpation, the swelling is purely scrotal and is confirmed by getting above the swelling. Although most children with swelling of the scrotum have either a hernia or hydrocele, other conditions must be considered. A thorough history and physical examination can often point to a specific diagnosis prior to or obviating the need for surgical exploration.

CHAPTER 401 Tetany

It is increased neuromuscular irritability due to low ionic calcium levels in blood. Clinical features include irritability, muscle cramps, paresthesia, dysphagia, and carpopedal spasm.

The wrist and elbow may become flexed, the fingers flexed at metacarpophalangeal joint but extended at terminal later phalangeal joint. Fingers all pressed together, with the thumb adducted into the palm of the hand **(Figs. 1A and B)**.

Latent tetany can be elicited by:

- *Trousseau sign:* Here sphygmomanometer cuff is inflated above systolic pressure. This precipitates the carpopedal spasm. This includes extension of interphalangeal joints. The flexed thumb lies in between index and middle finger. Pedal spasm is less frequently seen. Latent tetany is best diagnosed by this sign.
- *Chvostek sign:* Tapping the facial nerve in front of ear at its exit from the stylomastoid foramen leads to brief twitching of the facial muscles.
- *Erb sign:* Application of subthreshold electrical stimulation produces muscular contractions
- *Peroneal sign:* Tapping the Peronium at the neck of fibula produces plantar flexion and adduction.

CAUSES OF HYPOCALCEMIA

Most Common

- Chronic renal failure
- post operative (thyroidectomy and parathyroidism)

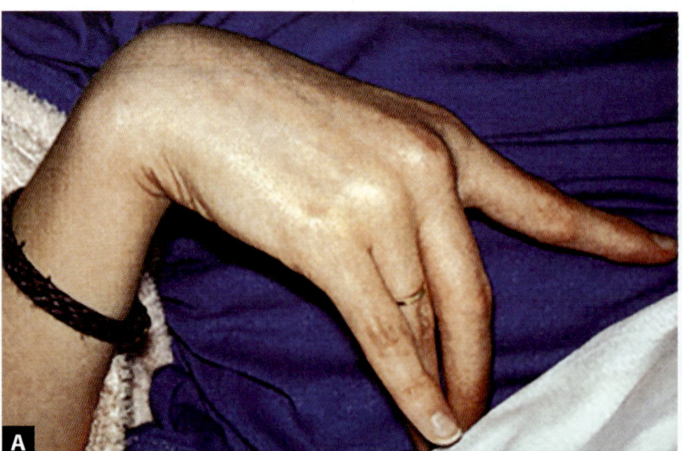
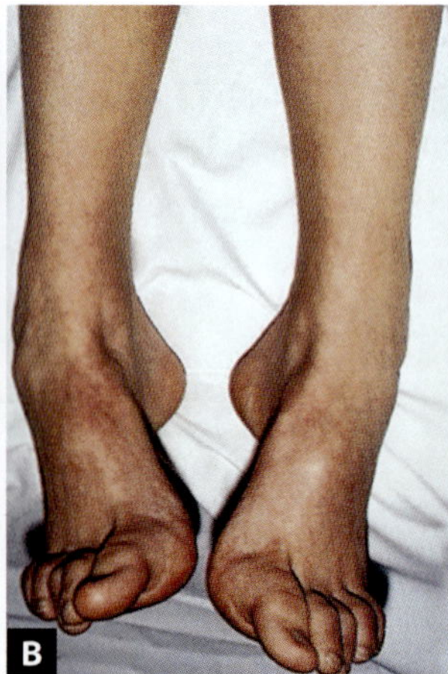

Figs. 1A and B: Tetany.

- Osteomalaria
- Rickets
- Persistent vomiting

Less Common

- Acute pancreatitis
- Alkalosis
- Magnesium deficiency
- Massive blood transfusion
- Vitamin D resistance
- Pseudo hypoparathyroidism
- Idiopathic hypoparathyroidism

Thoracocentesis

PLEURAL EFFUSION

The infant is placed supine. Gelco size F6, 17, or 19 is attached to a three-way tap. Then 20 mL is attached to it. This is inserted into the fourth intercostal space. In the mid-axillary line, large quantity of fluid can then slowly and safely be aspirated without disconnecting the syringe **(Fig. 1)**.

PNEUMOTHORAX

In an emergency situation with a tension pneumothorax, the chest should be tapped in the second and third space. This is done on the nipple line. The size of the needle is 21. The three-way tap is used. This will allow the repeated aspiration of the air without disconnecting the syringe from the needle or cannula.

This should always be followed by the insertion of thoracocentesis tube. Tube numbers FG10 or 12 should be used even in very small infants. A small nick is made in the skin with the scalpel. A track is made for trocar and cannula through the intercostal muscles. This requires fine mosquito forceps.

The cannula is then inserted 2–3 cm inside and connected to underseal drain. The pressure should be 10–20 cmH_2O suction pressure in all the cases tube must be held in place by suture. Skin incision is to be made airtight by dressing.

Care should be taken for preventing the air entry along its track. This is expected either during or following the removal of drain. This is done by having the purse-string suture placed in the sites.

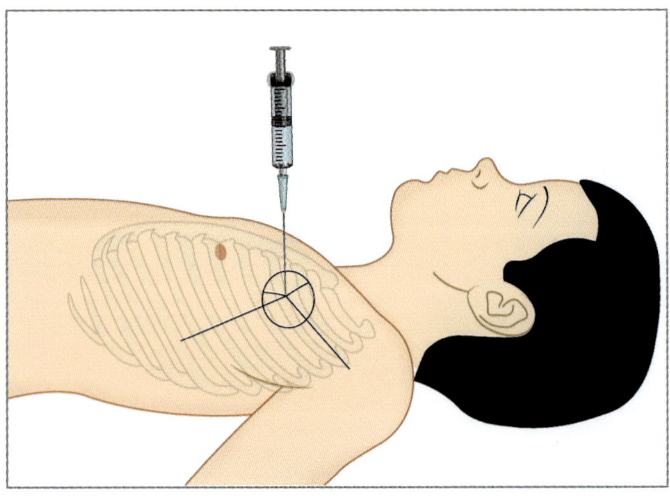

Fig. 1: Needle thoracocentesis.

403 CHAPTER

Thyroglossal Duct Cyst

A cyst may be located anywhere along the thyroglossal duct. Two-thirds of cysts are near the hyoid bone. They are typically in the midline, smooth, soft, and non-tender. Failure of regression of the thyroglossal duct may lead to cyst formation. On physical examination, the mass typically moves cephalad when the child sticks their tongue out **(Fig. 1)**. These lesions can typically be identified by history and physical examination alone. They are quite prone to infectious complications and require surgical excision. This excision requires resection of the midportion of the hyoid bone and ligation of the tract leading to the foramen cecum (Sistrunk procedure) to prevent future recurrence. One should attempt to identify the thyroid gland because 1–2% of the time the thyroglossal duct cyst may actually represent a lingual thyroid and removal will remove the entire thyroid tissue resulting in hypothyroidism.

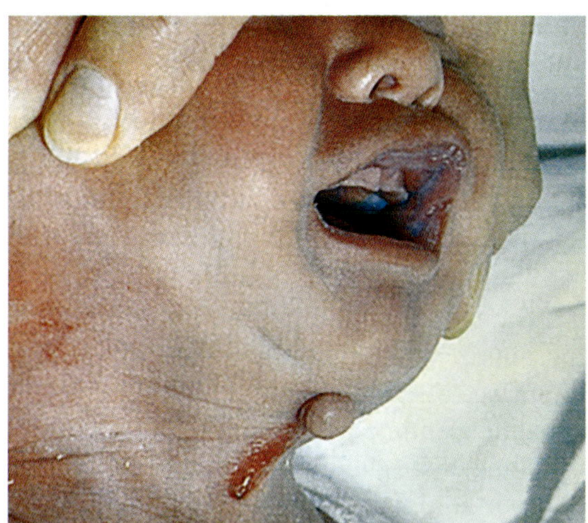

Fig. 1: Thyroglossal duct cyst.

CHAPTER 404

Thyroid Gland

The gland consists of two lobes connected by the isthmus, which lies in front of the second and third tracheal ring. In one-third of the children, a pyramidal lobe is felt, that extends upwards from the isthmus. The lobe is a remnant of the thyroglossal duct. Normal thyroid is not easily palpable but a small goiter or a nodule may be readily palpated.

METHOD OF PALPATION OF THYROID

The patient remains seated, and the examiner stands behind the patient. The thumbs of both hands are fixed at the root of the neck at the back, while the other four fingers palpate the gland on either side.

The isthmus is normally palpable one cm below the cricoid cartilage. The lobes are lateral to the trachea and medial to the sternomastoid muscle.

A slight retraction of this muscle permits better visualization and permits the fingertips of the hand to outline the surface of the lobe. When the patient swallows, the gland moves upward and so does the swelling of the gland. The diffuse swelling of the thyroid may be thyroiditis, or a goiter and a discrete thyroid mass is more likely to be a malignancy.

Retrosternal prolongation of the thyroid may be recognized by a dullness on percussion on the manubrium. When the patient is asked to swallow or cough. It is sometimes possible to feel the lower limit of the gland as it rises. At the end of the deglutation it ships back behind the sternum—plunging goiter.

Pressure symptoms are liable to be great, when the part or whole of the gland is in this position. Pressure on great veins is seen in the presence of dilated anastomotic skin vein over the upper anterior part of the thorax.

PRESSURE EFFECTS

- Pressure on trachea causing deviation or compression, or both with the varying degree of dyspnea and stridor.
- Pressure on esophagus causes dysphagia.
- Pressure on vein produces engorgement and setting up of anastomotic channel as a result of superior mediastinal obstruction from a large retrosternal gland.
- Pressure on nerves usually recurrent laryngeal nerves produces vocal cord palsy, alteration in voice, dyspnea, stridor, and brassy cough.
- Acute pressure symptoms may become aggravated by hemorrhage into the thyroid cyst.

HYPERTHYROIDISM

Primary hyperthyroidism is characterized by presence of symptoms of hyperthyroidism from the onset of disease **(Fig. 1)**. In secondary hyperthyroidism, symptoms develop after simple goiter has been present for a variable period.

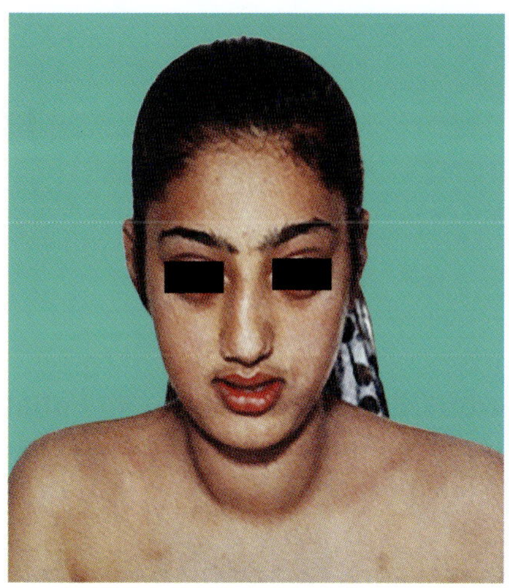

Fig. 1: Thyrotoxicosis.

Various eye signs are described in connection with exophthalmos:

Van Graef's sign:	Lagging behind the upper lid as the patient looks downward
Stellwag's sign:	Diminished frequency of blinking
Moebius sign:	Inability to maintain convergence for close vision
Dalrymple's sign:	• Retractable lids causing a wide palpebral opening • It is fairly constantly present but may be found in other conditions

Tics

It is spontaneous stereotyped muscle contraction. It involves the face. These scan be stopped momentarily by volition. They are often associated with obsessive compulsion disorder. Causes include encephalitis, head injury, Sydenham chorea, and carbon monoxide poisoning.

CHAPTER 406

Tinnitus

Tinnitus is a sound experience perceived by the child which originates within himself. In contrast to adults, children rarely complain of tinnitus unless specifically enquired.

- Subjective heard only by child/patient
- Objective heard by the examiner also enquire about
  - *Unilateral:*
    - Wax
    - Perforation
  - *Type of sound:*
    - Ringing
    - Vibratory, etc.
  - *Associated symptoms:*
    - Earache
    - Discharge

CAUSES

Vibratory

Vascular Disorder

- Arteriovenous malformation
- Carotid occlusive disease
- Aneurysm
- Venous hum
- Glomus tumor
- Dehiscent jugular bulb
- Persistent stapedial artery
- Abnormal mastoid emissary vein
- Arteriovenous fistula
- Benign intracranial hypertension
- Paget's disease.

Neuromuscular

- Palatal myoclonus
- Stapedial muscle spasm
- Tensor tympani muscle spasm
- Temporomandibular joint dysfunction

Miscellaneous

- Patulous eustachian tube
- Middle ear inflammation or cholesteatoma
- Spontaneous otoacoustic emissions (SOAEs)

Nonvibratory

Peripheral

- External auditory canal
- Middle ear
- Cochlea

Central

- Auditory nerve
- Brainstem
- Central auditory pathways

CHAPTER 407

Toe Walking

It is seen in spastic cerebral palsy, in normal children in early months of walking. In pathological condition there will be tightening of Achilles tendon and spasm of gastrocnemius. In normal children, toe walking is intermittent. They rest with their feet flat when they stop walking. Muscular dystrophy with proximal muscle weakness and tethered spinal cord are the causes of toe walking.

CHAPTER 408 Tongue

Fever, irritability, and regional lymphadenopathy usually precede intense inflammation of the gingiva. Pain accompanies the inflammation. Small vesicles erupt and then become shallow ulcers with red, elevated margins and gray craters. The gingiva, labial or buccal mucosa, soft palate, pharynx, sublingual mucosa, and tongue may be involved.

The tongue has been considered as an indicator of systemic disease. The tongue should be examined for anomalous malformations, color changes, white patches and ulcerations, tumors and transitory swellings, painful sensations and taste aberrations.

ANOMALIES

- *Macroglossia -acromegaly*
  - Cretinism
  - Mongolism
  - Lymphangioma
  - Hemangioma
  - Primary amyloidosis
  - Cystic hygroma
  - Angioedema
  - Endocrine dysfunction
- *Microglossia*
  - Isolated
  - Associated with Pierre Robin's syndrome.

Fissured Tongue

The tongue is asymptomatic and normal but crisscrossed by number of rounded deep folds. The sides of the fissures are devoid of papillae but otherwise the tongue is normally papillated.

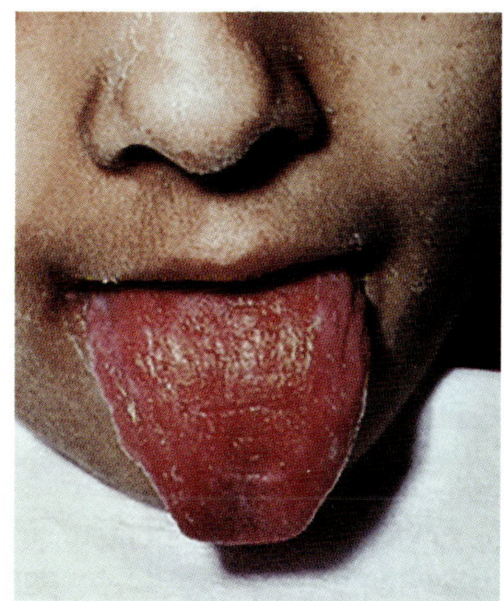

Fig. 1: Geographic tongue.

Geographic tongue or benign migratory glossitis A patch/patches of the tongue dorsum become depapillated. The patches heal on one side and progress on the another so that they "wander" over the tongue **(Fig. 1)**.

Small, red to purple spots form on the dorsal surface and edges of the tongue, gradually spread out, loose their papillae and form smooth, irregularly shaped, gray to white bordered, black and inflamed patches.

Coating of tongue can occur duc to many conditions like:

- High-fiber diet
- Mouth breathing

- Conditions causing xerostomia
- Infectious diseases
  - Pneumonia
  - Common cold
  - Enteric fever
  - Secondary mycoses due to antibiotics.
- General illness like
  - Diabetes
  - Polycythemia, etc.

Black hairy tongue presents as areas symmetrically involved about the midline of the tongue extending forward from the region of the circumvallate papillae due to overgrowth and staining of filiform papillae.

Tongue swellings may be generalized or may be confined to a region. If generalized they may stem from trauma, angioedema, and diffuse glossitis of uncommonly tumors. Local swellings may be due to lingual tonsillitis, mucocele, pyogenic granuloma, various cysts, or tumors.

The tongue should be palpated carefully if any swelling occurs and site, tenderness, temperature, mobility, consistency, etc., should be described.

The mucus membrane of the tongue is covered by filiform papillae and vary in length from 1 to 3 mm. These cover major portions on tongue. Fungiform papillae are found at the apex and along the lateral aspect of the tongue.

Very marked overgrowth of the filiform papillae produces black hairy tongue. This is a rare condition seen with anti-biotic therapy. Classical strawberry or raspberry tongue may be because of hypertrophy of fungiform papillae seen in scarlet fever.

The yeast candida albicans produces mucosal infection—the clinical picture—candidosis or oral thrush. Creamy white curd-like patches occur on the tongue and other areas of buccal mucosa. A raw bleeding area is revealed. When scrapped the lesion can be very painful. This is among sick infants, debilitated patients receiving high dose of corticosteroids and broad-spectrum antibiotics.

The tongue will appear blue in patients who are centrally cyanosed and pale in anemia patients. Many anemic patients however have a red and painful bald tongue. This is the consequence of complete atrophy of papillae. This may occur in iron deficiency anemia.

Acrodermatitis enteropathica is an autosomal recessive disorder related to zinc deficiency. Intra oral features include a white coating of a tongue and buccal mucosa with marked halitosis **(Fig. 2)**. There is chronic diarrhea, hair loss, severe dermatitis, and failure to thrive.

Swelling and enlargement of the tongue may be due to bite, stinge, and injury. It may be sometimes due to ingestion of serum, aspirin, and mercury. It may be symptoms of certain disease such as cretinism, acromegaly, mongolism, and myxedema.

Ranula and sublingual salivary gland calculus or cyst cause swelling that are beneath the front part of the tongue. This produces the bulging up one side of the floor of the mouth near the frenulum linguae. Ranula is a distended mucus gland.

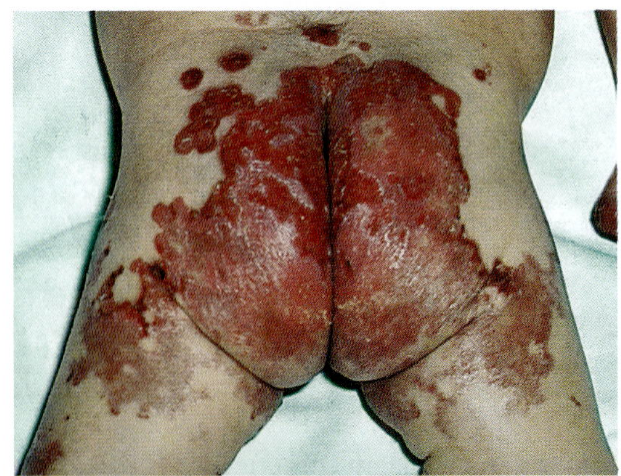

Fig. 2: Acrodermatitis enteropathica.

Suprahyoid cyst is situated at the root of the tongue posteriorly, when it arises from the remains of the embryo logical thyroglossal duct. Lipoma occurs infrequently in the tongue. Its lobulated form generally breaks surface and presents like a cluster of white cherries.

Hemorrhage into the substance of the tongue with swelling and inability to speak may result from blood disorders. These include leukemia, primary, or secondary thrombocytopenia.

Acute edema of the tongue may be due to severe stomatitis angioneurotic edema of tongue or Ludwig's angina. It is acute inflammatory condition caused by usually streptococcus. It affects the floor of mouth and tongue. It spreads rapidly through the deeper structures of the mouth, throat, and neck. Hence, it produces extreme swelling of the adjacent tissues.

Septic irritation of the mouth due to variety of causes such as decayed teeth, alkaline acids are accompanied by formation of small vesicles, which on bursting give rise to superficial ulcers. They are not limited to the tongue but also appear on the mucus membrane of the cheeks and gums.

Aphthous stomatitis occurs in febrile disease of childhood. It is characterized by the formation of whitish spots on the buccal mucus membrane, and superficial ulcers may be formed by shedding of the epithelium.

The ulcers of tongue occur during the course of general inflammation of mouth. The ulcers are found with chicken pox, pemphigus, and other conditions that may affect the buccal mucosa as well as the skin.

409 CHAPTER

Torticollis

Torticollis (wry neck) may be congenital or acquired. Most common reason is sternomastoid tumor (ischemic fibrosis in the sternomastoid muscle) may regress in 4–8 months' time, during this time torticollis or tilting of the head to the affected side may occur. This is often seen in a situation where there was difficulty in delivering after coming head in breech delivery.

OTHER CAUSES OF TORTICOLLIS

- Protective torticollis due to muscle spasm on the affected side-acute cervical adenitis
- Cervical Pott's disease
- Retropharyngeal abscess
- Subluxation of atlanto-occipital joint (nontraumatic)
- Cerebellar tumors such as astrocytoma (patient has tilting of the occiput to the affected side)

PROGNOSIS

Uncorrected torticollis may lead to facial asymmetry. The growth of the face on the affected side is diminished. Hence follow-up is essential.

CHAPTER 410

Tracheal Deviation

Palpation of the trachea in the neck may provide information about the position of the mediastinum, provided the thoracic cage is straight, and thyroid gland is not enlarged.

Displacement of the trachea from the midsternal line will usually signify disease of the pleura, lungs, or mediastinum. Deviation of the trachea away from the abnormal side will suggest volume displacement. This is seen with large pleural effusion, pneumothorax under tension, bullous emphysema, and rarely neoplasm.

Deviation toward the abnormal side suggests collapse of the underlying upper lobe or lung, fibrotic contracture of the lobe, pleural thickening, secondary to healed pulmonary tuberculosis.

The trachea will not be displaced by consolidation without the collapse of the underlying lung. The confirmatory chest radiograph should be taken if there is any clinical suspicion of lung or pleural disease.

411 CHAPTER

Tracheal Position

Tracheal can be assessed with the child in either the supine or upright position. Palpate as many normal tracheas in difficult childhood age groups as possible. The trachea is a mobile, easily displaced structure. In infants with short chubby necks, the exact location is difficult to ascertain. Your main purpose is to decide whether the trachea is shifted to the right or left, which would be associated with serious intrathoracic abnormalities such as pneumothorax or atelectasis.

The trachea extends downward from the lower border of the cricoid cartilage to the bifurcation into the two main bronchi. In normal individuals the upper half of the trachea lies in the midline of the neck, lower half of the neck, lower half of the trachea in the intrathoracic portion includes slightly to the right of the midline.

Trail sign: Undue prominence of the clavicular head of the sternomastoid muscle on one side, is usually indicative of tracheal displacement to that side.

Mechanism: The pretracheal fascia encloses the sternomastoid muscle and is in close contact with the tendon of the muscle. Tracheal displacement is reflected therefore in an increased tension of the sternomastoid muscle on the same side as that to which the mediastinum is pulled or pushed.

POSITION OF TRACHEA

In normal subjects the upper 4–5 cm of the trachea can be felt in the neck between the cricoid cartilage and the suprasternal notch.

Methods of palpation of trachea: With a little experience in tracheal palpation, it is possible to detect relatively small degrees of mediastinal shift.

Patient is made to sit or stand with head in midline and neck is slightly extended. Left hand of the examiner is used to fix the head in the midline. The tip of right index finger is placed in the suprasternal notch and gently slide in the midline which normally encounters trachea. In case of tracheal shift finger consistently slides off to the side of shift.

An alternative method of detecting tracheal deviation is to measure the space between the sternomastoid and trachea (trachea-sternomastoid space) by introducing index finger. This space is decreased to the side of tracheal deviation. This method is more suitable in children.

CHAPTER 412

Trendelenburg Test

To perform the test the patient stands on the unaffected leg and flexes the other knee to right angle. The pelvis should remain level or tilt up slightly on the non-weight bearing side. The patient then stands on the affected leg flexes the knee of other leg.

The positive sign indicates weakness in hip abductor muscles—gluteus medius and gluteus minimus. These findings can be associated with various hip abnormalities such as congenital hip dislocation, rheumatic arthritis, and osteoarthritis.

Tremor

RHYTHMIC AND REGULAR OSCILLATIONS OF A BODY PART

Types

- Resting tremors [3–5 cycles per second (CPS)] often seen in parkinsonism have low amplitude and regular frequency of five CPS, disappear during intentional movement and increases during emotional stress.
  There are two descriptive types:
  1. Pill rolling
  2. Drum beating
- Parkinsonism tremors are often associated with lead-pipe or cogwheel rigidity, over all bradykinesia, and akathisia (an irresistible need to move).
- Intentional (ataxic tremor) regular tremor of low or moderate amplitude that appears during intentional movement (Finger-Nose test).
- *Positional or postural tremor:* It occurs in maintaining a certain posture, e.g., holding head up or out stretching of hand. These are seen in cerebellar lesions or in their pathways. A combination of resting tremor, intention tremor, postural tremor constitutes "rubral tremor" due to a lesion in dentatorubral or dento-thalamic tract.
- Tremors of anxiety, hypoglycemia, and hyperthyroidism are fine and fast (10 CPS).

CLINICAL EVALUATION OF TREMORS

- Distribution (hand, jaws, tongue, head, trunk, and legs)
- Rate (3–12 CPS)
  - Physiological—10 CPS
  - Parkinsonism—5 CPS
- Amplitude (fine and coarse)
- *Relation to movement:* Intentional (cerebellar)
  - Posture—postural
  - Rest (resting—Parkinsonism)
  - End point tremor (Finger-Nose test—cerebellum)
- Relation to sleep and emotion—all disappear in sleep and increased during emotions
- Response to drugs
- Associated symptoms

Benign essential tremor: This is a mild and slowly progressive start on one side of the body may involve the other side within a period of 3 years. Hands are mainly involved but it can involve head, trunk, tongue, and legs. There will mildly gait disturbances.

Cerebellar tremor: This is other called as intention tremors occur in cerebellar lesions involving the hand. This is elicited by asking child to approach the object by hand.

Flapping tremor: These are irregular abrupt, brief loss of posture in outstretched hands. The patient is asked to stretch the hands forward with the hand dorsiflexed at wrist. The wing-beating movements at the wrist are seen.

Physiological tremor: These occur in normal children and are not significant.

Parkinsons tremor: It is classically seen as pill rolling movements of hand. It is increased by stress and emotion.

414 CHAPTER

Tuberous Sclerosis

It is inherited as an autosomal dominant trait. Two genes appear to cause the disorder. TSC1 is located on chromosome 9 TSC2 on chromosome 16p. Their gene products (hamartin for TSC1 and tuberin for TSC2) have tumor suppressive activity, which is dysfunctional in affected patients.

The more prominent features include seizure, mental retardation, autism, intracranial calcification tumors of various organs such as brain, heart, liver and kidneys, and skin lesions.

The characteristic skin lesion is the angiofibroma (adenoma sebaceum). These are erythematous papules distributed over the nose and malar region of the face. Hypomelanotic macule with irregular borders, termed as ash-leaf spots, are another common cutaneous lesion. These generally appear earlier than adenoma sebaceum and may be present at birth. They resemble vitiligo, but they are not completely devoid of melanin. Shagreen patch, a plaque of thickened skin with a cobblestone or orange-peel texture often seen on the dorsal aspect of trunk. Additional skin manifestation includes periungual fibroma and macular areas of hyperpigmentation.

CHAPTER 415 Umbilicus

The position of the umbilicus varies from infant to young adult. It is more toward the symphysis pubis at birth. It will be midway between xiphisternum and symphysis pubis, when the upper arm and lower arm equals.

Normally umbilicus is inverted. Flattened and everted is associated with ascites.

In the newborn, the umbilical stump dries up and falls by 4–6 days of life. Infection of umbilicus is suspected if umbilicus does not fall **(Fig. 1)**.

Umbilical polyp is related to the urachal and omphalomesenteric duct. It is associated with fecal or watery discharge. If small opening is present at the center of the lesion, then it is related to the urachus or an omphalomesenteric duct. The polyp will have a pedicle.

Umbilical granuloma is red granulation tissue present at the base of the umbilicus. It will have neither an opening nor a pedicle.

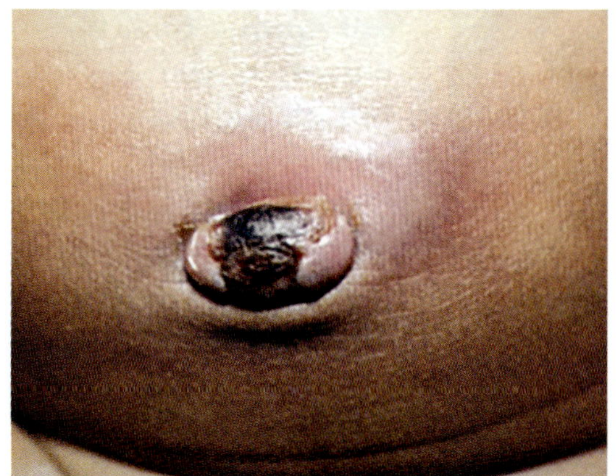

Fig. 1: Umbilical sepsis.

Discharge from the umbilicus could be urine, purulent or serosanguineous. It may be due to urachus, urachal cyst or patent omphalomesenteric duct.

Umbilical hernia is the defect present over an inch in diameter. Surgical treatment is required if it persists beyond 2 years. Omphalocele is a large hernia of the abdominal content into the base of the umbilicus, particularly into the presence of abdominal musculature.

UMBILICAL GRANULOMA

Umbilical granulomas are common in newborns and usually resolve spontaneously. If an umbilical granuloma persists, topical application of sliver nitrate produces chemical cauterization and desiccation. The granuloma is the result to residual umbilical cord tissue that persists after the cord separates. It can be a nuisance because the drainage that occurs can be somewhat purulent. Occasionally, such granulomas increase in size beyond the usual couple of millimeters in diameter to more than a centimeter in diameter **(Fig. 2)**. Large granulomas may require excision, but even these usually disappear with repeated topical applications of silver nitrate.

Persistent granulomas ultimately epithelialize to result in a tiny umbilical nodule at the base of the umbilicus. These nodules rarely increase in size and may result in an umbilical epidermoid inclusion cyst that requires surgical excision. Tiny persistent

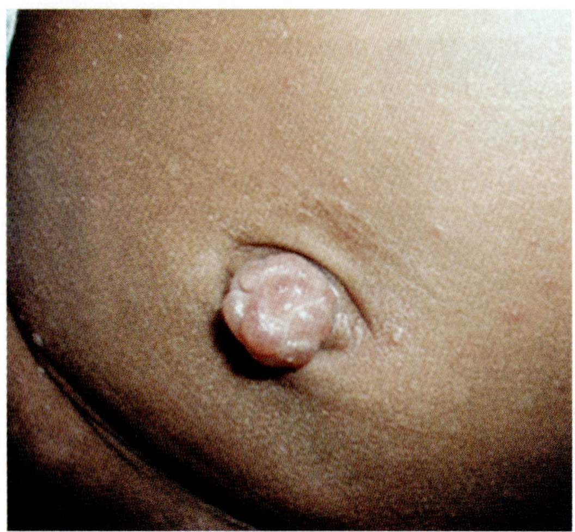

Fig. 2: Umbilical granuloma.

epithelial nodules at the base of the umbilicus should be left alone.

Occasionally, an umbilical granuloma will resist efforts at silver nitrate cauterization. Such a granuloma should be carefully evaluated because it may, in fact, represent a persistent ectopic (usually intestinal) mucosa rather than a granuloma, related to incomplete disappearance of the vitelline duct. Such a persistent mucosa demands careful evaluation to assess whether any deeper associated connections exist, such as an (uncommon) omphalomesenteric duct. A persistent mucosa ultimately will require excision; otherwise, it will continue to produce serous or mucous drainage.

CHAPTER 416

Umbilical Artery Catheterization

One of the arteries should be cut fresh with Wharton jelly. The orifice of the artery is gently teased open with the help of mosquito forceps. Edge of the artery and surrounding Wharton jelly is held with a pair of fine-toothed forceps. The artery catheter which is end holed PVC FG6 is used. Heparinized saline, i.e., 2 units/mL, is introduced. The cord stump should be pulled up toward the infant's head to strengthen the artery. False passage is the important cause of failure. Once this has been passed, it can be passed into the aorta.

Purse-string is put to immobilize around the umbilicus. Position is confirmed radiologically. Antibiotic powder is sprayed. Great care must be taken to ensure that air does not enter the catheter. Sometimes the tip of the catheter is required to advance into the internal iliac artery or beyond for adequate flow of arterial flood. The tip of the catheter should be advanced either to level T_{12} or T_{34} to avoid the celiac axis and renal vessels. Position should be checked radiologically.

UMBILICAL ARTERY CUT DOWN

If umbilical artery cannot be cannulated from the cut end of the stump, a small semi-circular incision is made below the umbilical stump. This contains umbilical arteries and urachus. The fascia is divided and urachus is identified as a glistening firm midline structure, umbilical artery lies on each side. The artery is cannulated with conventional umbilical artery catheterization.

CHAPTER 417

Umbilical Hernia

An umbilical hernia is a common finding. The incidence of this defect of the central fascia beneath the umbilicus is also higher in premature infants and those with congenital thyroid deficiency **(Figs. 1A and B)**. It is important to distinguish between this relatively benign fascial defect and the more serious defects of the somites that form the peritoneal, muscular, and ectodermal layers of the abdominal wall underlying the umbilicus, resulting in an omphalocele. In the latter condition, a portion of the intestine is located outside the abdominal wall. When large, the distinction is obvious; but in its mildest form, an omphalocele resembles a fixed hernia of the umbilicus.

True umbilical hernias usually require no therapy, and spontaneous resolution occurs within the first few years of life. Those that remain after 3 years old can be surgically repaired. Attempts to reduce the hernia with tape or coins are ineffective and may result in side effects, such as adhesive reaction/allergy. Incarceration is rare.

The most common condition of the abdominal wall is an umbilical hernia. This results from the failed closure of the fascial ring during the first few years of life. After desiccation of the umbilical vessels and urachus and separation of the umbilical remnant in the first month of life, the umbilical ring typically undergoes closure in the next 2–4 years. In some patients, this process is never completed. For unclear reasons, there appears to be strong familial and racial predilection for hernia development.

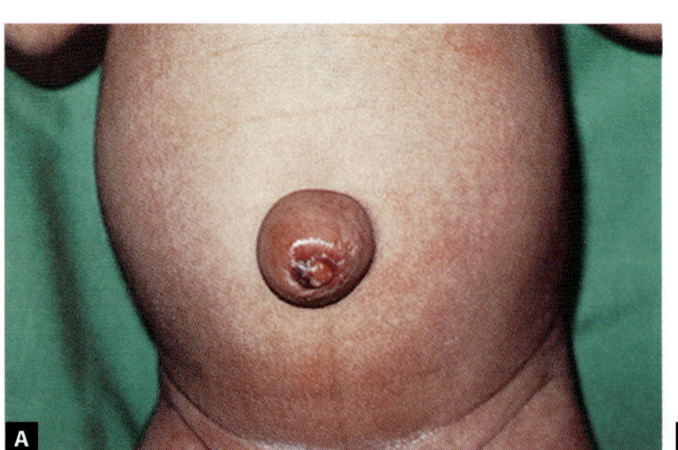

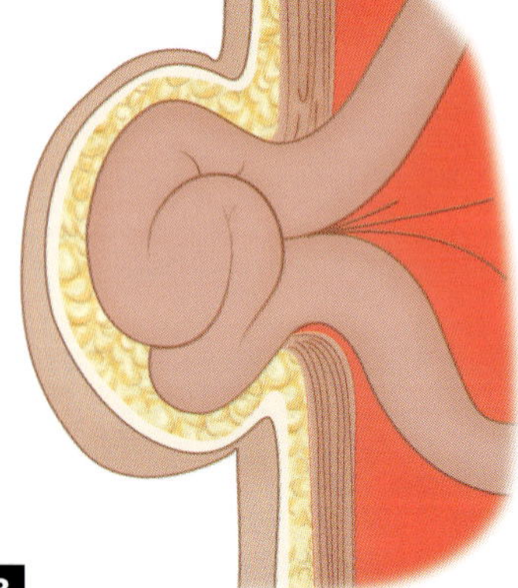

Figs. 1A and B: Umbilical hernia.

Because most of these lesions resolve spontaneously, and umbilical hernias rarely become incarcerated, repair is frequently deferred until the child's fifth birthday. Patients with hernias that are >2 cm in diameter, have a proboscoid or "elephant's trunk" appearance, or have a history of incarceration should not have their surgery delayed.

ABNORMAL UMBILICAL DISCHARGE

- *Serous:* Infection
- *Blood:* Granuloma
- *Pus:* Infection
- *Greenish:* Patent vitellointestinal duct
- *Urine:* Patent urachus—remnant omphalomesenteric duct
- *Feces:* Patent vitellointestinal duct

418 CHAPTER

Umbilical Vein Catheterization

Both the umbilical vein and the artery can be catheterized up to 7–10 days of the delivery. It is easier just after birth. Umbilical vein catheterization is rarely needed except for exchange transfusion or if umbilical artery catheterization fails **(Fig. 1)**.

Cord clamps or ligatures used to prevent bleeding at the time of delivery are removed. About 2-cm cord is to be exposed. Cord and surrounding skill are prepared with antiseptic and area is draped with a sterile towel.

The cord is cut 1 cm from the abdominal wall. The artery may spurt the blood. The whole cord is compressed between the fingers. There are two arteries and one vein. The vein is usually larger and lies open in an exposed cord. Vein has thin wall and an irregular outline. The arteries are usually smaller, thick walled, white and closed. Any clot present at the opening of the vein is removed.

The exposed or cut vein is held by one or two mosquito forceps. This helps to grip the edges of the vein. The catheter of the sized PVC FG6 filled with heparinized saline is used. The catheter can be gently introduced into the vein. Some obstruction is encountered when the catheter reaches the point where vein passes through the abdominal wall. At a depth of about 5–7 cm, the blood is easily withdrawn. The tip of the catheter is the portal sinus. The catheter can be passed from the portal sinus into the inferior vena cava through ductus venous within 24 hours of birth. Catheter can be passed to right atrium and then to left atrium. Radiological confirmation of the tip of the catheter is recommended. All these catheters should have a side hole.

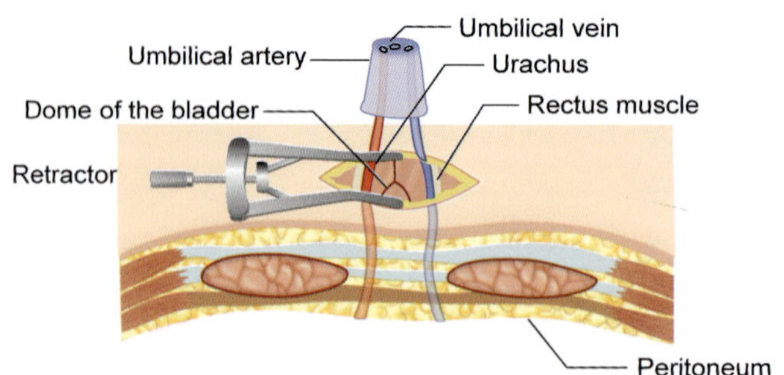

Fig. 1: Umbilical vein catheterization.

The catheter is connected to syringe according to the procedure intended by a 2- or 3-way tap. Maintenance drip at the rate of 1–2 mL/hour of dextrose or electrolyte is begun. The forceps are removed, and catheter is held in place by purse-string suture. Ligature around the cord stump, if there is bleeding around the catheter.

Catheters passing through the ductus venosus into the thorax is the consistent threat of air embolism. If the catheter cannot pass through the ductus, then its tip probably lies in comparatively slugging blood flow. Along with this hyperosmolar solution may produce risk of thrombotic complication. Hence catheter is placed for the shortest possible time.

There is a risk of arterial hemorrhage when removing the catheter. To prevent this ligature, the catheter should be divided. Dried and caked Wharton's jelly is removed. Umbilical stump is freshened. A black silk suture is inserted around the stump. When the catheter is removed, the sutures can be pulled tight. Catheter is withdrawn slowly. Before removing the final centimeter, a time of about 1–2 minutes is given for the vessel to get spasm proximally. Then the tip of the catheter is slowly removed and placed in transparent medium and sent for culture.

CHAPTER 419

Undescended Testes

The absence of palpable testes in scrotum indicates that the testes are undescended, atrophic, or retractile.

The process of testicular descent is regulated by an interaction among the genetic, hormonal, and mechanical factors, including testosterone, dihydrotestosterone, Müllerian-inhibiting factor, the gubernaculum, intra-abdominal pressure, and genitofemoral nerve. The gubernaculum distends inguinal canal and guides testes into scrotum. Following testicular descent, the patent process vaginalis (hernia sac) normally involutes.

The diagnosis of undescended testes depends upon the following points. One side of the scrotum is empty. Swelling in the outside, i.e., in superficial inguinal region or elsewhere. Sometimes it may result in acute pain secondary to inflammatory lesion or acute torsion of organ. The partially descended testicle is often accompanied by an inguinal hernia. The misplaced testes have the risk of malignant disease.

Treatment is surgical procedure done at 9–15 months of age. Surgical correction at 6 months is appropriate, because spontaneous descent will not be after 4 months of age. Most testes can be brought down to the scrotum with an orchiopexy. This involves an inguinal incision, mobilization of testis and spermatic cord, and correction of indirect inguinal hernia.

CHAPTER 420

Upper Limb

POLYDACTYLY

There are more than five fingers in the limbs. It can be congenital or familial. It is associated with Laurence-Moon-Biedl syndrome, Carpenter syndrome, Turner syndrome, and trisomy 13 **(Figs. 1A and B)**.

SYNDACTYLY

Syndactyly is a condition in which there is fusion of two or more digits. It is seen among Apert syndrome, Carpenter syndrome, Holt-Oram syndrome, trisomy 21,13 and 18, and Fanconi syndrome **(Figs. 2 and 3).**

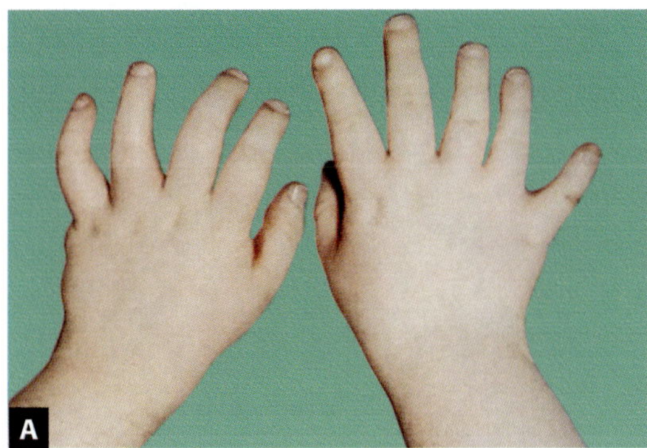

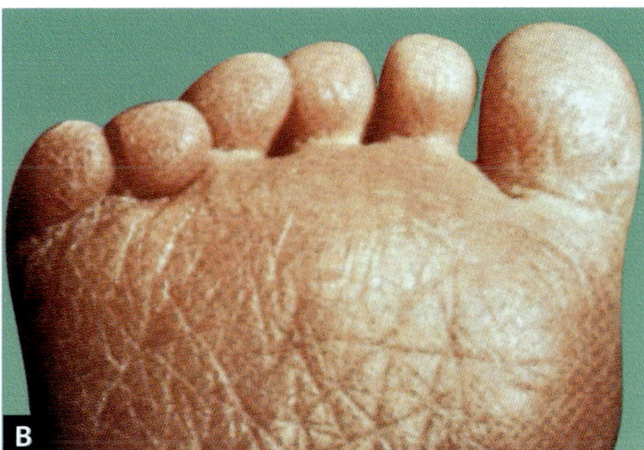

Figs. 1A and B: Polydactyly.

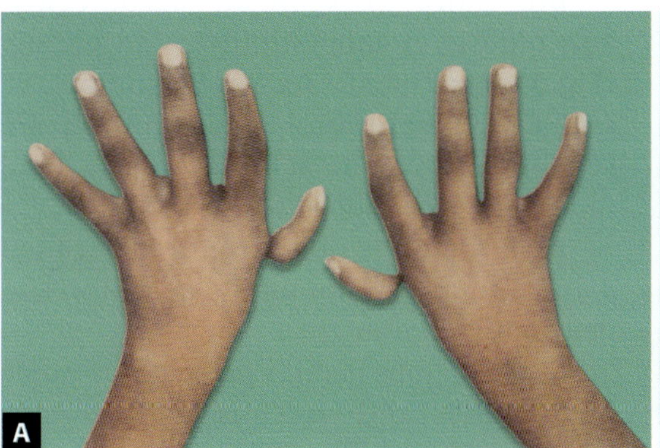

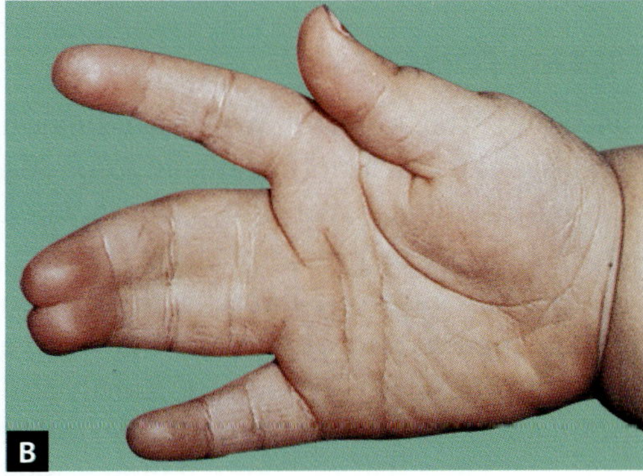

Figs. 2A and B: Syndactyly.

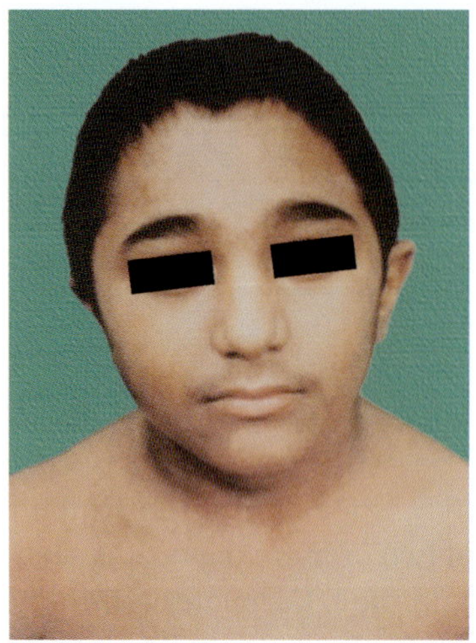

Fig. 3: Fanconi syndrome.

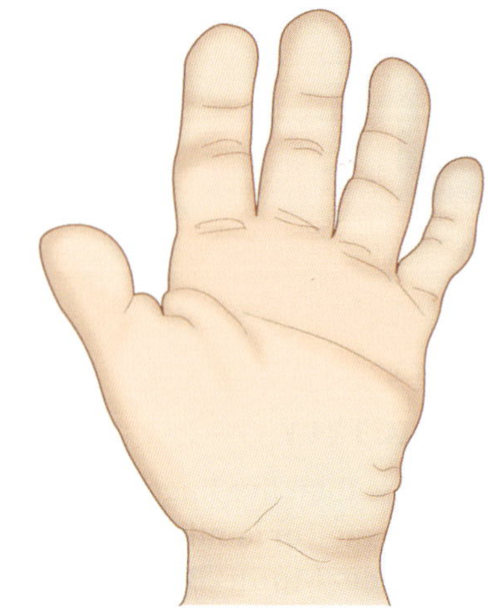

Fig. 4: Clinodactyly—incurving of fifth finger.

ARACHNODACTYLY

Here the fingers and toes are abnormally long and thin. It is associated with Marfan syndrome, hypogonadism, homocystinuria, and hypopituitarism.

CLINODACTYLY

Here the little finger is curved. Hypoplasia of the middle phalanx leads to the congenital deviation of little finger **(Fig. 4)**. It is seen in Down syndrome, Aarskog's syndrome, and de Lange syndrome.

CAMPTODACTYLY

It is congenital anterior-posterior flexion deformity at metacarpophalangeal joint and proximal interphalangeal joint. It is associated with trauma and neurological abnormality.

Ulnar deviation of hand is present in juvenile rheumatoid arthritis. Ulnar nerve paralysis produces extension of fourth and fifth finger at metacarpal joint and flexion at proximal interphalangeal joint. Radial aspect of the hand is hypoplastic in the Fanconi syndrome and Holt-Oram syndrome.

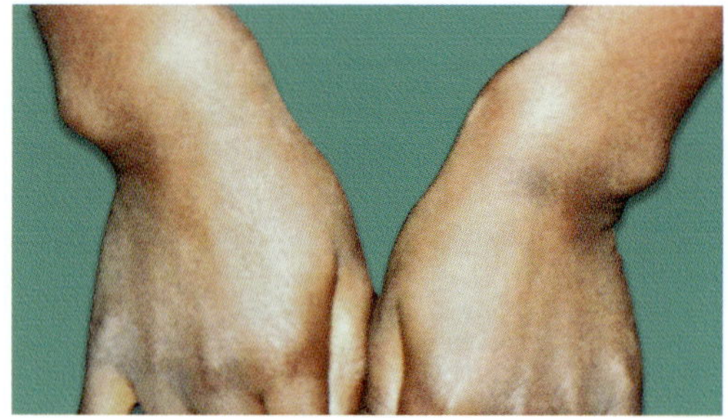

Fig. 5: Broad wrist.

Big hand is seen in acromegaly, amyloidosis, homocystinuria, and obesity **(Fig. 5)**. Small hand is seen in achondroplasia and Down syndrome. Short fingers are seen in cretinism, achondroplasia, and mucopolysaccharidosis **(Fig. 6)**.

Bifid thumb is present in translocation 3 and 13. Aplastic thumb is present in 13q deletion syndrome.

Erythematous palm is present in chronic liver disorders, thyrotoxicosis, and in juvenile rheumatoid arthritis. Pale palm indicates

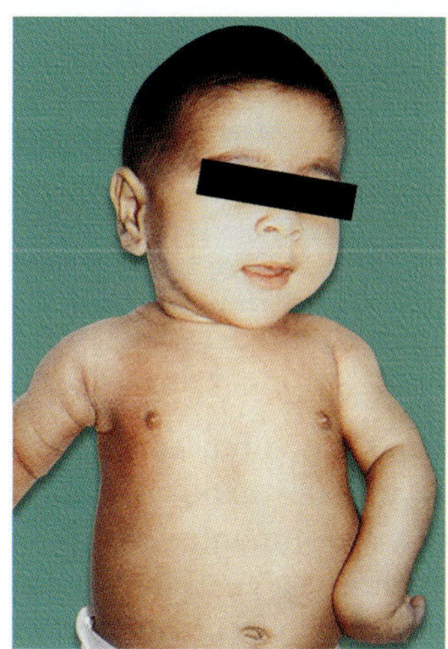

Fig. 6: Erb's palsy.

anemia. In Addison's disease, palm is pigmented.

Tremors and fasciculations are the involuntary movements present in the hand. Tremors are seen in anxiety, thyrotoxicosis. Fasciculation in hand is normal. Flapping tremors are present in liver failure, uremia and thiamine deficiency.

Simian-crease: A single palmar crease is present in 5% of normal newborn and 45% of Down syndrome. Hypoplasia of the middle phalanx in the fifth finger is present. This produces clinodactyly, i.e., deflection of the finger. Hands are short and broad. Gap between first and second toe is wide.

CHAPTER 421 Urticaria

Hypersensitivity reactions in which the skin is the major target organ are manifested clinically as diffuse erythema, urticaria, or angioedema **(Fig. 1)**. Most angioedema and urticaria are due to IgE-mediated type I hypersensitivity involving degranulation of mast cells and basophils from multiple triggers. However, non-IgE-mediated mechanisms can also cause degranulation of these cells through activation of other pathways, such as complement and immune complex formation. The end result is vascular permeability with edema in the dermis in urticaria and primarily in the subcutaneous tissues in angioedema. Although frequently seen in combination, urticaria and angioedema may also appear individually.

Urticaria is most frequently an acute disorder that resolves spontaneously. In children, it is often secondary to viral illnesses, allergen exposure (food, medication, or environmental), or idiopathic in nature. Typically, a good history looking for inciting exposures can identify a cause. When the duration exceeds 6 weeks, the condition is arbitrarily termed *chronic urticaria*. In contrast to acute urticaria, chronic urticaria is typically idiopathic in nature. Therefore, extensive workup looking for a cause is not helpful or warranted in the majority of chronic urticaria. In approximately one-third of these cases, an autoimmune etiology can be demonstrated, with evidence of an autoantibody to the IgE receptor on mast cells and basophils; thus, individuals experience degranulation of these cells in the absence of specific IgE to an allergen.

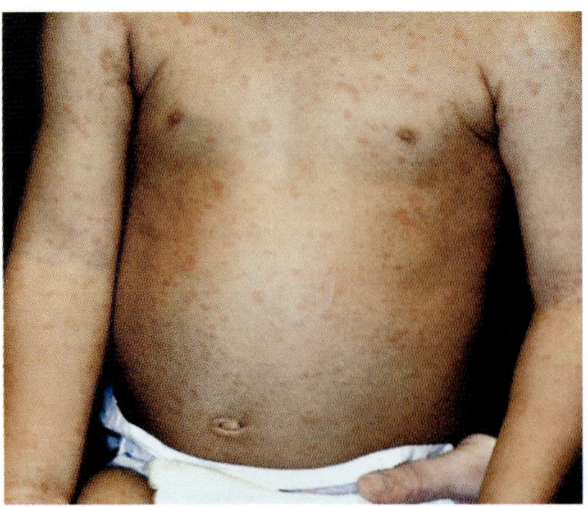

Fig. 1: Urticaria.

Urticarial lesions are well circumscribed, raised, palpable wheals that blanch with applied pressure. They are usually erythematous but may be pale or white with red halos. Typically, the lesions are intensely pruritic; however, in some instances the pruritus is mild. Angioedema is characterized by diffuse subcutaneous tissue swelling with normal or erythematous overlying skin. Angioedema may be more painful than pruritic. The face, hands, feet, and perineum are most commonly involved. Angioedema, unlike other types of edemas, is not gravity dependent. Skin involvement may be generalized or localized to body parts exposed to a provoking stimulus. In general, urticaria that is not associated with pain, respiratory or GI symptoms, or residual skin changes, and in which individual lesions are red/pink and last <24 hours, is benign and may be managed symptomatically.

A subgroup of urticarial disorders results from hypersensitivity to physical and mechanical factors. These include cold urticaria, pressure-induced urticaria and angioedema, aquagenic and solar urticaria, cholinergic, and exercise-induced urticaria. The history and distribution of lesions often help in identifying the source, which can then be confirmed by challenge.

Dermographism, translated literally as the "ability to write on the skin", is a form of trauma-induced pressure urticaria. It is elicited by stroking the skin with a fingernail or tongue blade. The initial white line secondary to reflex vasoconstriction is supplanted by pruritic, erythematous linear swelling, as seen in a classic wheal and flare reaction. The condition is chronic and the etiology unclear. Patients with dermographism suspected of having an atopic disorder must be skin tested with caution for specific IgE antibody, because all test results appear positive.

Uveitis

Uveitis is defined as inflammation of the uveal tissue of the eye, which includes the iris, ciliary body, and choroid. Inflammation can involve any or all of these structures, and terms such as iritis, iridocyclitis, choroiditis, and chorioretinitis are used to designate which portion of the uveal tissue is involved. Anatomic locations such as anterior, posterior, intermediate, or panuveitis are useful in determining etiology.

In iritis or "anterior uveitis", the eye is congested and painful (in contrast to a "posterior uveitis", or choroiditis, which simply blurs the vision).

It is suspected if the eyes appear large and protruding. The causes are:

- Hyperthyroidism
- Glaucoma
- Retro-orbital tumor
- Neurofibromatosis
- Lymphangioma
- Hemangioma

Juvenile idiopathic arthritis (JIA) is the most common cause of childhood anterior uveitis. JIA uveitis is most common in the pauciarticular form, when the onset occurs before the age of 7 years, and when the antinuclear antibody blood test is positive. Girls are at higher risk than boys; 10–15% of children with JIA develop uveitis and 10% of those who develop uveitis do so prior to the diagnosis of JIA. It is common for children with JIA to have no symptoms of inflammation in the eye. Despite the lack of symptoms, uveitis can cause severe vision loss due to the development of edema or deposition of calcium (band keratopathy) in the cornea or retinal edema.

A cataract and/or glaucoma may result from inflammation in the eye or chronic use of steroids used to quiet the inflammation. The pupil may have an irregular shape as a result of adhesions to the underlying lens (posterior synechiae). Visual impairment occurs in up to 40% of children with JIA uveitis and blindness occurs in 10% of affected eyes. For this reason, there are screening guidelines for the recommended frequency of eye examinations based on the risk factors that predispose patients with JIA to uveitis including category of arthritis (oligoarthritis vs. polyarthritis), age of onset of arthritis, presence of antinuclear antibody (ANA) positivity, and duration of disease.

The diagnosis of uveitis can be made from an eye examination. Because uveitis can be caused by infections, trauma, autoimmune disorders, and may be idiopathic, evaluation of the cause of the uveitis requires a thorough pediatric physical examination as well as supplementary radiologic and laboratory testing. A chest radiograph may demonstrate tuberculosis and sarcoidosis. Serologic evaluation may include tests for syphilis, sarcoidosis, JIA, Lyme disease, herpes, measles, and toxoplasmosis. In boys, haplotype testing for human leukocyte antigen B27 may be indicated because of the association between iritis and pauciarticular arthritis that may later evolve into ankylosing spondylitis.

SECTION 21

Vaginal Bleeding

The usual progression of puberty in females dictates that breast and uterine development begin about 2 years before the menses. When the rate of pubertal progression is accelerated, menses may start as early as 1–1.5 years after thelarche; if the rate is slow, menses may start perhaps 3–4 years after thelarche. In any case, vaginal bleeding is always a much later sign than breast development, and whenever vaginal bleeding occurs too early—especially if it ever occurs before breast development starts—it must be investigated thoroughly.

Causes of bleeding:

- Genital lesions
  - Vaginitis
  - Foreign body
  - Trauma
  - Tumors
- Endocrine changes
  - Estrogen ingestion
  - Precocious puberty
  - Hormone producing ovarian tumor

Varicocele

A varicocele consists of dilated veins of the pampiniform plexus of the spermatic cord. Varicoceles occur primarily on the left side and may be found before puberty. They may be bilateral.

Probably because of:

- Left spermatic vein is longer than the right.
- Left spermatic vein enters the left renal vein at a right angle.
- At times, the left testicular artery arches over the left renal vein to compress it.
- The left colon when loaded may press on the left testicular vein.

EXAMINATION

Ask the patient to stand, swelling appears and disappears when he lies down with the scrotum elevated. The impulse on cough will give a thrill. On palpation, it feels like a bag of worms. After occluding the superficial inguinal ring with the thumb, if the patient is asked to stand up, varicocele fills from below.

The postulated causes of varicocele vary from hormonal to hydrostatic. The postulated cause of testicular injury from varicocele varies from hormonal deficiencies to temperature effects. Most varicoceles decompress in the supine position. Those that do not decompress or those that present with acute onset on either side may lead to concern about lesions in the kidney or retroperitoneum causing obstruction to venous outflow and retroperitoneal ultrasound is recommended.

Most varicoceles are asymptomatic and are noted by the child incidentally or discovered on routine examination. Pain secondary to varicocele is uncommon, but a dull aching may occur in large varicoceles.

Infertility is found in approximately 33% of adults with varicoceles, and because semen analyses are not generally available in children, controversy has arisen over the proper management of adolescents. Ablating varicoceles in adolescents with testicular growth failure ipsilateral to the varicocele (>20% size discrepancy between testes), or in those with bilateral varicocele, is common practice. Semen analysis can be obtained in the patient to assess if abnormal semen parameters exist. In patients with minimal or no testicular atrophy, observation and serial measurements of testicular volume are indicated, with the option to perform varicocele ablation if ipsilateral testicular growth failure becomes evident.

CHAPTER 425 Venous Hum

- Most common type of innocent continuous murmur.
- It is usually present in children and in hyperkinetic conditions such as anemia, thyrotoxicosis, cirrhosis, arteriovenous (AV) fistula, post-exertion, and anxiety.

CHARACTERISTICS

- It is best heard in the right supraclavicular fossa but often quite loud below the clavicles.
- Hum is a blowing continuous murmur, typically loud in diastole.
- *Murmur is abolished by the following methods:*
  - Compressing the internal jugular veins
  - Patient turns head from the side to a midline position
  - Supine position
  - By performing Valsalva's maneuver

TIPS IN AUSCULTATING VENOUS HUM

- A preferable position for auscultation is sitting upright.
- Auscultation is done using a stethoscope bell and by the right hand of examiner.
- Left hand grasps the patient's chin from behind and pulls it gently to the left and upward.

Ventricular Puncture

This is rarely needed to confirm the intraventricular hemorrhage. It may be required for the intraventricular antibiotics in neonatal coliform meningitis. Computed tomography (CT) scan is used to assess the size of the ventricle. If the ventricular size is small, ventricular puncture should not be done.

The infant is wrapped and held supine with the crown of the head at the edge of the table. Edges of the anterior fontanelle are demarcated, the head is draped. Lumbar puncture needle is inserted at the lateral angle of the anterior fontanelle. Needle should be directed toward the plain of the inner canthus of opposite eye. The needle will get into the ventricle at the depth of 4–5 cm.

CHAPTER 427

Vernix Caseosa

The skin of the head and face of a newborn may exhibit a variety of changes. Most of them have little significance, but it is important to reassure the parents that they are normal and do not require treatment. At birth, the normal full-term infant is covered to varying degrees with vernix caseosa. The literal translation of this term from Latin is "cheesy varnish"—it is a greasy substance that protects the skin during the lengthy immersion that protects the skin during the immersion in amniotic fluid, much as the skin of a long-distance swimmer fluid, much as the skin of a long-distance swimmer is protected by having heavy grease applied to it. Vernix caseosa is the normal sebaceous secretion of the skin.

428 CHAPTER

Vertigo

The characteristic description of vertigo is the illusion of motion usually described as spinning or whirling. The perception of motion may be internal or external. The sensation is usually rotatory, but it can be linear.

The presence of associated symptoms may help locate the pathology to a central or peripheral cause of vertigo.

Fortunately, peripheral causes of vertigo are more common. Spontaneous nystagmus and abnormal head positions are symptoms associated more with peripheral causes of vertigo along with nausea, vomiting, sweating, faintness, and fright. Peripheral vertigo results in stimulation of the autonomic nervous system with resultant intense nausea, vomiting, pallor, and diaphoresis. If the dizziness occurs with abrupt changes in the position of the head, peripheral causes of vertigo should be suspected. Peripheral vertigo can be caused by the following—middle ear infections, paroxysmal positional vertigo, labyrinthitis, vestibular neuronitis, Ménière disease, or trauma. Patients suffering from acute ongoing peripheral vertigo appear very ill and very uncomfortable. Because middle ear infection can cause peripheral vertigo, some children seen with otitis media and vomiting may in fact have peripheral vertigo and secondary vomiting.

DIAGNOSIS

The history and physical examination results direct the diagnostic workup and indicate which tests need to be performed. Imaging studies important in the workup of the vertiginous patient include computed tomography and magnetic resonance imaging. Both techniques allow visualization of the inner ear and the labyrinthine apparatus, as well as the brainstem and cerebellum.

If an infectious cause is suspected, it may be useful to perform a lumbar puncture as long as increased intracranial pressure is not suspected. In the setting of trauma, the simple use of the pneumatic otoscope may allow the examiner to perform a "fistula test," reproducing or worsening the patient's symptoms because of an abnormal communication to the labyrinthine system. If hearing loss is a feature, audiometry and evoked response testing should be considered.

SUMMARY AND RED FLAGS

Vertigo is characterized by the perception of movement, particularly rotational movement, and can be a most distressing and incapacitating phenomenon. The history and examination should allow the examiner to distinguish between peripheral and central vestibular dysfunction.

In children and adolescents, peripheral vertigo is far more common than central vertigo. However, in certain at-risk populations, such as children with sickle cell disease, hemophilia, or congenital heart disease (especially children with right-to-left shunts or mixing lesions), and children receiving anticoagulation therapy, the central causes resulting from hemorrhagic and thromboembolic phenomena must be considered. Chronicity, persistence, vertical nystagmus, and signs of increased intracranial pressure are red flags. Because the diagnosis of vertigo requires that the patient be able to articulate the perception of movement, it is difficult to make this diagnosis in young children; the condition must be carefully distinguished from other movement impairments, especially disequilibrium.

CHAPTER 429 Visual Acuity

It is not possible to test visual acuity below 3–4 years of age.

Normal visual acuity

At birth: 3/60

At 6 months: 6/30

At 18 months: 6/9

At 2 years: 6/6

Features suggestive of child might not be able to see:

- No blinking response to flash of light
- No visual fixation to object/human face
- Nystagmus in an infant and young child

Blindness is very difficult to suspect <3 months of age. Partial loss of vision is called amblyopia and complete blindness is called as amaurosis. Blindness in children is caused by damage or lesion of visual pathways bilaterally.

CAUSES OF BLINDNESS

- Optic neuritis
- Retinitis pigmentosa
- Encephalitis
- Tuberculous meningitis
- Brain tumor
- Degenerative brain disease

Visual acuity is tested for distant vision and near vision.

Distant visual acuity is measured by using Snellen's chart. In the chart a series of letters of varying sizes are written in such a way that the top letter is visible to normal eye at 60 m. The subsequent lines are seen at 36, 24, 18, 9, 6, and 5 meters respectively. The visual acuity is recorded as d/D.

- *d:* Distance at which the letters are read.
- *D:* Distance at which the letters should be read.

The normal visual acuity is 6/6.

Visual acuity for the near vision or ordinary reading distance is assessed by Jaegar chart. The smallest print is N5. The nearest vision is recorded as the smallest type, which the child can read comfortably at a distance of 14 inches.

In infants, vision is tested by checking blinking response to bright light, turning of the head toward diffuse light or following colored moving ball or ring. Pupils may be dilated and fixed in optic atrophy. Pupillary response is normal in cortical blindness.

FEATURES OF CONGENITAL BLINDNESS

- Roving nystagmoid eye movements
- Persistence of squint beyond 6 months
- Absence of optico-kinetic nystagmus
- Lack of blink response to bright light or examiners hand
- Extra-sensitive to noise.

Visual Field

It cannot be tested precisely among infants and young children. Only gross assessment can be done by using some colorful objects. Any colorful object is moved in around the visual perimetry, and the response of the child is seen. The object is preferably placed from behind into the different quadrants of the field of vision.

Confrontation test is used in the older children, i.e., above map out the field of vision. Perimetry test is done only in children >9–10 years of age.

METHOD

The examiner sits opposite to the child at a distance of 1 m. To test the right eye, ask the child to cover the left eye with the left hand. Ask the child to look steadily into the examiner's left eye.

The examiner closes his right eye with his left eye. The examiner uses his left hand at its full length. Examiner brings his left hand with the moving finger from outward to inward, till the child notices the moving finger. That is the point of the field of the vision in that plane or direction. Like the examiner does in all directions, outward, downward, this same procedure is done and plotted with the other eye.

CAUSES OF CENTRAL SCOTOMA

- Meningitis
- Encephalitis
- Typhoid
- Mumps
- Measles
- Vitamin B_{12} deficiency
- Drugs—ethambutol
- Phenothiazine

CAUSES OF CONCENTRIC CONSTRICTION OF FIELD OF VISION

- Chronic papilledema
- Retinitis pigmentosa

Bitemporal hemianopsia is characteristically seen in craniopharyngioma producing lesions in the region of optic chiasma.

Homonymous hemianopia—temporal field of one eye and nasal field of opposite eye occurs due to lesions in optic radiation or visual cortex.

RED PIN TEST

This test outlines the central field of vision. This test is done by using a red pin head held up in the patient's field in the method described above. A central area of impaired vision (central scotoma) can be recognized by this method. This method allows the patient's visual field, including the size of the physiological blind spot, to be compared precisely with that of the examiner (assuming the examiner's vision is normal).

CHAPTER 431 Vitiligo

Vitiligo is an acquired disorder characterized by complete loss of the pigment of the involved skin. The condition often manifests during childhood and is believed to be linked to specific genetic mutations. Many authorities believe that vitiligo is an autoimmune process with circulating antibodies that destroy melanocytes. There is an increased incidence of autoimmune diseases in affected individuals and their families.

It is a common genetically determined patterned loss of pigmentation that follows the destruction of melanocytes. The lesions are oval/irregular ivory white patches surrounded by well-demarcated or hyperpigmented with convex border **(Fig. 1)**. Most of the patients have other autoimmune disorders.

Other features alopecia areata, ophthalmic abnormalities such as discrete depigmentation and pigment hyperplasia involving the choroid and retinal pigment epithelium, discrete atropic areas of the fundus, posterior chorioretinitis, and vitreous inflammation. Neurosensory hearing loss 20% of patients with melanoma has vitiligo.

The incidence of vitiligo in persons with diabetes mellitus is also higher than that in the general population.

The onset of vitiligo may be precipitated by sunburn or other trauma. Physical findings are usually sufficient for establishing the diagnosis. Well-demarcated depigmented macules and patches that are often bilateral and symmetric are distributed on the extremities, on the periorificial areas, and within skin folds. In some cases, depigmentation may have a segmental distribution. This variant is seen more commonly in children than in adults. The clinical course is unpredictable.

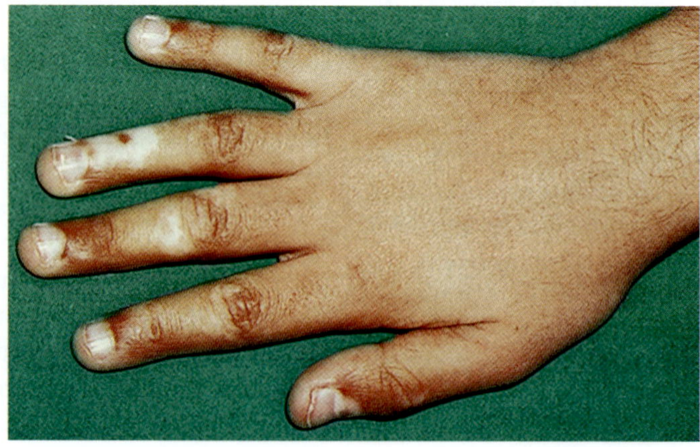

Fig. 1: Vitiligo.

Spontaneous complete repigmentation is unusual; however, partial repigmentation may be seen, especially within lesions of <2 years' duration. Repigmentation proceeds gradually and is more likely to occur in children than in adults.

In vitiligo, an acquired condition, there is partial to complete loss of pigmentation. Lesions consist of well-demarcated depigmented macules and patches that are usually seen in a characteristic distribution around the eyes, mouth, genitals, elbows, hands, and feet, although they may appear elsewhere, such as in a Koebnerized distribution in areas of prior friction or trauma. They enhance dramatically under a Wood lamp. Some patients may have halo nevi, which represents the same autoimmune reaction surrounding pigmented nevi. Spontaneous but slow repigmentation may occur from the edges of a lesion and around hair follicles (through which the pigment recurs first), resulting in a speckled appearance. Lesions on the head and neck repigment faster, because repigmentation occurs first through hair follicles and these areas have more numerous populations of hair follicles. Histologically, melanocytes are absent in areas of vitiligo, and evidence suggests that they have been destroyed by an autoimmune mechanism. In a small proportion of patients with vitiligo, other autoimmune conditions, such as alopecia areata, thyroiditis, diabetes, or pernicious anemia, can be detected concomitantly.

CHAPTER 432

Vocal Fremitus

Vocal fremitus occurs when sound vibration from the larynx passes down the bronchi. This causes the lungs and chest wall to vibrate. Intensity of fremitus is related to breathe sound intensity.

Increased tactile vocal fremitus is seen in consolidation and cavity. Decreased vocal fremitus is seen in pleural effusion, pneumothorax, fibrosis, bronchial obstruction, and pneumothorax.

433 CHAPTER

Vocal Resonance

Here the sounds are heard with the stethoscope over various parts of the chest during the act of phonation.

The patient is asked to repeat some syllables over and over again while the examiner auscultates the chest over the symmetric areas of chest. Vocal resonance is heard with chest piece of stethoscope. Decreased vocal resonance is heard in pleural effusion, pneumothorax thickened pleura, and emphysema.

Increased vocal resonance is seen in consolidatory and superficial lung cavity.

- *Bronchophony:* Here the spoken sounds appear loud and clear and close to ear. Individual syllables remain indistinguishable. It is normally audible over larynx and trachea. It is heard over pneumonic consolidation.
- *Whispering pectoriloque:* Vocal resonance is so much increased that even whispering from the patient is heard on the chest wall by stethoscope. It is seen in pneumonic consolidation with patent bronchus.
- *Aegophony:* Here the vocal resonance is increased, and intensity of spoken voice is increased and there is nasal quality. The quality of sound stimulates bleeding of goat. It is heard above the level of pleural effusion and pneumothorax.

  Vocal resonance of normal intensity generally conveys the impression of being produced just at the chest piece of the stethoscope. Various pulmonary pathologies alter the vocal resonance.
- *Increased VR:* When the vocal resonance is increased, it gives an impression that sound is nearer to the ear than at chest piece.
- *VR is increased in:*
  - Over areas of consolidation (solidified lung is a good conductor of sound vibrations).
  - Small superficial lung cavity.
- *Decreased VR is seen in:*
  - Pleural effusion
  - Pneumothorax
  - Thickened pleura
  - Emphysema

POST-TUSSIVE CREPITATIONS

These crepitations are audible after making the patient cough, while they are not audible during normal respiration.

It signifies presence of cavity which is filled with thick material which gets dislodged during coughing allowing air to bubble through the remaining fluid producing the crepitation. In small children crepitations that are not heard during quiet breathing may be heard after a bout of cry (post crying crepitations). They have the same significance as post-tussive crepitations.

CHAPTER 434

Vomiting

It is the forceful ejection of material from the upper gastrointestinal tract. True vomiting is often accompanied by nausea and retching.

Nausea is an unpleasant, vaguely epigastric or abdominal sensation accompanied by a variety of autonomic changes; decreases in gastric tone, contractions, secretion, and mucosal blood flow; increases in salivation, sweating, pupil diameter, and heart rate; and changes in respiratory rhythm. During nausea, retrograde peristalsis from the small intestine to the gastric antrum or generalized simultaneous contractions of antrum and duodenum may produce duodenogastric reflux.

Retching is defined as strong, involuntary efforts to vomit, which may be seen as preparatory maneuvers to vomiting. These efforts consist of spasmodic contractions of the diaphragm and abdominal wall at the same time that the lower esophageal sphincter relaxes. This sphincter is also pulled cephalad by contraction of the longitudinal muscles of the upper esophagus and may herniate through the diaphragmatic hiatus, preventing the increased intraabdominal pressure from augmenting the sphincter pressure. During retching, gastric material is moved into the esophagus by the combination of increased abdominal pressure and decreased intrathoracic pressure, but this material may be returned to the stomach by secondary (non-swallow) esophageal peristalsis.

Vomiting (emesis) differs from retching in that material is expelled from the mouth. This is fostered by relaxation of the diaphragm and reversal of intrathoracic pressure from negative to positive. The upper esophageal sphincter also relaxes, perhaps in response to the increase of intraluminal pressure in the esophagus.

Regurgitation is considered a form of gastroesophageal reflux and, as such, is caused predominantly by lower esophageal sphincter dysfunction. Although apparently effortless, it may be propelled by contraction of abdominal wall musculature; this propulsion perhaps distinguishes regurgitant from non-regurgitant reflux, which remains in the esophagus.

Rumination is similar to regurgitation in its effortless appearance and its probable propulsion by somatic muscle contraction. However, ruminated material is usually reswallowed rather than ejected from the mouth, and psychological or behavioral problems are considered the cause.

It may occur as a result of obstruction or partial obstruction of the gut lumen. Intra-abdominal pathologic, as well as metabolic systemic, psychogenic, and physiological condition such as pregnancy should be considered.

Obstruction of gastrointestinal tract at any level may result in vomiting. Obstruction may be mechanical. Mechanical obstruction may be secondary to narrowing of lumen.

- *Inflammation:* Acute gastritis and Crohn's disease
- *Fibrosis:* Healing inflammation and postsurgical
- *Neoplasia:* Adenocarcinoma, lymphoma, and polyp
- *Foreign body:* Worm infestation and trichobezoar

Small bowel obstruction occurs in adhesion, hernia, lymphoma, Henoch–Schönlein purpura, mesenteric adenitis.

Colonic causes of obstruction include diverticular disease, fecal impaction, invasive cancer, Hirschsprung's disease, and pelvic radiation therapy.

The causes responsible for both small and large intestine include Crohn's disease, anastomotic stricture, adenomatous polyps, and adenocarcinoma.

Recurrent chronic vomiting may be because of paresis of stomach and intestine. Paresis of stomach may be because of pancreatitis, diabetes, viral, postsurgical or due to retroperitoneal cancer such as lymphoma or pancreatic adenocarcinoma. Postsurgical ileus is the cause of paresis of intestine. It may occur because of periodic syndrome, volvulus and hernia, recurrent urinary tract infection and migraine. Vomiting is the clinical feature of intracranial pathology (space occupying lesions, meningitis, hydrocephalus, middle ear infection, and cerebrovascular accidents).

The presence of the vomiting center and chemoreceptor trigger zone in the medulla oblongata and fourth ventricle respectively. This is the cause of vomiting in systemic diseases such as sepsis, malaria, pyrexia, and diabetes ketoacidosis. Brain tumor may be important causes of daily effortless morning vomiting.

Infective causes of vomiting include food poisoning (*Staphylococcal aureus*), epidemic virus, viral and bacterial meningitis and syphilis.

Biliary and renal colic and appendicitis are associated with vomiting.

Complications of vomiting include Mallory–Weiss tear of the esophagus, rupture of esophagus, metabolic derangements such as hyperkalemia, alkalosis, secondary to renal correction of volume disturbances.

Vomiting may be benign nonorganic. This does not lead to dehydration or loss of weight. These infants do not regurgitate the whole of the food.

The features suggestive of organic vomiting include persistent vomiting with or without fever, excessive drowsiness, not taking feeds, marked abdominal distension, visible gastric peristalsis, bulging fontanelle, headache, convulsions, and palpable mass in the abdomen. In this case every effort should be made to find the cause.

Vomiting may be clinically insidious and projectile. Insidious vomiting is associated with nausea. Projectile vomiting is sudden is onset, no nausea. It is classically associated with pyloric obstruction and raised intracranial tension.

Vomiting is age related. Vomiting in newborn should rule out any correctable surgical cause. Vomiting is due to general causes rather than local cause in infants and early childhood. Gastroenteritis is the most common cause of vomiting in this age group. The other causes are tonsillitis, otitis media, urinary tract infection, and meningitis. In older children the possibility of migraine should be ruled out.

It may be site related. There will be excessive froth and choking on attempted feeds at birth in esophageal atresia and stenosis. It may not be possible to pass the nasogastric tube beyond the obstruction.

The child may vomit soon after the feed, vomitus may be curdled but not bile stained, if there is any obstruction at stomach. Vomitus may be bile stained, greenish if the obstruction is beyond the ampulla of Vater. Feculent vomiting suggests intestinal obstruction or paralytic ileus.

The cause of vomiting is often indicated by clinical settings and other organ specific symptoms and signs. The interval between the food intake and vomiting gives some clue to site of mechanical obstruction.

The presence of fever may indicate acute appendicitis, acute cholecystitis and systemic conditions such as tuberculosis, brucellosis, and urinary tract infection. Abdominal pain suggests pyelonephritis, pancreatitis, renal calculi, and peritonitis. Abdominal mass indicates pyloric or intestinal obstruction, pancreatic neoplasm, Chron's disease, perinephric abscess, and diverticulitis.

DIAGNOSIS

The investigation of vomiting aims to determine the underlying cause and its consequence (metabolic disturbance and aspiration pneumonia). General blood tests include CBC, urea, electrolytes, serum calcium/phosphate, serum amylase, serum glucose, and liver function tests.

Upper gastrointestinal pathology is most easily assessed by endoscopy. Colonoscopy can be attempted.

X-ray studies (contrast meal and enema) can be used to identify obstruction and paresis. This is best performed by using water soluble contrast.

Esophageal motility studies are useful in diagnosing achalasia or esophageal scleroderma. If no gastrointestinal or systemic cause is elicited, computed tomography (CT) scan/magnetic resonance imaging (MRI) of the head is done to rule out central nervous system (CNS) pathology.

Surgical causes of vomiting in infant should not be missed. Pyloric stenosis results in forcible vomiting, i.e., classically projectile, but not always in a baby who looks lean and hungry. The vomitus never contains a bile.

Bilious vomiting in an infant should always raise the possibility of intestinal obstruction. Malrotation should be excluded since delay may lead to massive gut necrosis.

The following conditions should be considered if the vomitus contains blood:

- Swallowed maternal blood from mother's cracked nipple.
- Late onset of hemorrhage disease of newborn.

Gross gastroesophageal reflux in newborn usually produces frequent nonforceful bringing back of small volumes of milk after feeds. This may even occur in overfed babies.

ORGANIC CAUSES OF VOMITING

- *Infection*
  - Gastroenteritis
  - Urinary tract infection
  - Otitis media
  - Respiratory infection
  - Meningitis
- *Gastrointestinal*
  - Gastroesophageal reflux
  - Hiatus hernia
  - Mechanical bowel obstruction
- *Metabolic*
  - Uremia
  - Diabetic ketoacidosis
  - Amino acidemias
  - Organic academia

GASTROINTESTINAL OBSTRUCTION

Esophageal Obstruction

Esophageal Atresia

Infants with esophageal atresia present at birth with a prenatal history of polyhydramnios and intolerance of initial feeding. The esophageal atresia is accompanied by a distal tracheoesophageal fistula in 85% of cases, by a proximal fistula in a small percentage, and by no fistula in the remainder. Esophageal atresia is associated with other anomalies in 15–50% of patients; cardiac, anorectal, and genitourinary defects are most common. 10% of all esophageal atresia patients and 25% of those without a fistula have the VATER or VACTERL (vertebral, anorectal, cardiac, tracheoesophageal, renal, radial, limb) association.

Esophageal Stenosis

Children with esophageal stenoses present in later infancy and occasionally in adulthood. Stenoses are divided into tracheobronchial rings that often contain cartilage, fibromuscular stenoses, and membranous webs. Diagnosis is by contrast radiography and may require pressure injections of contrast material if the stenosis is not tight.

Esophageal Strictures

Esophageal strictures are acquired lesions that may be caused by reflux esophagitis, but more commonly result from caustic ingestions (acid, alkali) or other causes. The strictures are best demonstrated with contrast radiography; endoscopic biopsies may be important for diagnosis of the etiology.

PYLORIC STENOSIS

Pyloric stenosis manifests with nonbilious projectile vomiting beginning at 2–3 weeks of age and increasing during the next month or so, usually in a firstborn male child. The vomitus may contain some blood, and propulsive gastric waves can be seen on the abdominal wall. Dehydration, poor weight gain, metabolic alkalosis, and mild jaundice are sometimes evident. A palpable "olive" in the epigastrium (felt best during or after feeding) represents the hypertrophied pyloric muscle.

Intestinal Obstruction

Rushes of bowel sounds associated with cramping and colic often indicate intestinal obstruction. Vomiting is a cardinal sign of intestinal obstruction, being more prominent in high small bowel obstruction than in low small bowel or colon obstruction. With high obstructions, vomiting is not feculent, the onset is often acute, and crampy pain may occur at frequent intervals; abdominal distention is minimal. With low obstructions, in contrast, the vomiting may be feculent and less acute in onset, the interval between cramping is longer, and distention is more notable. Identification of the site of obstruction is aided by the plain film and by other radiographic studies.

Infantile bilious vomiting is an important symptom of intestinal obstruction, which often signals a congenital gastrointestinal anomaly, particularly intestinal obstruction below the ampulla of Vater. Surgical consultation is needed early in these infants because they often require emergency therapy.

Duodenal Atresia, Stenosis, and Web: Annular Pancreas

The juxta-ampullary duodenum is susceptible to a cluster of obstructing congenital anomalies. Infants with complete duodenal obstruction, most commonly atresia, present with bilious vomiting and a radiographic "double bubble" sign. Associated prematurity (and polyhydramnios) or anomalies, including renal, cardiac, and vertebral defects occur in approximately 75% of infants; trisomy 21 is seen in about 50%.

Intestinal Strictures

Strictures produce partial obstruction of the gastrointestinal tract and may be located from the esophagus to the anus. They may occur post-surgically (anastomotic), may follow necrotizing enterocolitis, may be caused by Crohn disease, or may result from ingestion of nonsteroidal anti-inflammatory medications or high-dose pancreatic enzymes.

MALROTATION AND VOLVULUS

Volvulus is the twisting of a loop of bowel on the mesentery. Midgut volvulus occurs most often in the context of congenital intestinal malrotation, in which the small intestine is not normally fastened in place.

Volvulus is an extremely hazardous obstructing lesion. The luminal obstruction is closed at both ends, which leads to sepsis from rapidly proliferating and translocating bacteria. There is also vascular obstruction in which the root of the mesentery is twisted, which quickly produces ischemia of the small intestine.

Meckel Diverticulum

Meckel diverticula may cause obstructive vomiting by intussusception or by intestinal volvulus around a fibrous band. They may also cause vomiting by inflammatory changes, and they may bleed. This fibrous remnant of the omphalomesenteric duct is a small intestinal diverticulum.

Intussusception

Intussusceptum into distal intestine (intussuscipiens), causing both luminal obstruction, and mesenteric vascular compromise. Abdominal pain occurs in nearly all children with intussusception, whereas vomiting results in about 65%, and "currant-jelly stools" (from mucosal hemorrhage) occur in fewer than 20%. The pain is severe, crampy, and often contemporaneous with the vomiting. Between cramps, the child may be listless, may sleep, or may even play. Vomiting and bloody stools are more common in younger infants and in those with longer duration of symptoms. An abdominal mass is palpable in about 25% of patients.

Constipation, Meconium Plug, and Anal Stenosis

These distal colonic problems produce obstipation primarily, but if they are severe and persistent, vomiting may result. Rectal examination provides the diagnosis. Enemas, laxatives, dietary changes, and behavioral modification are useful in treating constipation, whereas surgery is usually necessary to treat anal atresia or stenosis. Infants with meconium plug syndrome need clinical follow-up to monitor for the presence of coexistent Hirschsprung disease.

GASTROINTESTINAL DYSMOTILITY

Achalasia

Achalasia, such as esophageal stenoses and strictures, produces effortless retrograde emptying of undigested food from the esophagus. Contrast radiography and esophageal manometry are needed for diagnosis.

Gastroesophageal Reflux

The apparently effortless *regurgitation* that represents gastroesophageal reflux in infants is of particular importance because (1) it is the most common cause of "vomiting" in infants; (2) physiologic reflux must be distinguished from reflux necessitating evaluation and therapy; and (3) the practitioner must be vigilant to avoid misdiagnosing other infantile vomiting diseases as reflux.

Lethal malrotation with volvulus, partially obstructing duodenal web, and metabolic disorders are three examples of such misdiagnoses. Children with primary neurologic disease may be more likely to regurgitate and suffer from reflux disease; it must be remembered that many metabolic disorders manifest both as neurologic dysfunction and as regurgitation.

Reflux typically is a benign feature in healthy infants that improves and resolves in a predictable manner as a function of growth, development, acquiring upright positions, and introducing some solids in the diet. In these infants, regurgitation will be effortless and will not have associated failure to gain weight, feeding problems, or airway symptoms.

Ileus

Paralytic ileus, typified by the postoperative ileus that follows most abdominal surgery, is very common. As in intestinal obstruction, intestinal contents fail to progress, causing abdominal pain and vomiting. Typically, the bowel sounds are decreased or absent; there may be abdominal distention. Other causes of ileus include unrelieved intestinal obstruction, peritonitis, intestinal ischemia, and sepsis. Signs of ileus may follow signs of intestinal obstruction; in this context, ileus is an ominous sign. Other causes of paralytic ileus are drugs (phenothiazines, narcotics, laxative abuse, and atropine), electrolyte disturbances (hypokalemia and hypercalcemia), endocrinopathies (hypothyroidism), or injuries (spinal fractures).

GASTROINTESTINAL INFLAMMATION

Esophagitis

Esophagitis may be associated with vomiting in the setting of eosinophilic esophagitis (EoE), where patients may also experience nausea and/or dysphagia. With regard to reflux disease, esophagitis is associated with vomiting, but it is usually not the primary cause.

Gastroenteritis

Gastroenteritis is a frequent cause of acute vomiting illness in childhood. The vomiting is often associated with diarrhea and sometimes with crampy abdominal pain or fever. Rotavirus, especially in infants, is notable for its prominent vomiting, which often precedes the diarrhea. "Food poisoning" also produces vomiting and diarrhea, often caused by bacterially derived toxin.

Peptic Ulcer Disease

The term *peptic ulcer disease* includes gastritis, gastric ulcer, duodenitis, and duodenal ulcer. In children, in contrast to adults, these disorders frequently cause vomiting. Defined causes for peptic ulcer disease include *Helicobacter pylori (H. pylori)* infections, bile reflux gastritis, nonsteroidal anti-inflammatory agents, and rare gastrin-secreting tumors (Zollinger-Ellison syndrome). Stress ulcers occur in the context of sepsis, burns, surgery, head trauma, and severe acute illness.

Meckel Diverticulitis

In addition to presenting as gastrointestinal obstruction, via volvulus or intussusception, Meckel diverticula may become inflamed and mimic appendicitis.

Mesenteric Adenitis

Mesenteric adenitis is often found on CT scans and refers to inflammation of lymph nodes in the mesentery. It is probably caused by viral (adenovirus and measles) or bacterial (*Yersinia enterocolitica*) infection, but the symptoms are similar enough to appendicitis that the diagnosis is usually not made before surgery. Ultrasonography can readily distinguish mesenteric adenitis from appendicitis.

Appendicitis

When vomiting occurs in appendicitis, it follows the periumbilical pain but may precede the localization of the pain to the McBurney point, two-thirds of the way between the umbilicus and the right anterior iliac spine. Before perforation, there is only occasional vomiting. After perforation, the fever may be higher; the child lies still with the right hip flexed, and vomiting may be more frequent and more feculent.

HEPATOBILIARY DISORDERS

Hepatitis

The presence of acute viral hepatitis is usually suspected in patients who have jaundice, but up to 50% of patients with hepatitis A are anicteric, and even those in whom jaundice develops have a pre-icteric prodrome lasting up to a week. In children with acute hepatitis, therefore, the presenting symptom may be vomiting, another reason for including liver enzymes in the screening evaluation of the ill-appearing vomiting child. The vomiting is often accompanied by fatigue, fever, headache, rhinorrhea, sore throat, and cough.

Biliary Colic and Cholecystitis

Biliary obstruction produces vomiting and abdominal pain in children; the vomiting is usually less severe and occurs later than that in pancreatitis. Biliary colic is visceral pain resulting from transient obstruction of the cystic duct, usually by a stone. In occasional patients, biliary dyskinesia causes these symptoms. Biliary colic produces several hours of steady, vaguely localized pain, often in the right upper quadrant; most patients also have vomiting. Episodes of biliary colic commonly recur at unpredictable intervals, from weeks to years. Acute cholecystitis may ensue if the obstruction persists and leads to inflammation of the gallbladder. The pain may localize more clearly to the right upper quadrant and may radiate to the back or shoulder.

Pancreatitis

Pancreatitis is usually associated with epigastric abdominal pain, which may radiate to the back. Elevated serum amylase and lipase levels usually confirm the diagnosis.

GYNECOLOGIC AND UROLOGIC DISORDERS

Pyelonephritis

High fever, chills, nausea, vomiting, and less often, diarrhea develop rapidly. There may be symptoms of cystitis with dysuria, frequency, urgency, and suprapubic pain. Costovertebral angle tenderness focuses the diagnosis on the urinary tract.

Ureteropelvic Junction Obstruction and Hydronephrosis

Ureteropelvic junction obstruction ("beer drinker's kidney," Dietl crisis) is caused by partial obstruction at the ureteropelvic junction and by the resulting hydronephrosis during fluid loading and diuresis.

Typically, the symptoms commence in the evening after an increased fluid intake, although the history of hyperhydration is often unclear. The child's pain and vomiting usually remit spontaneously in several hours, as dehydration gradually relieves the renal pelvic distention. Superimposed unilateral urinary tract infection may cause additional findings of fever, failure to thrive, and pyuria.

Renal Colic

Passage of a renal stone usually causes more pain than vomiting. Lateralized colicky pain, hematuria, and confirmatory radiologic studies assist the diagnosis.

Ovarian Torsion

Torsion of a normal ovary occasionally occurs in girls of any age, probably caused by laxity of adnexal supports. Repeated attacks of crampy, lower abdominal pain culminate in a final acute episode with severe retching and vomiting, an enlarged ovarian mass, and eventual signs of peritonitis.

RESPIRATORY DISORDERS

Sinusitis, Pharyngitis, and Otitis

Sinusitis may induce chronic, unexplained vomiting. The vomiting is more apt to occur in the morning and must be differentiated from serious intracranial processes. Sinus tenderness and sinus CT scans suggest the diagnosis, and a successful trial of antibiotic therapy confirms it. Less often, pharyngitis or otitis media may manifest acutely with nonspecific vomiting.

Pneumonia

Because pneumonia can also be caused by vomiting on the basis of aspiration, it is important to consider the direction of causality in children with pneumonia and vomiting. Aspiration of vomitus is particularly likely to occur in the context of obtundation or other neurologic dysfunction.

CENTRAL NERVOUS SYSTEM DISORDERS

Increased Intracranial Pressure

Various causes of increased intracranial pressure (e.g., tumors) induce vomiting, typically described as projectile but without retching. This description may be an oversimplification, but the occurrence on awakening and before eating is important information.

Abdominal Epilepsy

The diagnosis of abdominal epilepsy is suggested by recurrent episodes of nausea or vomiting, usually accompanied by abdominal pain and by symptoms suggesting its central nervous system origin, such as headache, dizziness, confusion, or temporary blindness. Patients may sleep after an episode.

435 CHAPTER Warts

WARTS (VERRUCAE)

These are intraepidermal tumors caused by human papilloma virus **(Fig. 1)**.

- *Verrucae vulgaris (common warts):* These appear predominantly on the dorsal surface of the hands or periungual region. They are round discrete flesh colored and later turn into larger with yellowish tan, grayish black, or brown lesion. With repeated trauma they get roughened with fine papillomatous surface.
- *Verrucae plana (flat warts):* Primarily occurs on face, neck, arms and legs, slightly elevated papules, smooth flesh colored to slightly tan or brownish, with a round or polygonal shape. Koebner effect is characteristic.
- *Verrucae plantaris (plantar warts):* It occurs on the plantar surfaces of feet generally overweight bearing regions, rough surfaced hard in consistency and often painful and tender.
- *Condylomata accuminata (genital warts):* They occur around mucocutaneous junction and intertriginous areas as soft flesh colored elongated sometimes pedunculated or polypoid nodules.

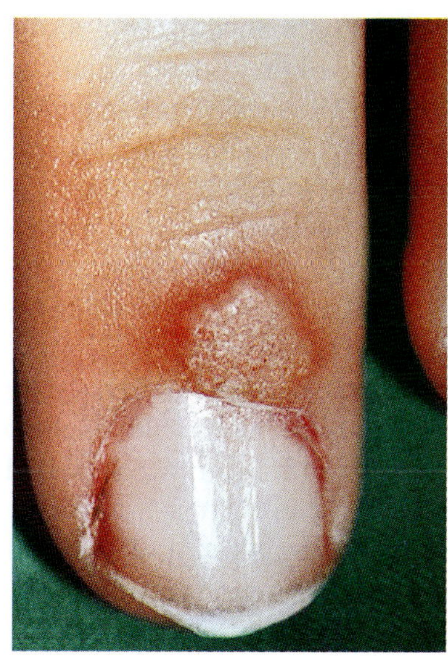

Fig. 1: Wart.

Warts can also be found on the trunk, oral and nasal mucosae, and conjunctivae. Anogenital lesions *(condylomata acuminata)* are usually associated with human papillomavirus (HPV) types 6 and 11, and the possibility of sexual abuse must be considered in children >3 years old (with no known obvious exposure to warts) who present with lesions at this site.

436 CHAPTER Weight

Infants and young children should be weighed with minimal dress. Infants should be weighed at the same time each day, ideally in the morning before being fed. Usually there will be a loss of weight in the first 10 days by 10% percent because of loss of extracellular fluid. Later newborns will gain 25–30 g/day till 3–5 months. Birth weight will double by 5 months and triple by 1 year.

Infants and younger children are weighed on platform type of electronic weighing scale **(Fig. 1)**. Older children are weighed on a standing type of upright scale. Measure the nearest 10 g for infants, and 100 g for children. Children who refuse to stand on a platform, mother and child should be weighed together and then mother alone. Then derive child's weight by subtracting the latter from the former.

It is the reliable indicator of nutritional status. Boys generally weigh more than girls up to the age of 10 years. During 12–13 years girls will weigh more than boys due to early pubertal growth spurt.

Formula to calculate the expected weight:

$$\text{3–12 months} = \frac{\text{Age in months} + 9}{2}$$

$$\text{1–6 years:} \quad \text{Age (year)} \times 2 + 8 \text{ kg}$$

$$\text{7–12 years:} \quad \frac{\text{Age (year)} \times 7 - 5 \text{ kg}}{2}$$

$$\text{Age (year)} \times 3 \text{ kg}$$

The indicative weight-for-height measurements for children up to 5 years of age are given in **Table 1**.

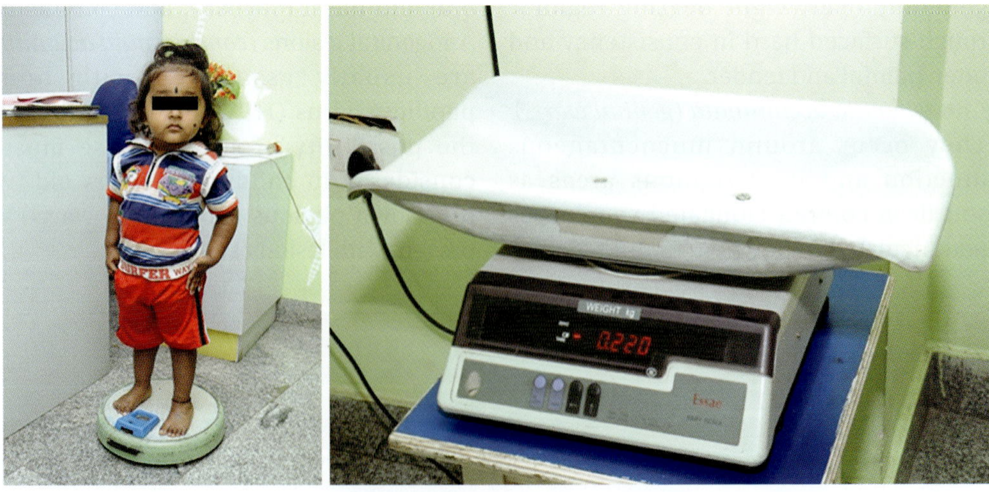

Fig. 1: Weighing machines.

TABLE 1: Weight-for-height measurements by age.

Age	*Increments*
	Weight increments per week
1–4 months	200 g
4–6 months	150 g
7–9 months	100 g
10–12 months	50–75 g
	Weight increments per week
1–2 years	2.5 kg
3–5 years	2.0 kg
	Length increments per week
1st year	25 cm
2nd year	12 cm
3rd year	9 cm
4th year	7 cm
5th year	6 cm

Chapter 437 Wheezing

Wheezing is defined as high-pitched musical sound of varying intensity, heard usually during expiratory phase, often without stethoscope and indicates obstruction to air passage from the lower part of trachea to bronchiole.

Wheezing occurs in children due to easy compression of soft passages, easy blockage of narrow passages, and plugging with mucous secretions of glands.

Pathogenic mechanisms leading on to wheezing

- Allergy
- Mechanical obstruction
- Aspiration
- Infection
- Genetic factors
- Miscellaneous

The factors responsible for the narrowing of airways include the mucosal edema, collection of large amount of secretions and bronchospasm. Bronchospasm occurs in smooth muscles of the airway. Hence, the bronchospasm does not occur in the infancy because of absence of smooth muscle. This wheeze in infants is due to secretion and mucosal edema. Increased susceptibility to these factors below 3 years in child make them more vulnerable to wheeze.

CAUSES OF WHEEZING

- *Reactive airway disease*
  - Asthma
  - Excessive induces asthma
  - Asthmatic bronchitis
- *Hypersensitive reaction*
  - Tropical eosinophilia
  - Visceral larva migrans
  - Allergic aspergillosis
- *Aspiration*
  - Foreign body
  - Tracheoesophageal fistula
  - Pharyngeal incoordination
- *Extrinsic compression*
  - Vascular ring
  - Enlarged lymph node
  - Mediastinal tumor
- *Cardiac failure*
- *Immotile cilia syndrome*

RATTLING

It is due to excessive secretion in the pharynx and tracheobronchial tree during breathing. Rattling may be normal if it is transient. If it is prolonged it is always pathological. It is present in asthma, bronchitis, and tracheobronchial stenosis.

STRIDOR

It indicates upper respiratory tract obstruction. It is accompanied by hoarseness, brassy cough, dyspnea, and inspiratory chest retraction. Accessary respiratory muscles are active.

CAUSES OF WHEEZE

- *Common causes*
  - Lower respiratory tract infection with wheeze

- Bronchiolitis
- Bronchitis
- Tropical eosinophilia
- Loeffler's syndrome
- Hyperreactive airway disease
- *Rare causes*
  - Cystic fibrosis
  - Foreign body inhalation
  - Pulmonary hemosiderosis
  - Tuberculosis
  - Mediastinal cyst/node
  - Pressure from enlarged mediastinal lymph node
- *Noninfectious causes of wheeze*
  - Aspiration pneumonitis
  - Bronchiolitis obliterans
  - Bronchopulmonary dysplasia
  - Ciliary dyskinesis
  - Congenital malformation
  - Cystic fibrosis
  - Foreign body aspiration
  - Vascular rings
  - Congenital cardiac anomalies

History should be taken to find out that the present wheeze is the first attack or any previous episodes of wheeze is present. Acute attack of wheeze in healthy child indicates foreign body aspiration in the lower respiratory tract. Isolated attack of wheezing may accompany bronchiolitis and bronchopneumonia. Congenital structural defects of lower respiratory tract may produce recurrent persistent wheeze from birth. Recurrent wheeze and recurrent bowel disturbances are seen in cystic fibrosis. In the developing countries, recurrent wheezing is often associated with tropical eosinophilia and hypereosinophilia accompanying ascariasis.

Magnitude of respiratory distress should be ascertained. The parameter that should be checked includes state of hydration, use of respiratory accessory muscles, temperature, and evidence of congestive cardiac failure. Evidence of respiratory acidosis, emphysema, and bronchiolitis, bronchopneumonia should be looked.

Presence of finger clubbing indicates chronic lung infection. Allergic rhinitis, eczema, and urticaria suggest bronchial asthma or asthmatic bronchitis. Mediastinal shift suggests foreign body aspiration. Cardiac conditions and features suggestive of congestive cardiac failure such as tachycardia, tachypnea and tender hepatomegaly should be examined.

Most will be tachypneic, using accessary muscles and will have expiratory wheeze. An alert playful child with audible wheeze is less worrying than the anxious or listless child who is too breathless to speak.

A chest X-ray may show evidence of hyperexpansion.

Although about one-third of children will have an episode of wheezing before they are 3 years old, most of them, i.e., 60% do not develop persistent wheezing. Risk factors for the persistent wheezing include:

- Positive maternal family history of asthma
- Atopic dermatitis
- Increased levels of immunoglobulin E (IgE)
- Rhinitis not associated with cold

Indications for chest X-ray

- Suspected pneumonia
- Suspected foreign aspiration
- Suspected CCF
- Marked asymmetry of breath sounds
- Marked respiratory distress
- History of trauma

Triggers for asthmatic bronchitis

- Upper respiratory tract infection (URTI)
- Changes in weather
- Vigorous exercise
- Allergic factor

Bibliography

1. Abend NS, Dlugos DJ. Medical treatment of pediatric status epilepticus. Semin Pediatr Neurol. 2010;17(7):242-6.
2. Aponte EP, Diehl N. Medical and surgical outcome in childhood glaucoma. J AAPOS. 2011;15(3):263-7.
3. Asthagiri AR, et al. Neurofibromatosis type 1. Lancet. 2009;373-5.
4. Bishara N, Clericuzo CL. Common dysmorphic syndromes in the NICU. NeoReviews. 2008;9:e29-e38.
5. Blair E. Epidemiology of the cerebral palsies. Orthop Clin Am. 2010;41:441-55.
6. Blanchette V. Childhood immune thrombocytopenic purpura: diagnosis and management. Pediatr Clin North Am. 2008; 55:393-420.
7. Bloomfield D. Secondary amenorrhea. Pediatr Rev. 2006;27(3):113-4.
8. Bry K. Newborn resuscitation and the lung. NeoReviews. 2008;9(11):e506-12.
9. Canty CA. Retinoblastoma: an overview for advanced practice. J Am Acad Nurse Pract. 2009;21(3):149-55.
10. Chou R, Dana T. Screening for visual impairment in children ages 1-5 years. Pediatrics. 2011;127(2):e442-79.
11. Cilliers A, Adler AJ, Saloojee H. Anti-inflammatory treatment for carditis in acute rheumatic fever. Cochrane Database Syst Rev. 2015;(5):CD003176.
12. Cohen LE. Idiopathic short stature: a clinical review. JAMA. 2014;311:1787-96.
13. Culbert TP, Benez GA. Integrative approaches to childhood constipation and encopresis. Pediatr Clin North Am. 2007; 54(6):927-47.
14. Davin JC, Coppo R. Henoch-Schonlein purpura nephritis in children. Nat Rev Nephrol. 2014;10(10):563-73.
15. De Silva NK. Breast disorders in female adolescent. Adolesc Med State Art Rev. 2012;23(1):34-52.
16. Dimario FJ Jr. Breath holding spells in childhood. Am J Dis Child. 1992;146:125.
17. Dobbs MB, Gurnett CA. Update on clubfoot: etiology and treatment. Clin Orthop Relat Res. 2009;467(5):1146-53.
18. Dubble AM, White DR. Laryngomalacia. Pediatr Clin Am. 2013;60:893-902.
19. Eisenberg JM. Evaluation and treatment of cryptorchidism. [online] Available from www.effectivehealthcare.ahrq.gov. [Last accessed June, 2025]
20. Elson TM, Ault BH, Jones DP, Chesney RW, Wyatt RJ. Poststreptococcal glomerulonephritis in children. Pediatr Nephrol. 2011;26(2):165-80.
21. Feldman AG, Sokol RJ. Neonatal cholestasis. Neoreviews. 2013;14(2):e63-73.
22. Fleck BW, McIntosh N. Retinopathy of prematurity: recent developments. NeoReviews. 2009;10:e20-30.
23. Gallagher PG. Abnormalities of erythrocyte membranes. Pediatr Clin North Am. 2013;60:1349-62.
24. Grover M. Functional abdominal pain. Curr Gastroenterol Rep. 2010;12(5):391-8.
25. Hanson CL, Hokanson JS. Etiology of chest pain in children and adolescents. WMJ. 2011;110(2):58-62.
26. Hegde AN, Mohan S, Pandya A. Imaging in infections of the head and neck. Neuroimaging Clin Am. 2012;22(4):727-54.

27. Hershey AD. Current approach to the diagnosis and management of pediatric migraine. Lancet Neurol. 2010;9:190-204.
28. Hung MH, Lin LH, Chen DF, Huang CS. Choledochal cysts in infants and children. Eur J Pediatr. 2011;170:1179-85.
29. Israel S. Platelet disorders in children, a diagnostic approach. Pediatr Blood Cancer. 2011;56:975-83.
30. Janus J, Moerschel S. Evaluation of anemia in children. Am Fam Physician. 2010;81:1462-71.
31. Kelly BP. Superficial fungal infection. Pediatr Rev. 2012;33(4):e22-37.
32. Kosnorsky GS. Idiopathic intracranial hypertension: pseudotumor cerebri. Headache. 2014;54(2):e11-14.
33. Lambert SM, Kolon TF. A practical approach to ambiguous genitalia in the newborn period. Urol Clin N Am. 2010;37(2):195-205.
34. Lauer BJ, Spector NJ. Hyperbilirubinemia in the newborn. Pediatr Rev. 2011;32:341-9.
35. Levi M. Guidelines for the diagnosis and management of the disseminated intravascular coagulation. Br J Hematol. 2009;145:24-33.
36. Lieberthal AS, Carroll AE, Chonmaitree T, Ganiats TG, Hoberman A, Jackson MA, et al. The diagnosis and management of otitis media. Pediatrics. 2013;133:346.
37. Lightdale JR, Gremse DA; Section on Gastroenterology, Hepatology, and Nutrition. Gastroesophageal reflux; management guidance for pediatrician. Pediatrics. 2013;131(5):e1684-95.
38. Mac Neill EC, Vashist S. Approach to syncope and altered mental status. Pediatr Clin North Am. 2013;60(5):1083-106.
39. Nordt CA, DiVasta AD. Gynecomastia in adolescent. Curr Opin Pediatr. 2008;20(4): 375-82.
40. O' Connor M, McDaniel N. Pediatric electrocardiogram, Part I. Am J Emerg Med. 2008;26(2):121-8.
41. Obermeyer RJ, Goretsky MJ. Chest wall deformities in pediatrics practice and surgery. Surg Clin North Am. 2012;92(3): 669-84.
42. Papendieck P, Chiesa A, Prieto L, Gruñeiro-Papendieck L. Thyroid disorders of neonates. J Pediatr Endocrinol Metab. 2009;22:547-53.
43. Pettit MA, Alex K, Mark F. Myocarditis. Pediatr Emerg Care. 2014;30(11):832-5.
44. Richter GT, Friedman AB. Hemangiomas and vascular malformations. Int J Pediatr. 2012;2012:645678.
45. Rintala RJ, Pakarinen MP. Long-term outcome of Hirschsprung's disease. Semin Pediatr Surg. 2012;21(4):336-43.
46. Robson WLM. Clinical practice. Evaluation and management of enuresis. N Engl J Med. 2009;360:1429-36.
47. Rosen R. Gastroesophageal reflux in infants. JAMA Pediatr. 2014;168(1):83-9.
48. Ruuskanen O, Lahti E. Viral pneumonia. Lancet. 2011;377:1264-75.
49. Shany E, Berger I. Neonatal electroencephalography: review of practical approach. J Child Neurol. 2011;26:341-55.
50. Shirly ED, Ain MC. Achondroplasia: manifestations and treatment. J Am Acad Orthop Surg. 2009;17(4):231-41.
51. Sivaswamy L. Approach to acute ataxia in children. Pediatr Am. 2014;43(4):e271-7.
52. Tamesis ME, Morellij JG. Vitiligo in childhood. Pediatr Dermatol. 2010;27:437.
53. Tugal-Tutkun I. Pediatric uveitis. J Ophthalmic Vis Res. 2011;6(4):256-69.
54. Warren JB, Anderson JM. Newborn respiratory disorders. Pediatr Rev. 2010;31:487.
55. Wipf JE, Lipsky BA, Hirschmann JV, Boyko EJ, Takasugi J, Peugeot RL, et al. Diagnosing pneumonia by physical examination. Arch Intern Med. 1999;159:1082-7.
56. Zumla A, Raviglione M, Hafner R, von Reyn CF. Tuberculosis. Engl J Med. 2013;368(8): 745-55.

Index

Page numbers followed by *b* refer to box, *f* refer to figure, and *t* refer to table.

A

B

C

F

G

H

I

J

K

L

M

N

O

P

Q

R

S

T

U

V

W

X

Y

Z